TEXTBOOK OF RHEUMATOLOGY

VOLUME 1

NERVOUS, CARDIOVASCULAR, RESPIRATORY, ENDOCRINE, AND RELATED SYSTEMS

Dr. Anand Anerao

ALLIED HEALTH PRESS

Textbook of Rheumatology Volume 1

Nervous, Cardiovascular, Respiratory, Endocrine, and Related Systems

Author: **Dr. Anand Anerao**

Allied Health Press
4164 Lakeshore Road
Burlington ON L7L 1A4
Canada
www.alliedhealthpress.com
Email: orders@arclereducation.com

ISBN: 978-1-77956-858-8

General Disclaimer:

This book is a summation of information from different sources and encompasses a wide range of medical conditions, the latest therapy methods, principals and techniques that are used in current practice, at the time of publication. This book offers general information with educational purposes, it is not to be applied or relied on for any diagnostic or treatment purposes. Please do not use the data/matter as a substitute for professional diagnosis and treatment. Please consult your healthcare provider or a licensed physician before making any healthcare queries or treatment choices. The medical information and research findings presented in this book are for educational purposes only and should not be used for the treatment of specific individual patients, as individual cases may vary. The author(s), editors(s) and publisher cannot be held accountable and make no guarantees that the information provided in this book will apply to each and individual patient. This book is meant to serve as a basic guideline and other relevant literature sources should be used for more specific information. This text can be a vital resource for students, trainees, and practitioners, covering essential topics. This book encompasses a wide range of medical conditions and the latest therapy options used in current practice. Through the utilization of many different medical studies this book provides the basics of different medical conditions, which can be used as a basic guide from where medical students, trainees and practitioners can extract necessary information. Further, some of the books have graphic images to explain anatomy for medical/educational purposes only. Hence, the book is intended for students or teachers/staff or individuals with a mature outlook looking to learn or enhance their knowledge.

Allied Health Press publishes wide variety of books and eBooks. For more information about Allied Health Press and its products, visit our website at www.alliedhealthpress.com

ABOUT THE AUTHOR

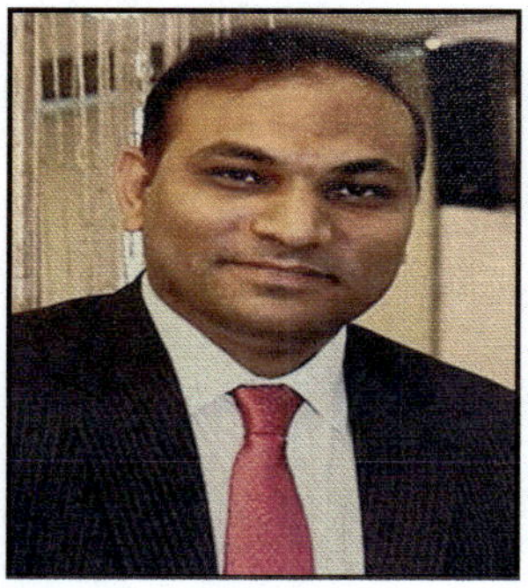

Dr. Anand Anerao is currently an Associate Professor at Parbhani Medical College. After completing his MBBS in 2001 from Indira Gandhi Medical College, Nagpur, he pursued his master's degree in Orthopedic Surgery from Shivaji University in 2007. Following his MS, he completed a fellowship in Arthroscopy from Kamineni Hospital, Hyderabad in 2009. He served as a Medical Officer at Sub-District Hospital, Gangakhed, for three years (2009-2012). Additionally, he has been in private practice for the past 18 years.

Brief Table of Contents

Getting Started with This Book

Chapter Openers

A list of Chapter Outline is presented providing a brief Introduction to what will be covered in the chapter.

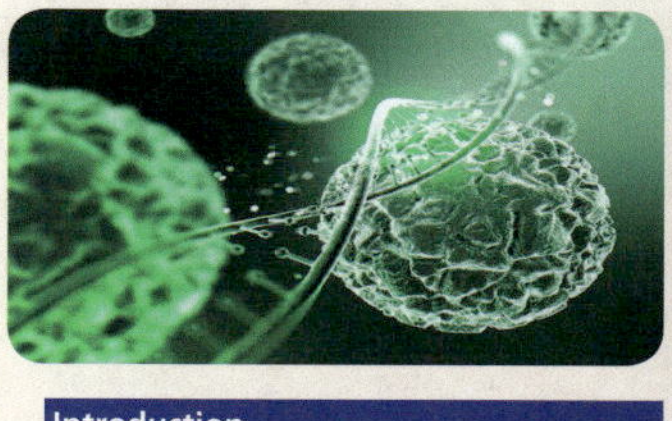

Introduction

Often referred to as the science of life, biology is a broad field of study aimed at comprehending the several kinds of life on Earth, from tiny creatures to sophisticated multicellular entities. Comprising several subfields, including molecular biology, ecology, and evolutionary biology, each of which advances our knowledge of living systems, this field clarifies the mechanisms controlling life events, including development, reproduction, and interaction with the surroundings, which is the central goal of biology. Moreover, biology fills in the void between the natural sciences and medicine by offering a necessary understanding of health, illness, and the interactions between organisms and their environments. Dealing with urgent global issues such as climate change, biodiversity loss, and new diseases depends on an awareness of these complex biological interactions, therefore highlighting the critical part biology plays in modern civilization. Fundamentally, biology explores and tests ideas about the living world using the scientific method. Through methodical observation and experimentation,

LEARNING OBJECTIVES

After studying this chapter, you will be able to:

1. Discuss the scientific method in biology;
2. Explain the cell theory;
3. Discuss the genetics and heredity;
4. Evolution and natural selection;
5. Focus on ecology and ecosystems;
6. Learn about human biology;
7. Evaluate the plant biology;
8. Explain the microbiology;
9. Focus on current trends in biology.

1.1. The Scientific Method in Biology

Learning Outcome

1. Describe the steps of the scientific method;
2. Focus on hypothesis formation;
3. Learn about experimental design.

Learning Outcomes

The beginning of each section of every chapter contains a set of Learning Outcomes that inform students of concepts they should understand. These outcomes help students understand what they should be able to do if they have mastered the material in that section.

Test Your Knowledge

Throughout each chapter, Test Your Knowledge cues you to note which topics have been covered and to self-test your understanding of the material presented.

Test Your Knowledge

1. Explain why correlation does not imply causation in scientific experiments.
2. How does the scientific method help reduce the influence of personal opinions in research?

Chapter Summary

The Summary Section appear at the end of each chapter and summarize main concepts covered throughout the chapter. These points provide key concepts in an engaging and meaningful way.

Summary

The investigation of biological principles highlights the importance of a comprehensive view of life by reflecting the intricate interactions that occur within living systems. The complexity of biology goes beyond individual species or systems, as this essay highlights; it also includes the interactions that mold ecosystems and affect biodiversity. Researchers can conduct in-depth analyses of metabolomic data using sophisticated technologies like MetaboAnalyst, which offer insights into the molecular mechanisms underlying these interactions. As demonstrated by the developments in MetaboAnalyst, for example, the integration of diverse omics data promotes a thorough understanding of metabolic pathways and helps identify important biological markers necessary for research on development and disease (Chong et al., 2018). Additionally, the phenomenon of ecological invasions is a key component of biological research and a vital field of study. The introduction of non-native species into unfamiliar habitats has significant ramifications and calls for multidisciplinary management strategies. Examining the origins and effects of these biological incursions, invasion science has become a crucial field that highlights the need to comprehend ecological dynamics and community interactions. As interest in biological invasions increases, new findings are emerging that put conventional ecological theories and practices to the test. The importance of incorporating various scientific viewpoints is shown by this developing discipline, which also highlights how invasive species shape ecosystems and advances our knowledge of ecological resilience (David et al., 2013). When taken as a whole, these discoveries from invasion science and metabolomics highlight the value of multidisciplinary biology research. Fostering cross-disciplinary collaboration and utilizing technological breakthroughs to improve our comprehension of intricate biological interactions are crucial as we look to the future of biological research. In addition to deepening our understanding of the complexities of life, this method lays the groundwork for tackling urgent environmental issues. Future studies can ensure the continued relevance of biology in a world that is constantly changing by acknowledging the interconnection of biological systems and opening the door to creative solutions that support sustainability and biodiversity conservation. We might imagine a thorough comprehension of life that serves both academia and society at large through ongoing investigation and integration of scientific knowledge.

Knowledge Assessment

The chapter includes material designed to review and reinforce each content. It includes Critical Thinking Questions to help test of your understanding of information presented in the chapter and Short answer Questions to review your understanding of the key concepts presented in the chapter.

Critical Thinking Questions

1. **Who is known as the "Father of Modern Biology"?**
   a. Aristotle
   b. Charles Darwin
   c. Gregor Mendel
   d. Louis Pasteur
2. **What is the basic unit of life?**
   a. Atom
   b. Molecule
   c. Cell
   d. Organism
3. **Which branch of biology studies the interaction of organisms with their environment?**
   a. Genetics
   b. Ecology
   c. Physiology
   d. Botany
4. **Which macromolecule is the main source of energy for living organisms?**
   a. Proteins
   b. Lipids
   c. Carbohydrates
   d. Nucleic acids
5. **DNA is primarily responsible for which function in living organisms?**
   a. Energy production
   b. Protein synthesis
   c. Storing genetic information
   d. Regulating body temperature

Short Answer Questions

1. What is biology, and why is it important to study biology?
2. What are the three main domains of life, and how are they different from one another?
3. Define homeostasis and give an example of how it works in living organisms.
4. What is the cell theory, and why is it fundamental to biology?
5. How do autotrophs and heterotrophs differ in the way they obtain energy?
6. What is the scientific method, and how is it applied in biological research?
7. Discuss how biology helps address global challenges such as climate change, disease, and food security.
8. Explain the levels of biological organization from the smallest unit to the largest. Provide examples at each level.
9. Describe the relationship between structure and function in biology, giving specific examples from cells or organs.
10. How has the discovery of genetics shaped our understanding of inheritance and variation among organisms?

Supplementary Materials

Key Terms: A list of key terms is given for quick reference

KEY TERMS FROM THIS CHAPTER

Annotation enrichment analysis	Biological structure	Cell
Cell theory	Cellular structure	Ecology
Ecosystems	Genetics	Human biology
Microbiology	Natural selection	Organism
Plant biology		

Further Resources: Recommendations for additional readings, websites, and multimedia resources.

References

1. Argelaguet, R., Velten, B., Arnol, D., Dietrich, S., Zenz, T., Marioni, J. C., Buettner, F., et al. (2018). Multi-omics factor analysis—A framework for unsupervised integration of multi-omics data sets. *Molecular Systems Biology, 14.* https://doi.org/10.15252/msb.20178124.
2. Bacher, S., Blackburn, T. M., Essl, F., & Genovesi, P. (2017). *Socio-Economic Impact Classification of Alien Taxa (SEICAT).* https://core.ac.uk/download/286567949.pdf (accessed on 8th March 2025).
3. Barnett, R., Brace, S., Cucchi, T., & Dobney, K. (2013). *Divergent Evolutionary Processes Associated with Colonization of Offshore Islands.* https://core.ac.uk/download/20664364.pdf (accessed on 8th March 2025).

Detailed Table of Contents

CHAPTER 2

Cells Involved in Autoimmune Diseases and Inflammation 29

CHAPTER 3

Effector Mechanisms in Autoimmunity and Inflammation 57

CHAPTER 10

Musculoskeletal Biopsy and Histopathology 235

CHAPTER 11

Clinical Pharmacology in Rheumatic Diseases 261

CHAPTER 12

LIST OF FIGURES

PREFACE

The study of rheumatologic disorders spans a broad and evolving landscape, encompassing immune system dysfunction, tissue pathology, and a spectrum of clinical manifestations that affect individuals across all age groups. These conditions are often chronic, with periods of flare-ups and remission, and they influence not only physical health but also emotional and social well-being. Advances in basic sciences, diagnostic imaging, molecular genetics, and targeted therapies have significantly transformed the approach to understanding and managing these diseases. However, a comprehensive foundation in anatomy, physiology, immunology, and pathology remains essential to interpret clinical signs accurately, initiate appropriate interventions, and evaluate treatment outcomes effectively.

Rheumatology brings together information from many fields, including immunology, genetics, pharmacology, and psychosocial medicine. This field demands a deep appreciation of both systemic processes and localized pathologies that impact joints, muscles, and connective tissues. Conditions such as rheumatoid arthritis, systemic lupus erythematosus, and vasculitides present a wide array of diagnostic and therapeutic challenges. These diseases often share overlapping features, making it crucial for healthcare professionals to rely on detailed assessments, laboratory support, imaging studies, and histopathological confirmation. As patient-centered care becomes increasingly important, attention to psychological and quality-of-life factors has emerged as an indispensable component of clinical rheumatology.

This book, *Textbook of Rheumatology Volume 1,* has been crafted to deliver the fundamental ideas and far-reaching information needed for students, clinicians, and scientists looking for an in-depth grasp of rheumatic diseases. This volume consolidates top subspecialists from many disciplines to submit a comprehensive and readable book. While the second book will continue some of the diseases and treatment strategies, this initial book is intended to present an integrated forum that summarizes the biological context, research models, and clinical paradigms of relevance to the subject. Every chapter has been authored with a view to balance scientific rigor and clinical usefulness so that the information presented is informative as well as practical.

Chapter 1 presents the structure and function of bones, joints, and connective tissue, which is essential for grasping how abnormalities arise in rheumatologic diseases. The chapter discusses the organization and mechanical properties of cartilage, synovial fluid, ligaments, and tendons, highlighting their contributions to musculoskeletal integrity and mobility. Understanding these foundational elements provides the baseline from which disease-related changes can be recognized and interpreted.

Chapter 2 focuses on the key immune cells implicated in autoimmunity and inflammatory processes. It outlines the roles of T cells, B-cells, macrophages, dendritic cells, and other leukocytes in normal immune surveillance as well as in pathogenic responses seen in autoimmune conditions. Their interactions with cytokines and chemokines are discussed with an emphasis on how dysregulation contributes to persistent inflammation and tissue injury.

Chapter 3 examines the mechanisms by which autoimmunity and inflammation produce clinical damage. It includes antigen presentation, molecular mimicry, loss of tolerance, and autoantibody formation, as well as cytokine network and complement pathway effects. The focus is on how each of the effector mechanisms plays a role in acute and chronic disease activity, paving the way to specific therapeutic interventions.

Chapter 4 discusses the differing clinical patterns and disease expressions seen across age groups, from pediatric populations to older adults. The chapter describes how hormonal and developmental factors control the onset, severity, and responsiveness to treatment of these syndromes disease, and provides comparative descriptions of juvenile idiopathic arthritis, adult-onset systemic lupus, and age-related syndromes like polymyalgia rheumatica.

Chapter 5 presents an integrated clinical method for evaluating patients with presumed rheumatic disease. History, physical exam, and functional status are stressed as essential. Patterns of complaints like swelling in the joints, morning stiffness, and extra-articular symptoms receive attention and serve to guide differential diagnosis and management recommendations.

Chapter 6 highlights the roles of genetic predisposition and environmental exposures in disease initiation and progression. The text explains how genetic variants, including HLA associations and non-HLA polymorphisms, interact with triggers such as infections, smoking, and microbiome changes. These interactions shape immune responses and modify disease trajectories, offering potential predictive tools and preventive strategies.

Chapter 7 discusses tissues commonly affected in rheumatic conditions, skin, blood vessels, serous membranes, and muscles, outlining how disease processes influence these components. Emphasis is placed on the morphological and functional alterations associated with inflammation, fibrosis, and ischemia, reinforcing the multisystemic nature of many rheumatic diseases.

Chapter 8 addresses the laboratory tests used in rheumatology, from basic hematological and biochemical profiles to advanced serologic and immunologic investigations. The chapter explains the principles behind autoantibody testing, acute phase reactants, and synovial fluid analysis. The reliability, limitations, and interpretative context of each test are explored in detail.

Chapter 9 provides a thorough overview of imaging modalities used in diagnosing and monitoring musculoskeletal disease. It compares conventional radiography, ultrasound, CT, MRI, and nuclear imaging in their application to joint, tendon, and spine assessment. Advances such as power Doppler ultrasound and whole-body MRI are introduced with illustrative examples to enhance understanding.

Chapter 10 centers on musculoskeletal biopsy and histopathological evaluation. It describes techniques for obtaining tissue samples from synovium, muscle, and skin and outlines how histology contributes to diagnosis and prognosis. Key histopathological features in various autoimmune and inflammatory conditions are presented to link clinical findings with microscopic changes.

Chapter 11 outlines pharmacologic principles and drug classes used in rheumatic disease management. This includes an overview of nonsteroidal anti-inflammatory drugs, corticosteroids, disease-modifying antirheumatic drugs, biologics, and emerging small molecules. The chapter discusses mechanisms of action, pharmacokinetics, side effects, and monitoring requirements to promote safe and effective prescribing practices.

Chapter 12 closes the volume with an examination of the psychosocial dimensions of rheumatic diseases. Topics include patient education, coping strategies, mental health issues such as depression and anxiety, and the role of social support networks. The impact of chronic illness on work, relationships, and quality of life is addressed with a view toward holistic patient care.

This text is intended for a wide audience that includes medical students, postgraduate trainees in internal medicine and rheumatology, practicing clinicians, physical and occupational therapists, and allied health professionals. It is equally valuable for researchers and educators who require a solid background in the mechanisms and diagnostic approaches associated with rheumatic disorders. Combining scientific rigor with clinical applicability, this volume serves both as a reference and a teaching tool for those seeking to deepen their knowledge and improve their practice in rheumatology.

STRUCTURE AND FUNCTION OF BONE, JOINTS, AND CONNECTIVE TISSUE

1

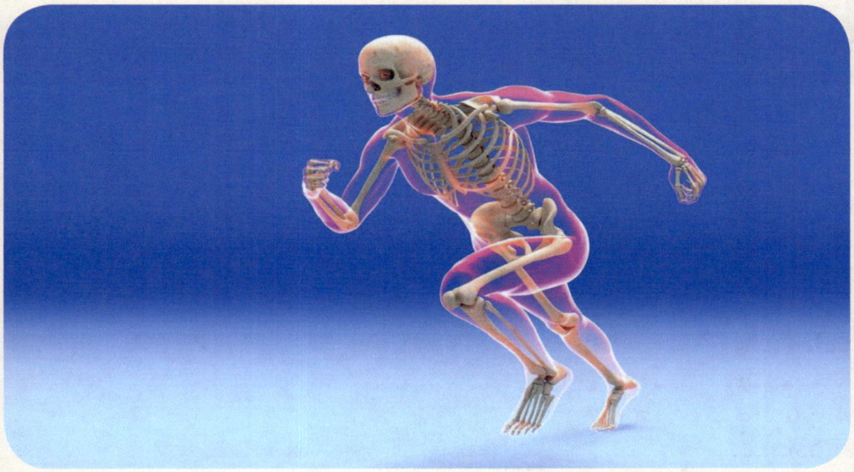

LEARNING OBJECTIVES

After studying this chapter, you will be able to:

1. Define the structure of bone;
2. Explain the function of bone;
3. Define the structure of joints;
4. Learn the function of joints.

Introduction

An understanding of bone structure and function, joints, and connective tissue is a basic aspect of human physiology and health. They are not only required to provide the support and enable movement but also to protect our vital organs and store minerals. The complexity of these interacting systems points toward a remarkable capacity to adjust, as described in recent research that provided the musculoskeletal system's inherent ability to modulate its structure and function to various stimuli. The versatility is particularly crucial in conditions such as prolonged periods of weightlessness, where the musculoskeletal system undergoes widespread unloading that may lead to functional impairment. Also, the advancement in bio-inspired robots has further validated the efficiency of compliant, flexible joints after human physiology, eliminating the brittleness of traditional mechanisms (Lessard et al., 2016). The following investigation will cover these critical aspects, highlighting the significance of understanding these biological models in health and technological progress.

1.1. Structure of Bone

Learning Outcome

1. Understand composition of bone tissue;
2. Explain types of bone;
3. Describe bone cells;
4. Reflect on bone matrix and mineralization;
5. Describe blood supply and innervation of bone;
6. Identify types of bones;
7. Describe bone remodeling process;
8. Describe role of hormones in bone structure;
9. Identify age-related changes in bone structure.

The bone structure is specifically designed to fulfill its multicategorical functions in the human body, providing mechanical support and a reservoir for minerals. Comprised mostly of a matrix of collagen fiber and mineral salt-rich, the bone tissue shows strong tensile strength and stiffness. As a result of the composite nature of the structure, bones can withstand many loads and maintain their form. The bone also expresses plasticity through its response to mechanical stress; it can change its density and architecture based on the loads it is exposed to, which is indicative of its plasticity. For instance, weightlessness induced by long-duration space flight provokes adaptive change in the musculoskeletal system, with possible structural injury. Such a dynamic nature underscores the importance of understanding bone physiology in health and disease, adding to a better appreciation of connective tissue and its wider implications for physical function (Figure 1.1).

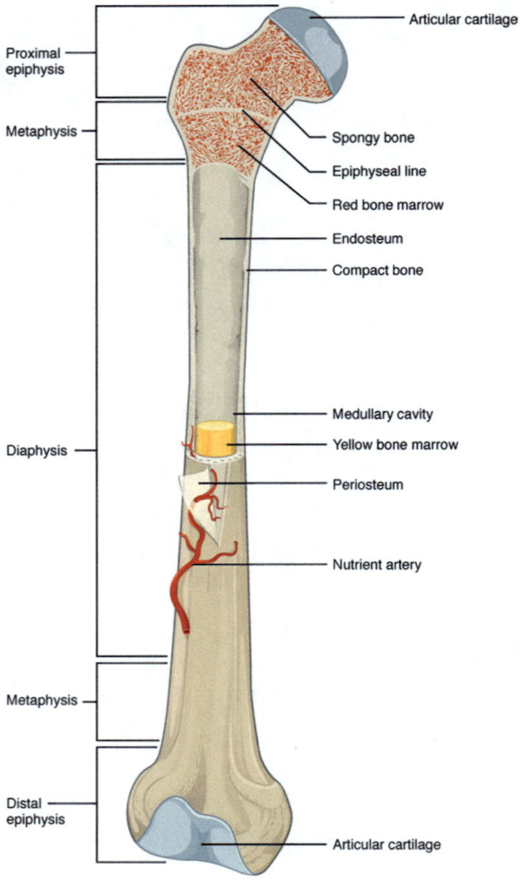

Figure 1.1. The structure of bone.

Source: https://pressbooks-dev.oer.hawaii.edu/anatomyandphysiology/wp-content/uploads/sites/29/2017/09/603_Anatomy_of_a_Long_Bone.jpg..

1.1.1. Composition of Bone Tissue

The composition of bone tissue is a complex interaction of organic and inorganic components that enables it to perform and continue to be structurally intact. Comprising approximately 30% organic material in the form of collagen fibers, bone tissue provides bones with flexibility and tensile strength. The remaining 70% consists of inorganic minerals, primarily hydroxyapatite, contributing to bone hardness and resistance to compressive forces. The unique structure enables bones to withstand a range of mechanical forces without being overly cumbersome. Furthermore, bone is also marked by a dynamic cellular milieu, composed of osteoblasts, osteocytes, and osteoclasts, which play significant roles in the continuous processes of bone remodeling and repair. Besides, the musculoskeletal system plasticity demonstrates that overloading, as during weightlessness, can have a detrimental effect on bone strength and density due to the lack of mechanical stress, yet again emphasizing the need for interventions to protect the bone under the conditions of change (Burgin et al., 2013). The intricate relationship between composition and function again puts into perspective the importance of bone in the structure and function of the skeleton.

1.1.2. Types of Bone: Compact vs. Spongy

There are two types of bones that constitute the skeletal system: compact and spongy bone, both with some definite structural and functional functions. Compact bone, which is dense in appearance, forms the outer layer of the bones, providing them with strength and support through stress. Such bone is organized into osteons, or Haversian systems, which provide for the delivery of nutrients and the removal of waste products through a canal system. Spongy bone, found principally at the ends of the long bones and in the interior of others, is spongy in nature to reduce weight but contribute to strength. Such a trabecular structure is required to contain bone marrow, within which hematopoiesis occurs. The relationship of compact and spongy bone represents a unique example of structural organization working together with functional demand within the bone structure, as explained in the overall model of bone structure and physiology (Cozart et al., 2017; Rahardjo et al., 2018) (Figure 1.2).

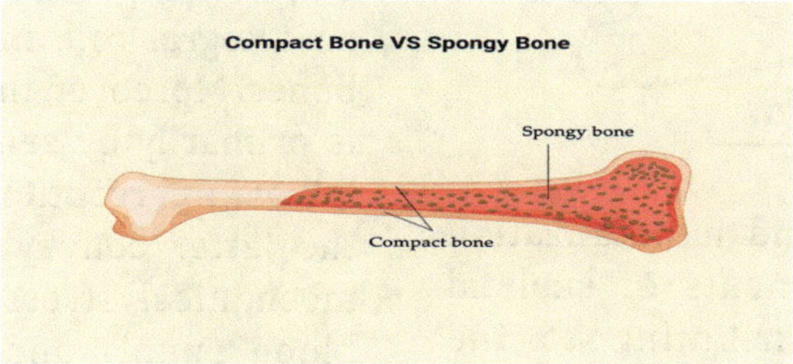

Figure 1.2. The skeletal system comprises two distinct types of bone: compact and spongy bone, each serving unique structural and functional roles.

Source: https://knyamed.com/cdn/shop/articles/Compact-Bone-VS-Spongy-Bone.jpg?v=1711457463..

1.1.3. Bone Cells: Osteoblasts, Osteocytes, and Osteoclasts

The dynamic intercellular interactions of bone cells—osteoblasts, osteocytes, and osteoclasts—play a critical role in the integrity and homeostasis of the skeleton. Osteoblasts, the bone-forming cells, create and secrete the extracellular matrix for mineralization to take place. Trapped in the matrix, they transform into osteocytes and are mechanosensors, which in turn respond to both osteoblasts and osteoclasts for regulating processes involved in bone remodeling. Osteoclasts play a crucial role in bone resorption, breaking down mineralized tissue to release calcium and phosphate into the bloodstream. This intricate balance relies on regulation by connexins, influencing differentiation and function of these cells; for instance, connexin43 plays a significant role in osteoblast and osteoclast function, and connexin37 plays a significant role in osteoclast differentiation (Plotkin et al., 2015). These collaborative efforts are meant to emphasize the significance of interactions between bone cells in developing therapeutic regimens for bone disorders (García et al., 2021).

1.1.4. Bone Matrix and Mineralization

Bone matrix and mineralization are essential components of skeletal function and health that make up the integrity of bones and the musculoskeletal system overall. Bone matrix is composed primarily of collagen fibers for tensile strength and a dense mineral phase with high hydroxyapatite concentration, a crystalline structure that enables bones to withstand compressive loads.

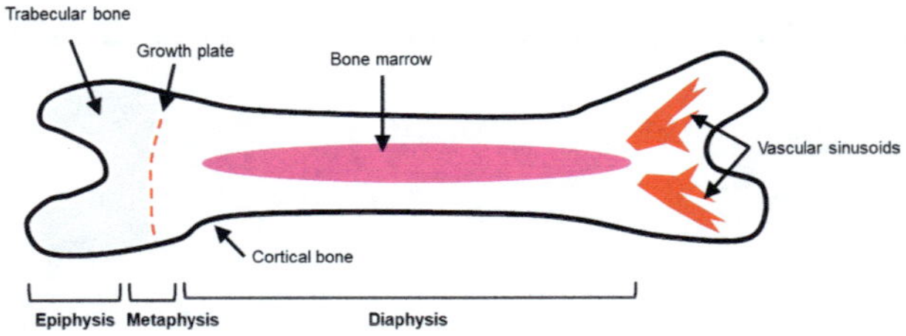

Figure 1.3. Bone matrix and mineralization represent essential components of skeletal health and function, contributing to the structural integrity of bones and the overall musculoskeletal system.

Source: https://pub.mdpi-res.com/cancers/cancers-11-01020/article_deploy/html/images/cancers-11-01020-g001.png?1564746519.

Mineralization is a dynamic process of depositing minerals such as calcium and phosphate into this matrix that is necessary to maintain bones strong and dense. Interference in the mineralization of this process can lead to pathological conditions such as osteoporosis, where the balance between bone formation and bone resorption is impaired. Studies have revealed that some molecular pathways that are involved in the regulation of mineralization, such as the role of equilibrative nucleoside transporter 1 (ENT1), possess the capacity to influence ectopic calcification and degenerative connective tissue changes, thereby portraying the complexity of bone homeostasis (Warraich, 2013) (Figure 1.3).

1.1.5. Blood Supply and Innervation of Bone

Bone innervation and blood supply are crucial to maintaining its health and functional ability and have a direct impact on the general skeletal system physiology. Bone tissue is highly vascular, with the majority of its blood supply provided by the periosteal arteries that penetrate into the bone and branch into smaller vessels for the purpose of removing waste and supplying nutrients. Nutrient arteries entering through the nutrient foramina provide the interior of the bone with essential resources needed by bone cells, particularly osteocytes, which play an integral role in repairing and maintaining bones. Moreover, the innervation of bone, which is primarily by sensory nerve fibers, is crucial for pain perception and mechanotransduction, the latter conveying the bone's response to mechanical stresses. Such synergy between blood supply and innervation indicates the complexity of bone as a living tissue, necessary both for structural support and for metabolic needs (Larson, 1996; Cozart et al., 2017).

1.1.6. Types of Bones: Long, Short, Flat, and Irregular

The human skeleton is divided into four basic bone categories: long, short, flat, and irregular, each with a special structural and functional role. The long bones, such as the femur and humerus, are named by their length and play a central role in weight support and locomotion and offer muscular attachment and ease of motion. Short bones like the carpals and the tarsals provide support and stability but only allow a minor amount of motion, which is required for dexterity in situations such as the wrists and ankles. Flat bones like the ribs and the cranial bones are utilized for protection, guarding the vital organs and providing attachment surfaces for muscles. Irregular bones, such as pelvic bones and vertebrae, consist of complex shapes that are adapted to specific functions, ranging from support to shielding the spinal cord. This difference among the bone types indicates the complex structure of the skeleton that accommodates different types of movements and operations critical for human life (Anton du Plessis et al., 2021; Benedetti et al., 2021) (Figure 1.4).

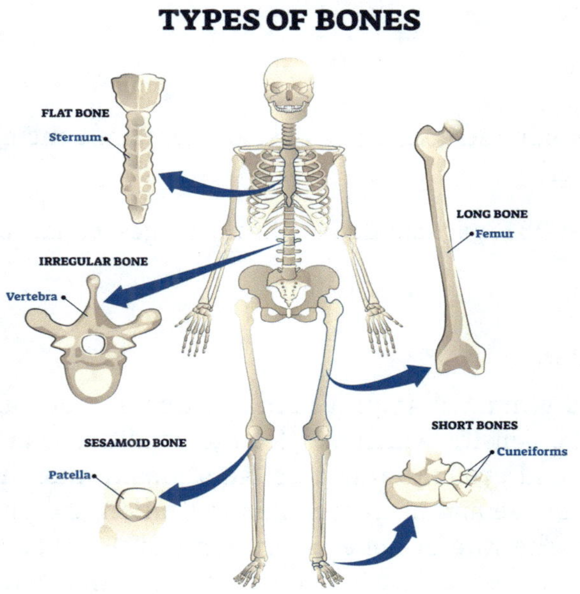

Figure 1.4. The human skeleton is composed of four primary types of bones: long, short, flat, and irregular, each serving distinct structural and functional purposes.

Source: https://ptinstitute.co.uk/wp-content/uploads/2021/05/IMAGE_3_Bone_Classifications_-Converted-scaled.jpg.

1.1.7. Bone Remodeling Process

The bone remodeling process is a crucial physiological process that ensures bone integrity and mechanical strength throughout the life of a person. This complex process is the combined activity of osteoclasts, which break down bone tissue, and osteoblasts, which form new bone. These cellular dynamic processes enable the skeletal system to adapt to various mechanical stresses and to heal micro-damage from normal use. Strangely enough, bone remodeling rates are heavily influenced by hormonal regulation and mechanical loading, suggesting the highly interdependent nature of these factors and skeletal health. Bone remodeling dysregulation may cause diseases like osteoporosis, where the equilibrium is tipped towards over-resorption, resulting in brittle bones. Furthermore, the process of remodeling is akin to processes in tendinopathy, in which turnover of collagen is disrupted, as indicated by type III collagen and metalloproteinases overexpression, suggesting that insight into such mechanisms is essential in the prevention of degenerative disease (Beeson et al., 2009; McCormick et al., 2008).

1.1.8. Role of Hormones in Bone Structure

Hormones play a significant role in the regulation of bone structure and growth, both in the establishment and preservation of skeletal integrity. Estrogen, in particular, is vital to osteogenesis as it maintains bone density and structure by promoting osteoblastic action and inhibiting osteoclastic action, resulting in bone resorption. Hormonal control extends even to bones to affect other structures in connective tissues such as tendons and ligaments. Interestingly, while estrogen stimulates muscle size and strength, it also decreases tendon and ligament rigidity, potentially with a negative effect on the risk of injury in female athletes, as indicated in Baar et al. (2018). Additionally, bone formation mechanisms through intramembranous and endochondral ossifications can be affected by hormone levels, further emphasizing the complex interplay of hormonal balance and bone health, as indicated in Rahardjo et al. (2018). This intricate interaction indicates the key role that hormones have in bone structure and related connective tissues (Figure 1.5).

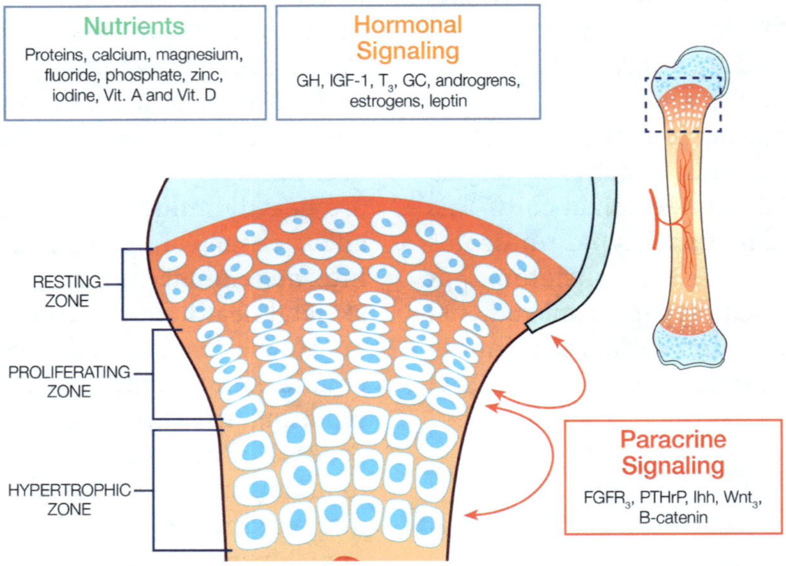

Figure 1.5. Hormones play a critical role in regulating bone structure and development, influencing both the formation and maintenance of skeletal integrity.

Source: https://www.mdpi.com/children/children-11-00817/article_deploy/html/images/children-11-00817-g001.png.

1.1.9. Age-related Changes in Bone Structure

As one ages, extensive changes in the bone structure ultimately impact both function and overall skeletal integrity. These changes include reduced bone density, which may lead to conditions such as osteoporosis, making the bones more susceptible and prone to fractures. Additionally, there is a loss of bone quality with microarchitectural compromise and decreased mineralization, thereby increasing the susceptibility of skeletal frameworks. The rate of bone resorption has a tendency to surpass that of bone formation due to a decline in osteoblast activity in combination with amplified osteoclast activity. Interestingly, the biochemical mechanisms of these alterations are yet to be fully explored, with ongoing studies suggesting that proinflammatory cytokines could be pivotal in mediating bone metabolism alterations during aging (Riley, 2004). Furthermore, these aging alterations in the bone have the ability to induce altered functional stresses on adjacent structures, such as periodontal ligaments, hence inducing complex biomechanical adaptations in associated tissues (Lee et al., 2013).

Test Your Knowledge

1. What are the main parts of a long bone?
2. What is the function of the periosteum?

1.2. Function of Bone

Learning Outcome

1. Explain how bone supports and shapes the body;
2. Explain the defense of important organs;
3. Prioritize movement and leverage;
4. Explain mineral storage and homeostasis;
5. Understand blood cell production in bone marrow;
6. Prioritize energy storage in bone adipocytes;
7. Know the function in endocrine function;
8. Explain the effect of exercise on bone function;
9. Prioritize pathological bone function conditions.

Bones serve critical functions beyond acting as structural support for the body; they are dynamic tissues and also perform major roles in many physiological functions. Among these are serving as protective coverings to the vital organs, facilitating movement through joints, and storing minerals like calcium and phosphorus. Bones are also involved in the process of hematopoiesis since they harbor bone marrow where blood cells are formed.

Current evidence indicates that bone's cellular and molecular reactions to mechanical loading are critical to understand with the aim of understanding bone disease and health. As an example, research into the bone-periodontal ligament-cementum complex reveals that changes in these tissues create enormous changes in bone function, reflecting on the deeply interconnected relationship between mechanical forces and bone remodeling processes (Riley, 2004; Lee et al., 2013). Hence, the multilateral role of bone highlights its significance in the health and homeostasis of the body as a whole (Figure 1.6).

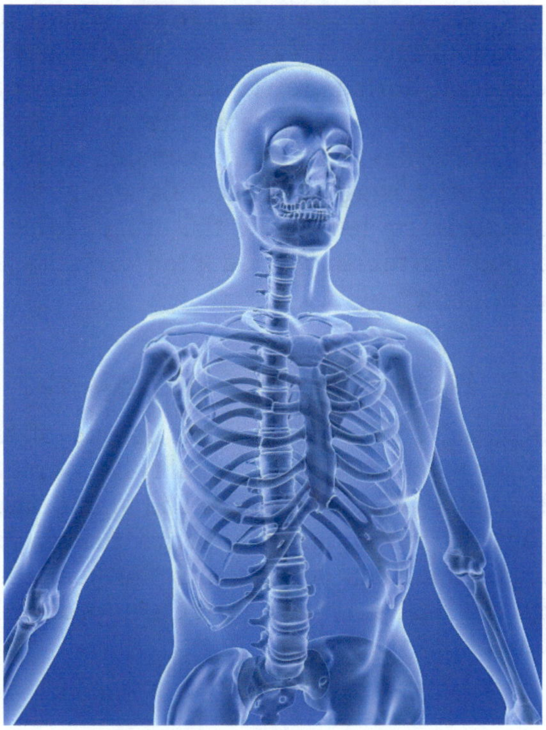

Figure 1.6. Bones serve critical functions beyond mere structural support for the body; they are dynamic tissues that play vital roles in various physiological processes.

Source: https://cdn.mos.cms.futurecdn.net/mGfKXFfhxXuLuoCT8ZnuxZ-1200-80.jpg.

1.2.1. Support and Shape of the Body

The intricate structure of bone, joints, and connective tissue forms the foundation for support and shape in the human body. Bones provide stability and bodily support, allowing the upright stance and aiding locomotion through their joint articulation. It not only houses and protects vital organs but also serves as a reservoir for minerals employed for the maintenance of the body. The active state of bone is further highlighted by developmental processes described in Abzhanov et al. (2019), where cranial neural crest mesenchyme influences the morphology and integration of various tissues such that skeletal frameworks adapt to functional demands. Also, the function of mobility exercises, particularly in adolescents during growth stages, as identified in Rouvali (2016), indicates the necessity of maintaining flexibility and functional integrity in such stabilizing structures. Generally, these characteristics detail how the architecture of the body is thoroughly adapted for stability and flexibility.

1.2.2. Protection of Vital Organs

Protection of the vital organs is one of the primary functions of the skeletal system, greatly helped along by the structure and organization of bones, joints, and connective tissue. The ribcage, for example, encloses the heart and lungs and has a very robust but elastic protection against bodily injury.

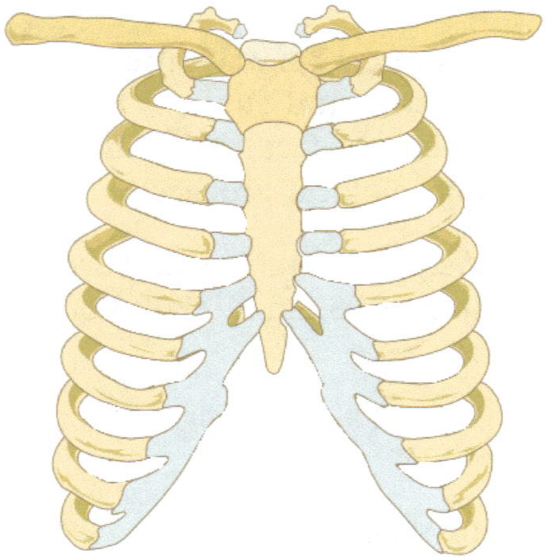

Figure 1.7. The rib cage, for example, encases the heart and lungs, providing a sturdy yet flexible barrier against physical trauma.

Source: https://upload.wikimedia.org/wikipedia/commons/d/d1/Rib_cage.gif.

The pelvis similarly guards organs of the lower abdominal cavity, an instance of the structural function of bone in protecting vulnerable tissues. Besides, other types of connective tissue , such as cartilage, also play a crucial role in offering strength and function to joints that connect bones to each other, as well as safeguarding organs from impaired motion. It is also critical to observe that injury to the musculoskeletal system will increase the risk of damage to important organs and therefore, should also involve thorough investigations after trauma (Alsheikhly et al., 2018). As a whole, the bony framework is not only for structural support but also for being a vital protector of the body's most vulnerable parts (Patwardhan, 2008) (Figure 1.7).

1.2.3. Movement and Leverage

It is important to understand the movement dynamics and leverage within the human musculoskeletal structure so as to comprehend its function and structure as a whole. Bones, joints, and connective tissues all unite to create a structure that supports complicated movement—essentially levers to optimize performance and reduce energy usage. The leverage caused by bones allows for muscle contractions to produce sufficient movement in the body. As highlighted in cranial structure, disturbances in the molecular and cellular systems can affect both form as well as function, that is, how these factors contribute in adaptive evolution of movement (Abzhanov et al., 2019). In addition, hyaluronic acid is crucial in providing effective joint lubrication that is vital in facilitating smooth and effective movement under stress mechanics (Ashrafi et al., 2024). Thus, the interaction between structure and function illustrated by movement and leverage is to impress upon us the importance of an optimally integrated musculoskeletal system in maintaining both mobility and overall health.

1.2.4. Mineral Storage and Homeostasis

The role of bone in the storage and homeostasis of minerals plays a pivotal function in maintaining overall physiological balance in the human body.

Bones serve as reservoirs for essential minerals, primarily calcium and phosphorus, required for various metabolic processes, including muscle contraction and conduction of nerve impulses. As mineral status varies, the body implements complicated regulatory processes, under strict control of hormones like parathyroid hormone and calcitonin, to ensure homeostasis. These hormones facilitate the release or deposition of minerals based on demand, illustrating the dynamic character of bone tissue. New evidence indicates that loaded conditions altered, such as in the case of ligature-induced periodontitis, can exert a strong effect on the bone's mineral metabolism, which means that mechanical stress affects cellular reaction concerning bone remodeling and mineralization (Lee et al., 2013). In addition, interaction between mechanical and neuroendocrine components accounts for the enhanced complexity of bone health, particularly in obese populations (Reeves et al., 2014) (Figure 1.8).

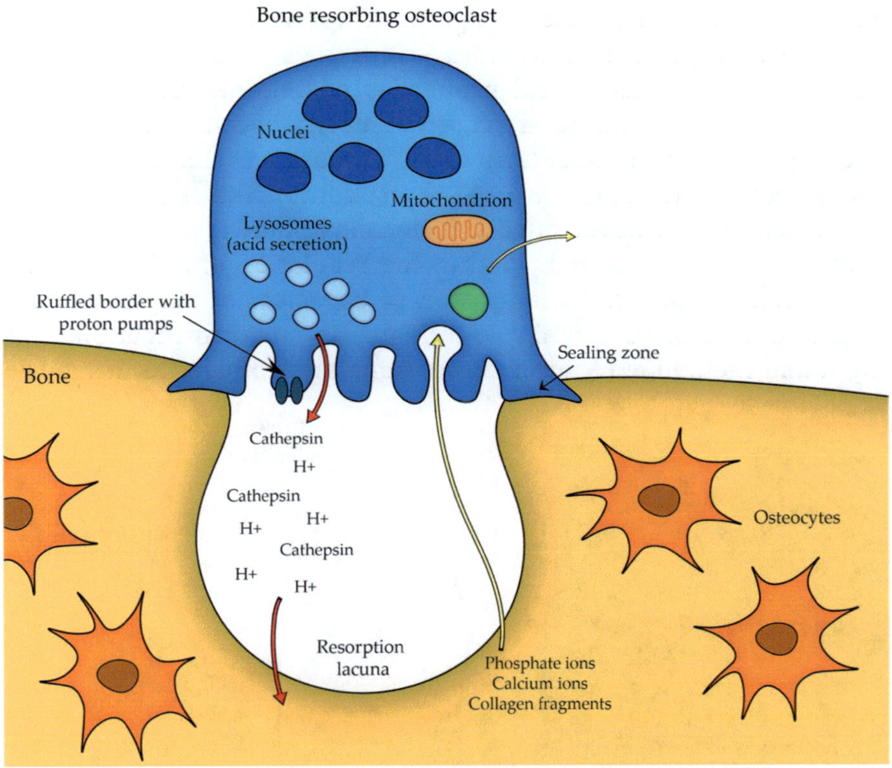

Figure 1.8. The role of bone in mineral storage and homeostasis is critical for maintaining overall physiological balance within the human body.

Source: https://www.mdpi.com/cells/cells-12-02576/article_deploy/html/images/cells-12-02576-g002.png.

1.2.5. Blood Cell Production in Bone Marrow

Production of blood cells in the bone marrow, an important process known as hematopoiesis, highlights the intricate association of bone structure with its multifarious functions. Located within the cavities of certain of the bones, such as the vertebrae and pelvis, is the bone marrow, which is the site of the primary production of the red blood cells, white blood cells, and platelets.

This functioning activity not only maintains the oxygen-carrying capacity and immune status of the body but also highlights the role of the bone matrix in hematopoietic stem cell support. Surprisingly, synovial tissue homeostasis diseases , such as rheumatoid arthritis are capable of affecting bone marrow function through the regulation of immune cell recruitment, as reflected by the increased prevalence of pro-inflammatory macrophages during disease activity (Kurowska-Stolarska & Alivernini, 2017). Thus, blood cell generation in bone marrow needs to be known to value more general meanings of bone health on whole-body physiology and disease states like ankylosing spondylitis (Owen et al., 2017).

1.2.6. Energy Storage in Adipocytes of Bone

The relationship between energy storage in bone adipocytes and structural outcomes reveals a complex relationship of biological processes significant for valuing bone physiology. Adipocytes, traditionally associated with peripheral fat storage in tissues, also inhabit the bone marrow and influence metabolic as well as mechanical properties of bone. Recent findings document that cortical bone strength is elevated due to increased adiposity because of obesity and suggest that the accumulated energy in such adipocytes may be a causative factor for bone adaptation and remodeling to mechanical load (Reeves et al., 2014). In addition, the effect of abnormal metabolism and obesity also impacts bone turnover rates and signaling pathways, demonstrating how skeletal integrity should be maintained since it is vital in the regulation of adipocyte function (Adam et al., 2012). Therefore, bone adipocytes' energy storage capacity not only serves as a reservoir for systemic metabolism but also plays a vital role in regulating the coordination of balance between mechanical strength and metabolic requirement of bone and connective tissue (Figure 1.9).

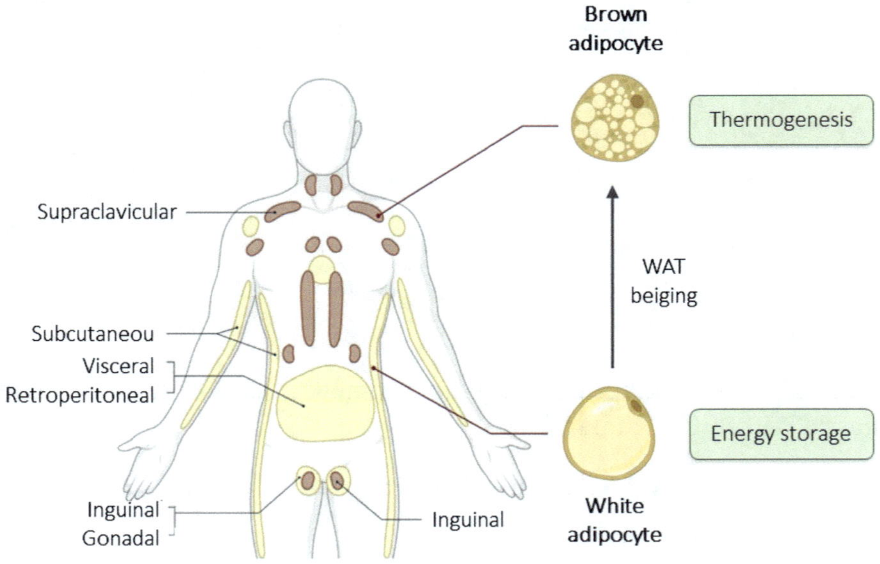

Figure 1.9. Adipocytes, traditionally associated with fat storage in peripheral tissues, also inhabit the bone marrow, influencing both metabolic and mechanical properties of bone.

Source: https://www.mdpi.com/cells/cells-13-00380/article_deploy/html/images/cells-13-00380-g001.png.

1.2.7. Role in Endocrine Function

The complex interrelationship of the musculoskeletal system and endocrine activity plays an essential role in assisting the homeostasis of the body as a whole. In addition to providing structural support, bones, joints, and connective tissue play an important role in endocrine control through their secretion of hormones and signaling molecules. As an illustration, osteoblasts secrete the hormone osteocalcin, which has an impact on insulin sensitivity and the metabolism of fat, thus pointing to the intersection between bone health and metabolic regulation. In addition, through the experience of mechanical loading and unloading, such as with long periods of weightlessness faced when going into space, the adaptive traits of bone and muscle tissue illustrate how sensitive they are to endocrine signals that control growth and repair processes. Understanding these dynamics is paramount, as testified to by some of the more mature concepts in Ayurveda, where a balance of bodily dhātus will determine functional health, relating structure and endocrine function in an integrated manner (Patwardhan, 2008).

1.2.8. Impact of Physical Activity on Bone Function

Physical exercise plays an important role in the maintenance and enhancement of bone function through a process known as mechanotransduction, where mechanical stress on bones results in bone remodeling and growth. Resistance and weight-bearing exercises on a daily basis guarantee the development of bone mineral density, reducing the risk of osteoporosis and fractures at advanced age.

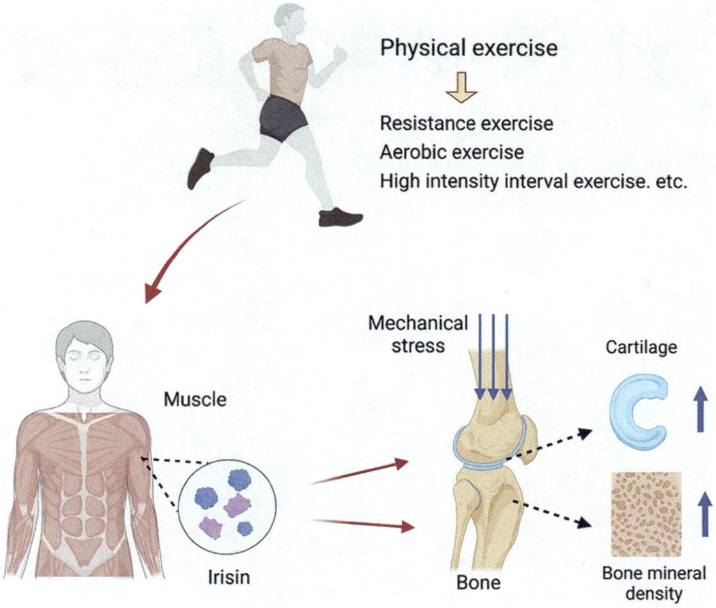

Figure 1.10. Physical activity plays a crucial role in maintaining and enhancing bone function, primarily through a process known as mechanotransduction, where mechanical stress applied to bones stimulates bone remodeling and growth.

Source: https://www.frontiersin.org/files/Articles/934406/fnagi-14-934406-HTML/image_m/fnagi-14-934406-g001.jpg.

On the contrary, prolonged sedentary living can lead to harmful changes in bone structure and strength, as indicated by experiments showing the extreme negative effects of prolonged weightlessness on the musculoskeletal system, proving the plasticity of bone structure in response to load. In addition, patients with diseases like ankylosing spondylitis (AS) tend to have compromised bone function, for which there is a need to engage in non-impact exercises to ensure mobility and avoid further deterioration of the joint structures (Owen et al., 2017). Thus, the inclusion of regular physical activity in daily lifestyles is integral to ensuring optimal bone health and the general musculoskeletal integrity (Figure 1.10).

1.2.9. Pathological Conditions Affecting Bone Function

Pathological conditions that impact bone function are critical to the stability of the skeletal system and have a direct impact on mobility and overall health. Osteoarthritis, for instance, is defined by degenerative change in the synovial joints that not only compromises structural integrity but also initiates proteolytic activity that degrades the extracellular matrix, as typified by complex interactions among matrix metalloproteinases (MMPs) and other proteases (Buttle et al., 2008). These biochemical disturbances can lead to increased bone turnover and architectural changes that increase pain and functional impairment. Besides, research has emphasized addressing these ailments through appropriate methodologies taking into account a number of factors, including biomechanical stress and skeletal preservation in fossil groups (Becker et al., 2019). Deeper knowledge of these pathologic mechanisms is paramount for designing effective treatment protocols and improvement in the quality of life for individuals suffering from such debilitating illnesses.

Test Your Knowledge

1. List and briefly describe the five major functions of bone.
2. How does bone contribute to regulating calcium homeostasis?

1.3. Structure of Joints

Learning Outcome

1. Gain understanding of the classification of joints;
2. Learn synovial joint anatomy;
3. Describe joint capsules, ligaments;
4. Explain the structure of articular cartilage;
5. Highlight synovial fluid and function;
6. Discuss the bursae's role in joint function;
7. Understand stability vs. mobility in the joint structure;
8. Know age changes in joint structure;
9. Identify common joint injury and structural implications.

Joint structure is at the foundation of joint function and skeletal mechanics overall. Joints, or their classification into synovial, fibrous, and cartilaginous types, possess unique architectural forms that are appropriate to their functions in motion and stability. Synovial joints, for instance, and their joint capsules and synovial fluid, provide optimum mobility with smooth movement between nearby bones. Subchondral bone density response in these joints reflects the chronic mechanical stresses that they experience, which may lead to significant variation in structural integrity in aged populations (Bullough et al., 1993). Secondly, the effect of pathological conditions, such as periodontal disease, illustrates that change in the periodontal ligament and cementum has direct implications for joint function and well-being. This emphasizes the role of joint structure in providing both functional mobility and structural stability within the skeleton (Lee et al., 2013).

1.3.1. Classification of Joints: Fibrous, Cartilaginous, Synovial

Knowing the classification of joints is critical for understanding their structural and functional roles in the human body. Three primary forms of joints can be categorized based on them: fibrous, cartilaginous, and synovial. Fibrous joints, such as sutures in the skull, have little or no movement and are characterized by dense connective tissue that holds together neighboring bones. Cartilaginous joints, such as intervertebral discs, have little movement and are employed to absorb shocks while providing support. Synovial joints, the most movable, contain intricate structures , such as cartilage, ligaments, and synovial fluid, which enable movement and reduce friction. Microscopic and macroscopic features of these joints highlight their functional importance: fibrous joints provide stability, cartilaginous joints provide flexibility, and synovial joints enable a considerable degree of motion, hence showcasing the functional interdependence between form and function in the human musculoskeletal system (Patil et al., 2020) (Figure 1.11).

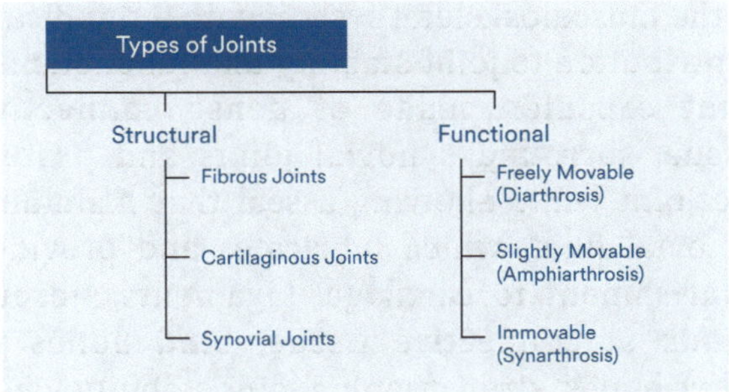

Figure 1.11. Joints can be categorized into three primary types: fibrous, cartilaginous, and synovial.

Source: https://cdn.shopify.com/s/files/1/0606/7313/0669/files/Understanding_Joint_Health_2.jpg?v=1712142046.

1.3.2. Anatomy of Synovial Joints

Synovial joints are a complex structural component of the human skeletal system, characterized by their sophisticated architecture that allows for a variety of movements. Synovial joints have several key structures, including the synovial membrane, which produces the synovial fluid, acting as a lubricant to minimize friction between joint movements. The presence of articular cartilage, a form of specialized connective tissue, also adds to shock-absorbing capacity required in weight-bearing function. Synovial joints are likewise usually stabilized by ligaments and tendons, adding to structural dependability while allowing flexibility. The interaction of these anatomical structures not only permits locomotion but is also involved in joint durability against wear and tear in general. It is essential to know the anatomy of synovial joints, as dysfunctions in these areas may lead to severe disorders, such as those in the case of ankylosing spondylitis, that involve several systems of the body (Cozart et al., 2017; Owen et al., 2017).

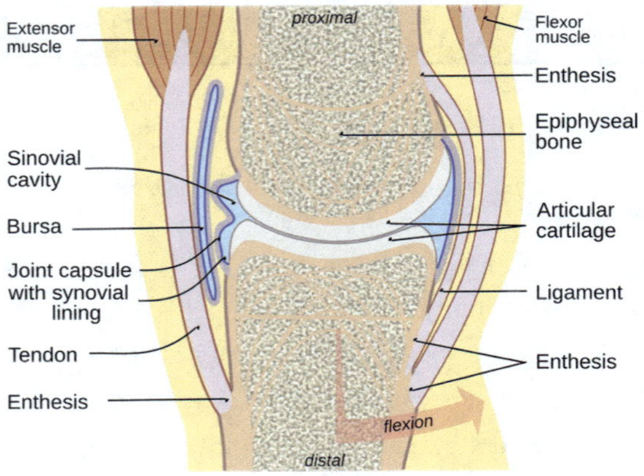

Figure 1.12. Joint capsules and ligaments are crucial components of the musculoskeletal system, contributing significantly to the stability and functionality of joints.

Source: https://upload.wikimedia.org/wikipedia/commons/thumb/7/7f/Joint.svg/1200px-Joint.svg.png.

1.3.3. Joint Capsules and Ligaments

Joint capsules and ligaments are basic structures of the musculoskeletal system with a significant contribution to joint stability and functionality. Joint capsules, made of dense connective tissue, surround synovial joints and protect the joint while allowing a seal that maintains synovial fluid, which lubricates and provides nourishment to cartilage. Ligaments, fibrous bands of connective tissue, bind bones to other bones, strengthening joint stability while allowing a certain amount of movement. They are tendon-like in structure, with a complicated matrix of collagen fibers providing elasticity and tensile strength (Karahan et al., 2019).

In addition, the overlying fascia also plays the role of supporting and compartmentalizing the musculoskeletal structures, a sign of how these tissues are interrelated (Hetherington et al., 2019). Along with joint capsules and ligaments, they permit movement as well as safeguard against injury, emphasizing their structural role in the body's overall integrity (Figure 1.12).

1.3.4. Articular Cartilage Structure

Articular cartilage is a specialized connective tissue with an important function in joint function through the provision of a smooth, lubricated surface for articulation and transmission of loads across the joint during movement. Articular cartilage is structurally composed of hyaline cartilage, which consists of chondrocytes surrounded by an extracellular matrix containing collagen fibers, proteoglycans, and water. This novel organization is also the cause of the tissues' enhanced mechanical behavior, like resilience and flexibility. Recent advances in imaging technologies, e.g., polarized-light techniques for optical imaging, have unlocked the knowledge of articular cartilage's microstructural characteristics and allowed insight into what happens when it is under healthy and pathological loads. Such developments also provide promise for tissue-engineering therapies to cartilage pathology, since they provide significant information for the establishment of successful therapeutic treatments for pathologies like osteoarthritis

(Matcher, 2009). Understanding the intricate organization of articular cartilage is therefore essential in advancing both clinical practices and studies on joint function (Burgin et al., 2013).

1.3.5. Synovial Fluid and Its Functions

Synovial fluid plays a critical role in the general synovial joint operation, serving not just as a lubricant but also as a medium of exchange for nutrients and tissue homeostasis.

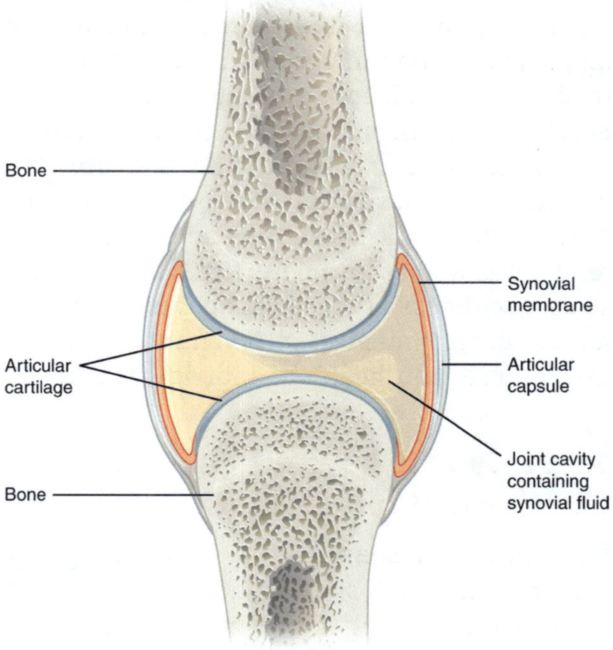

Figure 1.13. Synovial fluid plays a crucial role in the overall function of synovial joints, serving not only as a lubricant but also as a medium for nutrient exchange and tissue homeostasis.

Source: https://pressbooks-dev.oer.hawaii.edu/anatomyandphysiology/wp-content/uploads/sites/29/2017/09/907_Synovial_Joints.jpg.

The synovial fluid is viscous in composition and significantly reduces the friction between articular cartilages with movements of joints, thereby avoiding wear and tear. In addition, synovial fluid contains high concentrations of hyaluronic acid and lubricin, the origin of its specific rheology, thus making it an even more effective lubricant (Krause, 2008). Apart from its mechanical functions, synovial fluid also serves as a reservoir for certain immune cells, e.g., macrophages that maintain tissue homeostasis. Recent research has shown that these resident macrophages, in addition to infiltrating leukocytes in conditions of inflammation, are critical for maintaining joint health, especially where this involves rheumatoid arthritis, as they regulate inflammatory reactions (Kurowska-Stolarska & Alivernini, 2017). As such, it is important to appreciate the multidimensional functions of synovial fluid to understand joint stability and disease (Figure 1.13).

1.3.6. Role of Bursae in Joint Function

Bursae play a crucial role in joint function by their smooth movement and prevention of friction between various tissues, particularly bone and muscle. The small fluid-filled sacs act as shock-absorbing cushions that relieve pressure upon the movement of tendons or muscles over bony prominences during joint use. This is particularly evident in joints of high mobility , such as the knee and the shoulder, where wear and inflammation are caused by repetitive motion. Interestingly, the synovial membrane structure, which is involved in bursae development, is distinct from that of the fibrous capsule, suggesting that bursae occur as independent structures in the joint apparatus (Hyc et al., 2014). Therefore, functioning bursae in a normal state are essential not only for the function of a joint but also for overall musculoskeletal integrity. The function of bursae can provide insight into the pathophysiology of pathologies , such as bursitis, where joint mechanics is destabilized by inflammation (Abujarour et al., 2018).

1.3.7. Stability vs. Mobility in Joint Structure

The interaction between mobility and stability in joint structure is a biomechanical principle underlying both function and vulnerability to injury. Joints are designed to weigh these two opposing values; some structures, the hip joint, lean towards stability by virtue of deep sockets and robust ligaments and others, the shoulder joint, prefer mobility but lose stability. This delicate balance is also shaped by the surrounding myofascial tissues, which also provide stabilizing support through mechanisms of passive tension referred to as human resting myofascial tone (HRMT). Evidence suggests that this passive stiffness plays an important role in maintaining an upright posture and dynamic stability with movement and therefore linking joint structure with stability and mobility (Masi et al., 2010). Furthermore, biomechanical model developments explain how these principles are being transferred in a clinical setting, and our understanding of movement and rehabilitation is enhanced (Harris et al., 2012) (Figure 1.14).

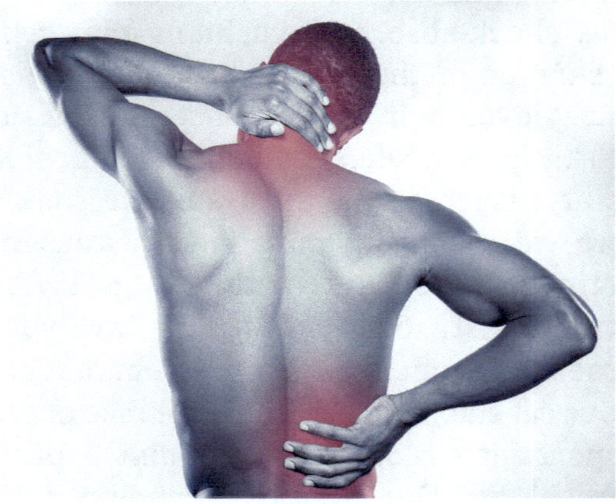

Figure 1.14. The relationship between stability and mobility in joint structure is a fundamental aspect of biomechanics, influencing both functionality and the potential for injury.

Source: https://mainstaymedical.com/wp-content/uploads/2023/02/Images-2023-02-28T141434.632.jpg.

1.3.8. Age-related Changes in Joint Structure

With increasing age, structural modification of the joints becomes a major factor in mobility and function. Such age-related alterations include cartilage weakening, which, due to reduced extracellular matrix production, thins and becomes less viscoelastic to eventually impair joint functioning. Additionally, the reduction of synovial fluid production leads to reduced lubrication, hence increased friction upon movement. These variations are most apparent in the instance of tendinopathy, where age-related biochemical alterations may affect tendon integrity and repair, making tendons more vulnerable to injury (Riley, 2004). Furthermore, hormones , such as estrogen play a key role in maintaining the integrity of connective tissue, and their diminishment during aging will accelerate deterioration in tendons as well as ligaments (Baar et al., 2018). Thus, awareness of these changes is important for the development of interventions that aim to preserve joint health as individuals age.

1.3.9. Common Joint Injuries and Their Structural Implications

Joint injury is shared by a broad range of activities, including sporting activities and daily activities, and joint injury has the ability to greatly alter the structural make-up of associated tissues. A classic case is a rotator cuff tear, which involves partial or complete disruption of the tendons that surround the shoulder. The injury predisposes one to agonizing pain and mobility constraints, curbing one's quality of life. As one ages, the prevalence of such injury increases, as degenerative changes are the causative factors (Loccisano et al., 2016). Parallel with this, metatarsal stress fractures are a high percentage of running and dancing athletic injuries among athletes, underscoring the importance of mechanical forces to joint health (Arditi, 2024). Structural implications of these injuries need to be recognized since they aid in the development of effective treatment modalities and prevention techniques, and this eventually results in an enhanced functional capacity of joints and connective tissue (Figure 1.15).

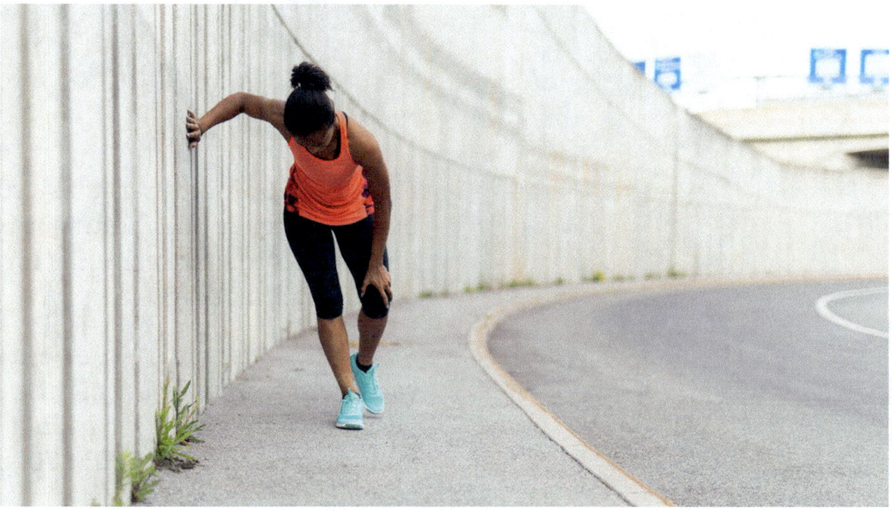

Figure 1.15. Joint injuries are prevalent across various activities, ranging from athletic endeavors to daily tasks, and these injuries can significantly alter the structural integrity of associated tissues.

Source: https://post.healthline.com/wp-content/uploads/2020/07/Female_Running_Pain_1296x728-header-1296x729.jpg.

Test Your Knowledge

1. What are the three types of structures that make up joints?
2. Describe the components of a synovial joint.

1.4. Function of Joints

Learning Outcome

1. Understand facilitating movement;
2. Explain load distribution and shock absorption;
3. Discuss range of motion and flexibility;
4. Focus on joint stability and support;
5. Discuss role in posture and balance;
6. Learn the effect of joint function on global mobility;
7. Discuss the effect of muscle-tendon interactions;
8. Discuss joint function in sports and physical activities;
9. Understand pathologies of joint function.

Joints are essential interfaces between bones that facilitate varied movements required for everyday functioning and global mobility. Functionally, they are of different types, like synovial, cartilaginous, and fibrous joints, with each of them having its own specific advantage as far as flexibility and stability are concerned. Synovial joints, like knee and elbow joints, are all the more important due to their ability to facilitate free movement with additional support from the ligaments and rich synovial fluid that greases the joint surface.

This lubrication is important as it minimizes wear and friction on the articular cartilage, enhancing joint longevity. Joint health, however, is inseparable from the health of tendons and the extracellular matrix, which can be affected in tendinopathy. This also emphasizes the need for ongoing research in an effort to understand the mechanics of the joint better, and the role of metalloproteinases in maintaining healthy tendons, since these factors are necessary for joint function (Abbaszade et al., 2005; Burgin et al., 2013) (Figure 1.16).

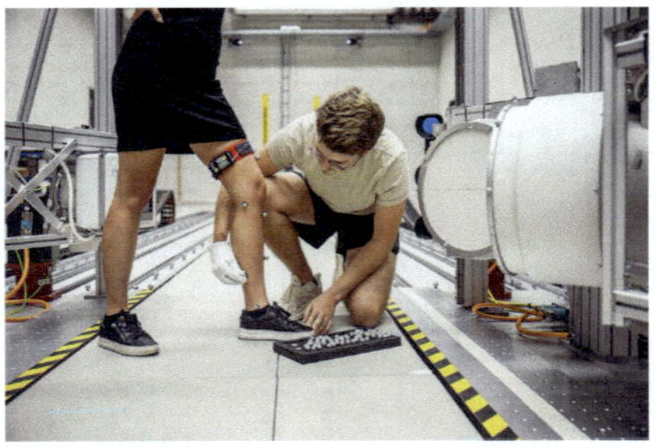

Figure 1.16. Joints serve as crucial interfaces between bones, facilitating a wide range of movements that are essential for daily activities and overall mobility.

Source: https://movement.ethz.ch/research/clinical-movement-biomechanics/_jcr_content/par/image/image.imageformat.930.1991756270.jpg.

1.4.1. Facilitating Movement

The intricate interaction among bone, joints, and connective tissue is necessary to facilitate human movement, which is based on structural organization and functional dynamics of these tissues. The skeletal system is the support structure that maintains body weight and facilitates movement through joint articulation. To this end, tendons and ligaments are dynamic collaborators in maintaining stability and flexibility, allowing a variety of movement and preventing damage. These relationships must be understood; variation between molecular and cellular processes can influence the diversity of movements, as is illustrated through developmental disorders resulting in structural deformities in the skeletal framework (Abzhanov et al., 2019). Besides that, conditions , such as metatarsal stress fractures also show the immediate impact that mechanical loading and the structure of trabecular bone have on movement and injury susceptibility (Arditi, 2024). A sound knowledge of these mechanisms thus serves as the foundation of future advancements in rehabilitation treatment and injury prevention.

1.4.2. Load Distribution and Shock Absorption

The complex bone, joint, and connective tissue architecture is responsible for shock absorption and load distribution required for musculoskeletal health. Bone structures are not merely passive frameworks; they also possess dynamic qualities that enable them to absorb and dampen the forces of function during various activities.

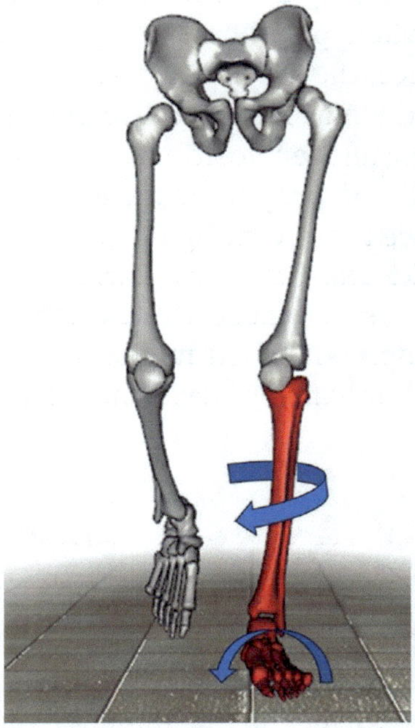

Figure 1.17. Load distribution and shock absorption.

Source: https://www.jisakos.com/cms/10.1016/j.jisako.2024.100381/asset/9fee254b-e0f0-4607-9b97-f6f59ac8cf5a/main.assets/gr3_lrg.jpg.

For instance, cartilage in the articular surfaces of synovial joints is designed to withstand severe stress, whereas it distributes loads evenly onto joint surfaces. Current evidence has also been shown to reveal extensive differences in mechanical and structural cartilage properties among various joints with varying shock absorption and load distribution capability (Beeson et al., 2009). In further studies, the anatomy of the animal digital pads, including horses and elephants, shows how different morphologies affect internal stress and pressure responses to loading, with the implications for shock-absorbing structure relevance in preventing pathologies due to excessive stress (Henry et al., 2014) (Figure 1.17).

1.4.3. Range of Motion and Flexibility

The mechanisms of range of motion and flexibility are directly linked with the structural features of bones, joints, and connective tissues, all of which play significant roles in human movement. Range of motion is the amount of movement that takes place at a joint, and flexibility is the ability of muscles and tendons to elongate and enable this movement. Studies have shown, individuals with generalized joint hypermobility have a much broader range of motion, according to findings aligned with the Beighton hypermobility criteria and maximum mandibular opening (Thomas et al., 1993). Additionally, flexibility can be enhanced with some stretching techniques that are used to maintain or improve joint motion, with benefits for healthy persons and athletes who recover from injury (Tirado et al., 2010). Thus, it is essential to understand the dynamic between these factors in the design of successful training and rehabilitation programmes, maximizing musculoskeletal function.

1.4.4. Joint Stability and Support

The joint stability and support theory is inextricably linked with the structural and functional dynamics of bone, joints, and connective tissues. Superior joint stability is grounded in a sophisticated interplay of passive and active support systems like ligaments, tendons, and the myofascial system. The myofascial tissues form interconnected networks of tensile tensions that provide essential stabilizing support and control movement throughout the body. Important, the process of HRMT is evidence of how passive tensions in muscles have an essential role in maintaining balanced postures, thereby enhancing joint stability during both static and dynamic exercises (Masi et al., 2010). More than this, knowledge of disease pathogenesis , such as tendinopathy, underlines the importance of molecular integrity of the tendon matrix for joint stabilization (Riley, 2004). In general, the complex biomechanics of such structures demonstrate the centrality of their function in maintaining joint integrity and maximizing functional movement (Figure 1.18).

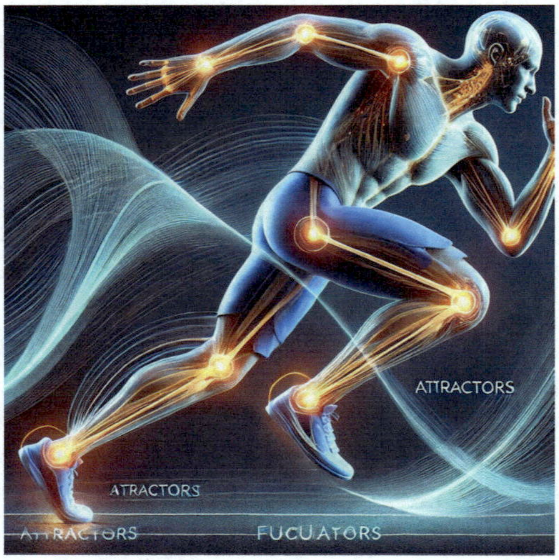

Figure 1.18. Effective joint stability is achieved through a sophisticated interplay of passive and active support mechanisms, including ligaments, tendons, and the myofascial system.

Source: https://substackcdn.com/image/fetch/f_auto,q_auto:good,fl_progressive:steep/https%3A%2F%2Fsubstack-post-media.s3.amazonaws.com%2Fpublic%2Fimages%2F471d571c-40f7-4ead-aa9c-198169d325db_1024x1024.webp.

1.4.5. Role in Posture and Balance

The role of bone, joint, and connective tissue in posture and balance is essential to human mobility and stability. The skeletal structure, referred to as Asthi Sharira in Ayurvedic terms, provides adequate support and protection to the body, forming the basis of proper movement. Alignment of the joints and spine is necessary because otherwise they will lead to musculoskeletal disorders that will severely affect one's ability to balance and perform day-to-day activities. Muscle tissues, or Peshi Sharira, work with the skeletal system to regulate and stabilize movements; this adjustment is most important during activities of fine motor skills, such as when playing a stringed instrument. For instance, the particular stances adopted by violins and violas result in discomfort or injury due to their uneven positions, underscoring the importance of proper posture consciousness and balance in preventing performance-related musculoskeletal disorders (Carroll et al., 2020). An awareness of these associations enhances the development of strategies for preventing injury and enhancing performance (Chatore et al., 2024).

1.4.6. Impact of Joint Function on Overall Mobility

Joint function is essential to overall mobility, as it has a direct effect on the body's ability to perform a variety of movements required to perform daily activities. Smooth, coordinated movement is facilitated by functioning joints, while their dysfunction can produce dramatic limitations in more than just mobility, but also quality of life. Arthritis and other diseases can erode joint integrity, causing pain and inflammation that restricts movement, demonstrating the complex interaction between joint health and overall function. The frequency of musculoskeletal trauma, responsible for nearly 30% of all charges for work-related trauma compensation, highlights the importance of maintaining firm joint function to prevent long-term mobility disability (Alsheikhly et al., 2018). Furthermore, biomechanics provides a greater understanding of how various forces impact and interact in and around joints during exercise and trauma, allowing for more effective rehabilitation methods to be discovered for those afflicted (Harris et al., 2012). As such, joint function needs to be preserved in order for mobility and general physical well-being to persist (Figure 1.19).

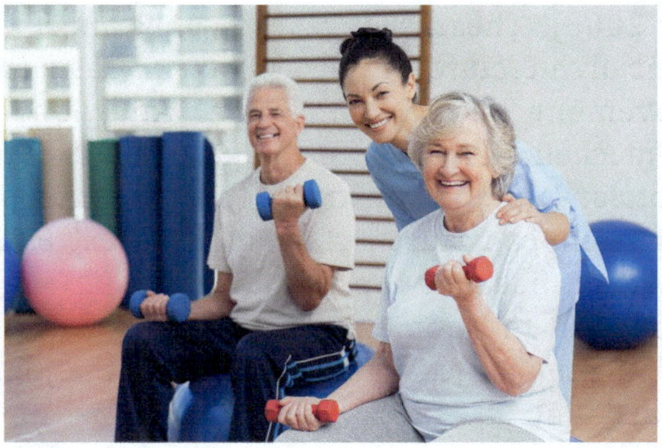

Figure 1.19. Well-functioning joints facilitate smooth and coordinated motion, while their dysfunction can lead to significant restrictions, impairing not only mobility but also quality of life.

Source: https://cdn-cmdne.nitrocdn.com/hNJckCstFVQjUckKaelcVKoVJrzdTVkW/assets/images/optimized/rev-e2e9498/www.provocollege.edu/wp-content/uploads/2024/02/shutterstock_256067746-scaled.jpg.

1.4.7. Influence of Muscle-tendon Interactions

Muscle-tendon interactions play a fundamental role in the mechanics of movement, influencing both the musculoskeletal system's structural competence and functional capacity. Tendons, as the connecting point between bone and muscle, enable the force generated by muscle contractions to be transmitted to the skeletal system, thus facilitating movement and stability. This dynamic process is most visibly apparent with high-stress exercise, where tendon integrity is purely essential. As recent research indicates, tendinopathy—a degenerative joint disease of the tendons—begins as an underlying process of matrix remodeling driven by several biochemical factors, including matrix metalloproteinases (Riley et al., 2005). Additionally, muscle-tendon unit organizational complexity is in close relation with developmental phenomena, namely the signaling communication between various tissue types, including mesenchymal cells, which define anatomical organization while being calibrated to biomechanical forces (Abzhanov et al., 2019). Thus, an awareness of the interactions between muscle and tendon is necessary in order to comprehend normal biomechanics and the pathophysiology of musculoskeletal trauma.

1.4.8. Joint Function in Sports and Physical Activities

The role of joints in facilitating movement during sports and physical activity cannot be exaggerated, as they are principal points of articulation between bones, which provide a range of motion necessary for athletic function. Each joint is individually adapted to permit certain movements while equaling flexibility and stability.

Synovial joints, for instance, with their fluid-filled cavities, enable high mobility, which comes in handy during dynamic sports involving sudden changes of direction. However, the mechanical strains placed upon joints can lead to issues , such as tendinopathy, where tendons break down and inhibit their ability to transfer force effectively. This condition, typically caused by overuse or faulty technique, underscores the importance of respecting joint function and health in sport situations (Riley, 2004). New evidence on the molecular mechanisms of tendon pathology underscores the importance of measures to maintain joint health and encourage long-term athletic function (Riley et al., 2005) (Figure 1.20).

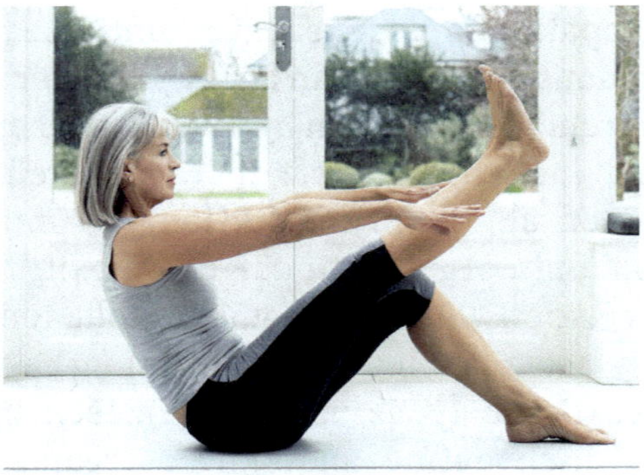

Figure 1.20. Joint function in sports and physical activities.

Source: https://coloradopaincare.com/wp-content/uploads/2019/02/how-your-joints-benefit-from-exercise-blog-colorado-pain-care.jpg.

1.4.9. Pathologies Affecting Joint Function

The complexity of joint function is most often challenged by pathologies that highlight the interdependence of the various tissues responsible for joint mechanics. Interestingly, synovial joint pathologies can lead to severe morbidity from proteolytic activity-mediated degenerative change controlled by MMPs and other proteases accountable for weakening the extracellular matrix required for ideal articulation and tissue homeostasis (Buttle et al., 2008). These changes not only affect the joint architecture but also result in restricted movement and chronic pain. Additionally, biomechanical malalignment, particularly of the subtalar joint, demonstrates the way improper alignment can cause a chain of lower extremity injuries because abnormal subtalar joint pronation or supination can change patterns of walking and exaggerate stress on the joints (Martin et al., 1995). Appreciation of these pathologies emphasizes the need for optimal assessment and intervention to decrease the impact of joint dysfunction on physical health.

Test Your Knowledge

1. What are the three functional categories of joints by type of movement?
2. How do joints help body movement?

Summary

The intricacy of bone, joint, and connective tissue attests not only to their structural significance but also to their functional pliability to various mechanical requirements. The knowledge of this relationship provides a deeper insight into human anatomy as well as biomedical engineering advancements. For instance, the development of robotic joints based on bio-mimicry indicates how mimicking human anatomical structures' compliance and elasticity can avoid mechanical failure for tensegrity systems because they have the potential to absorb impact due to unexpected loads elegantly (Lessard et al., 2016). Additionally, studies on the bone-periodontal ligament-cementum complex highlight the dynamic nature of such tissues in response to pathological stimuli, demonstrating structural and functional adaptability of connective tissue under tension (Lee et al., 2013). Such studies reinforce the need for structural solidity and functional resistance for the maintenance of general health and guide new approaches towards rehabilitation and prosthetic device design.

A thorough understanding of bone structure and function, joint structure and function, and connective tissue structure and function shows their complex interrelation in the musculoskeletal system. Salient points of discussion are the role of bone as a dynamic organ, not only supporting but also functional in metabolic processes via mineral regulation and cytokine release, as indicated by results in models of periodontitis where bone and soft tissue interactions were major contributors to disease development and healing response (Lee et al., 2013). In addition, the diverse morphology of connective tissues enables them to adapt and cater to various mechanical needs, as illustrated in studies on bat wing membranes with specialist features for flying behavior (Fenton et al., 2017). Lastly, such arguments promote the significance of biomechanical properties and tissue flexibility in maintaining overall functional integrity in the skeletal system.

KEY TERMS FROM THIS CHAPTER

- Bone structure
- Connective tissue
- Health
- Minerals
- Functional impairment
- Human physiology
- Haversian systems
- Hematopoiesis
- Joints
- Physiology
- Vital organs
- Stimuli
- Flexible joints
- Compact bone
- Spongy bone
- Osteoblasts

Critical Thinking Questions

1. **Which of the following is NOT a function of the skeletal system?**
   a. Support
   b. Blood cell production
   c. Hormone regulation
   d. Movement
2. **The hard outer layer of bone is called:**
   a. Spongy bone
   b. Bone marrow
   c. Compact bone
   d. Periosteum
3. **Which bone cell is responsible for forming new bone?**
   a. Osteoclast
   b. Osteoblast
   c. Osteocyte
   d. Chondrocyte
4. **What is the name of the process where bone is formed from cartilage?**
   a. Osteolysis
   b. Endochondral ossification
   c. Intramembranous ossification
   d. Calcification
5. **Which type of joint is freely movable?**
   a. Synarthrosis
   b. Amphiarthrosis
   c. Diarthrosis
   d. Symphysis

Short Answer Questions

1. Discuss the differences between compact and spongy bone.
2. Compare and contrast the structure and function of fibrous, cartilaginous, and synovial joints.
3. What are the reasons for joint stability?
4. Explain bone remodeling and the role of osteoblasts and osteoclasts.
5. Explain the roles of tendons and ligaments during joint movement.
6. What is the function of cartilage in joints?

Answers to Critical Thinking Questions

1. (c); 2. (c); 3. (b); 4. (b); 5. (c)

References

1. Abbaszade, I., Akeson, W. H., Alfredson, H., Amiel, D., Archambault, J., Astrom, M., Bank, R. A., et al. (2005). Gene expression and matrix turnover in overused and damaged tendons. https://core.ac.uk/download/2776591.pdf (accessed on 17th June 2025).

2. Abril García, D., Crespo Lora, V., Galindo Moreno, P. A., Hernández Cortés, P., et al. (2021). Expression of *Musashi-1* increases in bone healing. https://core.ac.uk/download/427405735.pdf (accessed on 17th June 2025).

3. Abujarour, M., Allt, G., Archer, D., Arikawa-Hirasawa, E., Asari, A., Bakopoulou, A., Bertoni, L., et al. (2018). Concise review: Stem/progenitor cell proteoglycans decorated with 7-D-4, 4-C-3, and 3-B-3(-) chondroitin sulfate motifs are morphogenetic markers of tissue development. https://core.ac.uk/download/161526959.pdf (accessed on 17th June 2025).

4. Abzhanov, A., Abzhanov, A., Abzhanov, A., Baggiolini, A., Baroffio, A., Beverdam, A., Chevallier, A., et al. (2019). Molecular and cellular mechanisms underlying the evolution of form and function in the amniote jaw. https://core.ac.uk/download/323079229.pdf (accessed on 17th June 2025).

5. Adam, C. (2012). Endogenous musculoskeletal tissue engineering–A focused perspective. https://core.ac.uk/download/10908942.pdf (accessed on 17th June 2025).

6. S. Lessard et al., "A bio-inspired tensegrity manipulator with multi-DOF, structurally compliant joints," 2016 IEEE/RSJ International Conference on Intelligent Robots and Systems (IROS), Daejeon, Korea (South), 2016, pp. 5515-5520, doi: 10.1109/IROS.2016.7759811. keywords: {Manipulators;Biological system modeling;Shoulder;Joints;Muscles;Elbow},

7. (accessed on 17th June 2025).

8. Kurowska-Stolarska, M., & Alivernini, S. (2017). Synovial tissue macrophages: friend or foe?. *RMD open*, *3*(2), e000527. https://doi.org/10.1136/rmdopen-2017-000527 (accessed on 17th June 2025).

9. Alsheikhly, A. S., & Alsheikhly, M. S. (2018). Musculoskeletal injuries: Types and management protocols for emergency care. https://core.ac.uk/download/322440204.pdf (accessed on 17th June 2025).

10. Anton du Plessis, Razavi, N., Benedetti, M., Murchio, S., Leary, M., Watson, M., Bhate, D., et al. (2021). Properties and applications of additively manufactured metallic cellular materials: A review. *Progress in Materials Science, 125*, 100918–100918. https://doi.org/10.1016/j.pmatsci.2021.100918 (accessed on 17th June 2025).

11. Arditi, F. (2024). Comparative analysis of FEM models with homogeneous and structured bone in the foot-ankle complex for the study of stress fractures in the first metatarsal. https://core.ac.uk/download/604158603.pdf (accessed on 17th June 2025).

12. Ashrafi, H., Baseer, A. Q., Hassand, M. H., Hejran, S., et al. (2024). The importance of hyaluronic acid in biological systems. https://core.ac.uk/download/603903802.pdf (accessed on 17th June 2025).

13. Burgin, L. V., Edelsten, L., & Aspden, R. M. (2014). The mechanical and material properties of elderly human articular cartilage subject to impact and slow loading. *Medical engineering & physics*, *36*(2), 226–232. https://doi.org/10.1016/j.medengphy.2013.11.002(accessed on 17th June 2025).

14. Baar, K., & Chidi-Ogbolu, N. (2018). Effect of estrogen on musculoskeletal performance and injury risk. https://core.ac.uk/download/323069599.pdf (accessed on 17th June 2025).
15. Becker, S. K. (2019). Osteoarthritis, entheses, and long bone cross-sectional geometry in the Andes: Usage, history, and future directions. https://core.ac.uk/download/323311202.pdf (accessed on 17th June 2025).
16. Beeson, P., & Hendren, L. (2009). A review of the differences between normal and osteoarthritis articular cartilage in human knee and ankle joints. https://core.ac.uk/download/9696220.pdf (accessed on 17th June 2025).
17. Benedetti, M., Anton du Plessis, R., Ritchie, R. O., Dallago, M., Razavi, N., & Berto, F. (2021). Architected cellular materials: A review on their mechanical properties towards fatigue-tolerant design and fabrication. *Materials Science and Engineering: R: Reports, 144*, 100606–100606. https://doi.org/10.1016/j.mser.2021.100606 (accessed on 17th June 2025).
18. Bullough, P., Bullough, M., Bullough, T., Byers, P., Carter, D., Cowin, S., Fick, J., et al. (1993). People in different age groups show different hip-joint morphology. https://core.ac.uk/download/12168631.pdf (accessed on 17th June 2025).
19. Buttle, D., Jones, G. C., & Riley, G. P. (2008). The role of proteases in pathologies of the synovial joint. https://core.ac.uk/download/2776586.pdf (accessed on 17th June 2025).
20. Carroll, L. (2020). The unique demands of playing posture on youth violinists and violists. https://core.ac.uk/download/345182745.pdf (accessed on 17th June 2025).
21. Chatore, V. M., Chavhan, N. S., & Patki, S. R. (2024). Physiological importance of *Asthi* and *Peshi Sharira*: An Ayurveda and modern perspective. https://core.ac.uk/download/604048742.pdf (accessed on 17th June 2025).
22. Cozart, D., Hesse, D., Nichols, R., Szymik, M., et al. (2017). *UGA Anatomy and Physiology 1 Lab Manual* (3rd ed.). https://core.ac.uk/download/217306564.pdf (accessed on 17th June 2025).
23. Masi, A. T., Nair, K., Evans, T., & Ghandour, Y. (2010). Clinical, biomechanical, and physiological translational interpretations of human resting myofascial tone or tension. *International journal of therapeutic massage & bodywork, 3*(4), 16–28. https://doi.org/10.3822/ijtmb.v3i4.104 (accessed on 17th June 2025).
24. Fenton, M. B., Gray, P., Holbrook, K. A., Humphry, G. M., Maisonneuve, P., Meyer, W., Schumacher, S., et al. (2017). Diversity in the organization of elastin bundles and intramembranous muscles in bat wings. https://core.ac.uk/download/76981004.pdf (accessed on 17th June 2025).
25. (accessed on 17th June 2025).
26. García Tirado, J., & Pacheco Arajol, L. (2010). On the application of stretching to healthy and injured sportsmen and women. https://core.ac.uk/download/39043932.pdf (accessed on 17th June 2025).
27. Harris, G. F., & Slavens, B. A. (2012). *Biomechanics.* https://core.ac.uk/download/213080657.pdf (accessed on 17th June 2025).
28. Henry, V., Hildebrandt, T., Hutchinson, J. R., Panagiotopoulou, O., et al. (2014). Regional variation in digital cushion pressure in the forefeet of horses and elephants. https://core.ac.uk/download/159067743.pdf (accessed on 17th June 2025).
29. Hetherington, C. S. (2019). *Myofascial Release.* https://core.ac.uk/download/289198166.pdf (accessed on 17th June 2025).

30. Hyc, A., Jankowska-Steifer, E., Moskalewski, S., Osiecka-Iwan, A., et al. (2014). Synovial membrane asks for independence. https://core.ac.uk/download/268450388.pdf (accessed on 17th June 2025).

31. Karahan, N., Kaya, M., & Yılmaz, B. (2019). Tendon structure and classification. https://core.ac.uk/download/322441362.pdf (accessed on 17th June 2025).

32. Krause, W. J., II. (2008). *Joints.* https://core.ac.uk/download/62754357.pdf (accessed on 17th June 2025).

33. Larson, J. A. (1996). *Functional Human Anatomy Lab Manual* (4th ed.). https://core.ac.uk/download/643693577.pdf (accessed on 17th June 2025).

34. Loccisano, A. (2016). Platelet-rich plasma for the treatment of partial rotator cuff tears. https://open.bu.edu/bitstream/2144/14355/9/Loccisano_bu_0017N_10415.pdf (accessed on 17th June 2025).

35. Martin, D. (1995). The role of foot biomechanics in lower extremity pathologies. https://core.ac.uk/download/235073870.pdf (accessed on 17th June 2025).

36. Matcher, S. J. (2009). A review of some recent developments in polarization-sensitive optical imaging techniques for the study of articular cartilage. https://core.ac.uk/download/50699.pdf (accessed on 17th June 2025).

37. McCormick, A., Drummond, A. H., Banes, A. J., Bamji, A. N., Corps, A. N., Corps, A. N., Corps, A. N., et al. (2008). Tendinopathy—from basic science to treatment. https://core.ac.uk/download/2756893.pdf (accessed on 17th June 2025).

38. Owen, H. L. (2017). A review of ankylosing spondylitis. https://core.ac.uk/download/158970001.pdf (accessed on 17th June 2025).

39. Paraskevas, G. K. (2011). Human ligaments classification: A new proposal. https://core.ac.uk/download/268450373.pdf (accessed on 17th June 2025).

40. Patil, R. K., & Jadhav, T. A. (2020). A critical review on *Sandhi Sharir* with special reference to *Upamana Pramana*. https://core.ac.uk/download/478521845.pdf (accessed on 17th June 2025).

41. Kishor Patwardhan, Concepts of Human Physiology in Ayurveda, in 'Sowarigpa and Ayurveda', published by Central Institute of Higher Tibetan Studies, Sarnath, Varanasi. Samyak Vak Series-14, Editor: Pabitra Kumar Roy (2008), Page No.53 to 73. ISBN: 978-81-87127-76-5(accessed on 17th June 2025).

42. Plotkin, L. I., & Stains, J. P. (2015). Connexins and pannexins in the skeleton: Gap junctions, hemichannels and more. https://core.ac.uk/download/84831119.pdf (accessed on 17th June 2025).

43. Rahardjo, P., & Setiawati, R. (2018). Bone development and growth. https://core.ac.uk/download/322440382.pdf (accessed on 17th June 2025).

44. Reeves, N. M. (2014). Augmenting functional adaptation: Does obesity have a systemic effect on bone strength properties in humans? https://core.ac.uk/download/268768139.pdf (accessed on 17th June 2025).

45. Riley, G. P. (2004). The pathogenesis of tendinopathy: A molecular perspective. https://core.ac.uk/download/2776643.pdf (accessed on 17th June 2025).

46. Rouvali, J. (2016). Online network mobility exercises for male hockey players during an adolescent growth spurt. https://core.ac.uk/download/38135602.pdf (accessed on 17th June 2025).
47. Thomas, T. D. (1993). Systemic joint hypermobility and maximum mandibular opening. https://core.ac.uk/download/235074166.pdf (accessed on 17th June 2025).
48. Warraich, S. (2013). Ectopic mineralization of spinal tissues in mice lacking equilibrate nucleoside transporter 1. https://core.ac.uk/download/61637591.pdf (accessed on 17th June 2025).

CELLS INVOLVED IN AUTOIMMUNE DISEASES AND INFLAMMATION

2

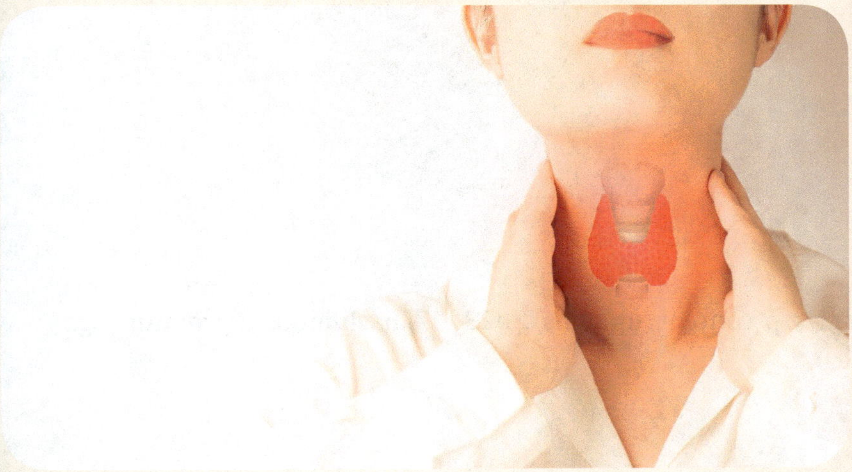

LEARNING OBJECTIVES

After studying this chapter, you will be able to:

1. Identify cell types that cause autoimmune diseases;
2. Explain mechanisms of autoimmunity;
3. Emphasize inflammation in autoimmune diseases;
4. Discuss current research and treatment strategies employed.

Introduction

Autoimmune diseases are a complex interaction between environmental influences and genetic predispositions in which the immune system mistakenly attacks healthy tissues. The thyroid itself is often involved in autoimmunity, seen in autoimmune thyroid diseases (AITDs) like Graves' disease and *Hashimotos thyroiditis*, which are significantly more prevalent among females because of hormones and underlying inflammatory conditions (Merrill & Mu, 2015).

Moreover, the contribution of infectious agents cannot be ignored, as they may play essential roles as precipitating factors for the development of autoimmune diseases. Experiments proved that infection caused by bacteria and viruses may induce or exacerbate autoimmune responses through mechanisms , such as molecular mimicry, bystander activation, and release of pro-inflammatory mediators (Delogu et al., 2011). Recognition of such interactions is important in the development of targeted treatments and prevention of autoimmune diseases, highlighting the importance of an extensive analysis of the immune cells and pathways involved in such complex diseases (Figure 2.1).

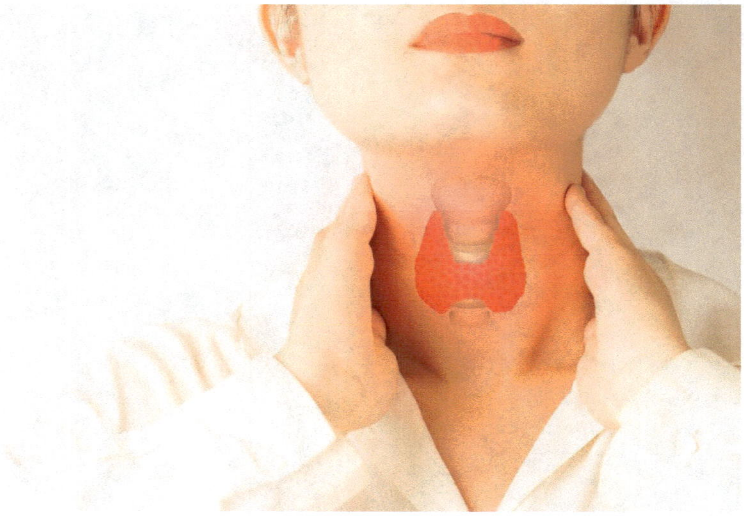

Figure 2.1. Hashimoto's thyroiditis.

Source: https://www.happiesthealth.com/wp-content/uploads/2023/07/hashimoto-thyroiditis.jpg.

2.1. Types of Cells Involved in Autoimmune Diseases

Learning Outcome

1. Comprehend T cells and their role;
2. Explain B-cells and the process of antibody formation;
3. Discuss dendritic cells as antigen-presenting cells;
4. Explain macrophages and their roles;
5. Inquire into natural killer (NK) cells in autoimmune reactions;
6. Know regulatory T cells and immune regulation;
7. Explain mast cells and their role in inflammation;
8. Inquire into neutrophils in autoimmune pathology;
9. Discuss eosinophils and their role in some autoimmune diseases.

Autoimmune diseases are characterized by a deregulated immune response, consisting predominantly of a mix of immune cells responsible for tissue damage and disease progression. At the core of this process lie the T lymphocytes and, even more specifically, a subset known as effector memory T (T-EM) cells, which play a critical role in orchestrating inflammation and tissue injury in autoimmune pathologies. These T-EM cells secrete pro-inflammatory cytokines that enable the recruitment of other immune cells, including macrophages and B-cells, to aid in inflammation (Abdulahad et al., 2014).

In addition, an impairment of regulatory T cells may weaken their ability to execute anti-inflammatory functions, thereby enhancing autoimmune activity. In other contexts, e.g., immune-mediated inner ear disease, the activity of such immune cells produces symptoms like hearing loss, complementing the clinical manifestation of autoimmune systemic disorders (Ralli et al., 2018). Understanding these cellular migrations is fundamental to the development of particular therapeutic strategies.

2.1.1. T Cells and their Role

Amongst all varieties of immune cells, T cells are pivotal in the regulation and worsening of autoimmune disorders. These lymphocytes, particularly the CD4$^+$ T helper cells, are components of the adaptive immune response, differentiating into subsets that have the capacity to either cause inflammation or augment immune tolerance. In conditions , such as rheumatoid arthritis, activation of T cell subsets leads to synovial inflammation and joint damage, as depicted in recent studies (Chaplain et al., 2019). In addition, GM-CSF, which is produced by T cell, is involved in the pathogenetic events in several inflammatory disorders, including rheumatoid arthritis and multiple sclerosis (Adorini et al., 2019).

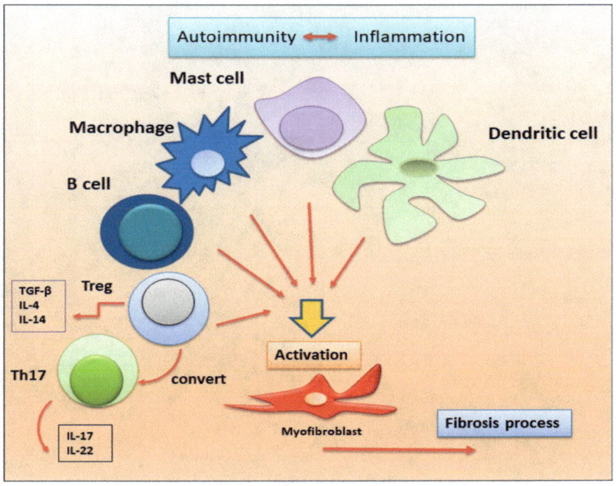

Figure 2.2. Among the various immune cell types, T cells play a pivotal role in the regulation and exacerbation of autoimmune diseases.

Source: https://pub.mdpi-res.com/jcm/jcm-12-03801/article_deploy/html/images/jcm-12-03801-g003.png?1685956983.

The well-regulated balance of T cell function and their interaction with the other immune cells highlights their central function in autoimmune pathology, providing promises for selective therapeutic strategies in modifying their function in preventing symptoms and disease progression (Figure 2.2).

2.1.2. B-cells and Antibody Production

B-cells play a central role in the immune system with respect to the production of antibodies that play a critical role in pathogen recognition and neutralization. In the setting of autoimmune disease, these cells inadvertently produce autoantibodies against self-antigens, causing tissue inflammation and destruction. A good example is autoimmune thyroid disease , such as Hashimoto's thyroiditis, where the production of anti-thyroid antibodies is a defining feature of the disease and indicates a basic flaw in normal immune regulation (Merrill & Mu, 2015). Dysregulation of a single cytokine, such as GM-CSF, but one that further complicates the imbalance in influencing B-cell proliferation and activation and, therefore, amplifying the autoimmune response. The cytokine has been shown to induce or suppress autoimmune pathology, depending on the nature of the immune response setting (Adorini et al., 2019). Such mechanisms must be thoroughly understood so that drugs can be specifically engineered to rebalance B-cell activity in autoimmune diseases.

2.1.3. Dendritic Cells as Antigen-presenting Cells

In the intricate universe of immune responses, dendritic cells (DCs) are key antigen-presenting cells that bridge innate and adaptive immunity.

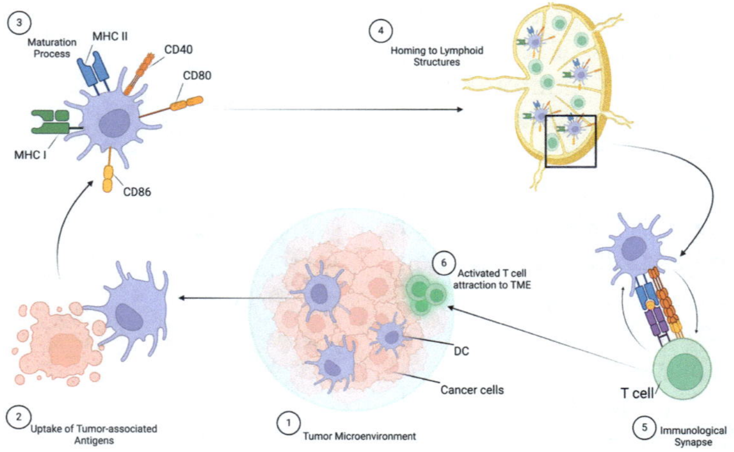

Figure 2.3. Dendritic cells and anti-neoplastic response. The anti-neoplastic immune response initiated by intra-tumoral DCs relies on a sequential process, beginning with the recognition, uptake, and processing of tumor-associated antigens. Subsequently, DCs undergo a maturation process characterized by the upregulation of MHC class I and class II molecules, increased expression of costimulatory molecules, such as CD40, CD80, CD86, and, finally, their homing to lymph nodes or lymphoid structures to encounter and activate T cells. This process will result in the eradication of tumor cells.

Source: https://www.mdpi.com/biomedicines/biomedicines-12-01240/article_deploy/html/images/biomedicines-12-01240-g001.png.

These cells are key to capturing, processing, and presenting antigens to T cells and ultimately initiating and modulating immune responses. Their ability to act as tissue sentinels makes it possible for them to activate naïve T cells, something particularly relevant in autoimmune disease, where immune function dysregulation leads to tissue damage. Furthermore, dendritic cells are impacted by many cytokines, including GM-CSF, that can influence maturation and function in autoimmune disorders like rheumatoid arthritis and multiple sclerosis, as outlined in recent research (Adorini et al., 2019). In alopecia areata and other disorders, abnormal lymphocytic infiltration of follicles highlights the role of DCs in the mediation of autoimmune attack, the pathology of disease, and as therapeutic targets (Simakou et al., 2019) (Figure 2.3).

2.1.4. Macrophages and Their Functions

Macrophages play a key role in the initiation and resolution of inflammation and serve as crucial regulators of the immune response to infection while also being involved in tissue repair processes. These pleiotropic cells are able to take on many distinct phenotypes, most typically being referred to as M1 and M2 macrophages depending on the cytokine environment. M1 macrophages are inflammatory, releasing factors that enable pathogen destruction, while M2 macrophages participate in anti-inflammatory responses and tissue healing. In autoimmune conditions, e.g., Rheumatoid Arthritis (RA), dysregulation of macrophage activity is emphasized; M1 macrophages incessantly drive inflammatory processes, causing tissue malfunction and damage (Alivernini et al., 2018). This anti-inflammatory vs. pro-inflammatory imbalance is further exacerbated by underlying chronic conditions , such as obesity, where the invading macrophages turn the immune response from its beneficial state to an undesirable, inflammatory state, increasing the risk for consequent complications (Crowe et al., 2017). Thus, macrophage dynamics are a crucial concept to understand when designing therapeutic interventions.

2.1.5. Natural Killer (NK) Cells in Autoimmune Responses

NK cells play an important part in immunity, particularly in the case of their function within autoimmune disease and inflammation. Innate lymphocytes are distinguished by their ability to recognize and destroy abnormal cells, but their dysregulation will additionally accelerate autoimmune diseases. Recent evidence suggests that NK cells contribute to the development of autoimmune disease by controlling the proliferation and activity of other immune cells, including *T lymphocytes* and macrophages, which are essential in sustaining inflammatory reactions (Abdulahad et al., 2014). In Primary Sjogren syndrome (pSS) and related disorders, NK cells, particularly invariant natural killer T cells (iNKT), are involved in orchestrating the immune response and modulating cytokine environments that can enhance clinical manifestations (Barbera et al., 2019). Knowledge of protective immunity and autoimmune pathology functions of NK cells is vital in the design of selective therapies capable of mitigating autoimmune attacks while preserving essential immune functions (Figure 2.4).

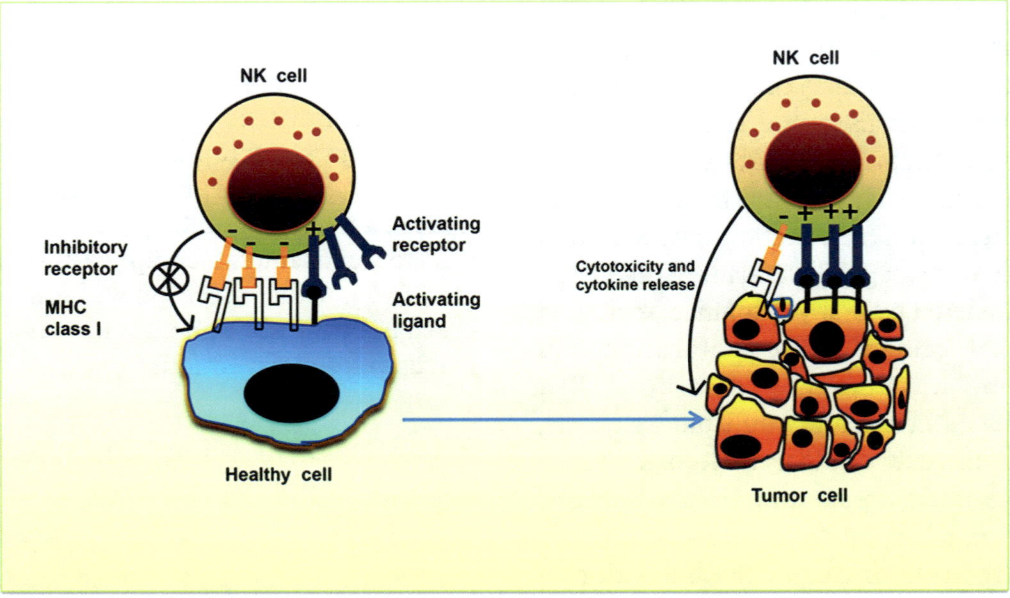

Figure 2.4. Natural killer (NK) cells play a pivotal role in the immune response, particularly concerning their involvement in autoimmune diseases and inflammation.

Source: https://www.frontiersin.org/files/Articles/290728/fimmu-08-01124-HTML/image_m/fimmu-08-01124-g001.jpg.

2.1.6. Regulatory T Cells (Tregs) and Immune Regulation

Tregs also play a central role in immune homeostasis and prevention of autoimmunity and play a role in functioning as moderators of the immune response. They suppress the activation of autoreactive lymphocytes, thereby preventing excessive inflammation resulting in tissue damage and autoimmune diseases. The functional capacity of Tregs can be regulated by a number of factors, including cytokines and environmental signals. In chronic inflammatory conditions, such as multiple sclerosis and rheumatoid arthritis, the balance between effector T cells and Tregs is disrupted, leading to pathogenic immune responses. Moreover, the contribution of cytokines , such as granulocyte-macrophage colony-stimulating factor (GM-CSF) illustrates the intricacy of the regulation of the immune response; in certain autoimmune diseases, GM-CSF promotes pro-inflammatory functions, but in others, protective functions are also played by GM-CSF (Adorini et al., 2019). This duality of immunity underlines the necessity of extremely precise Treg modulation in order to restore balance and avoid autoimmune disease (Sfera et al., 2018).

2.1.7. Mast Cells and Their Involvement in Inflammation

Mast cells are critical in organizing inflammatory responses, particularly when it comes to autoimmune diseases. These cells, located at the immune system-environment interfaces, are responsible for initiating and maintaining inflammatory cascades through the release of cytokines, histamine, and proteases. In autoimmune diseases, mast cells contribute to tissue injury through the maintenance of a pro-inflammatory microenvironment, which enhances local and systemic inflammation. Interestingly, research has revealed an opposite correlation of parasitic infection with incidence of autoimmune disease, with the implication that helminth-derived immunomodulatory products can modulate activation of mast cells and consequently inhibit inflammatory processes. This relationship is in line with the Hygiene Hypothesis, which postulates that decreased exposure to certain pathogens, e.g., parasitic worms, can lead to dysregulated immune reactions and ultimately enhance vulnerability to autoimmune diseases (Al-Riyami et al., 2010, 2014) (Figure 2.5).

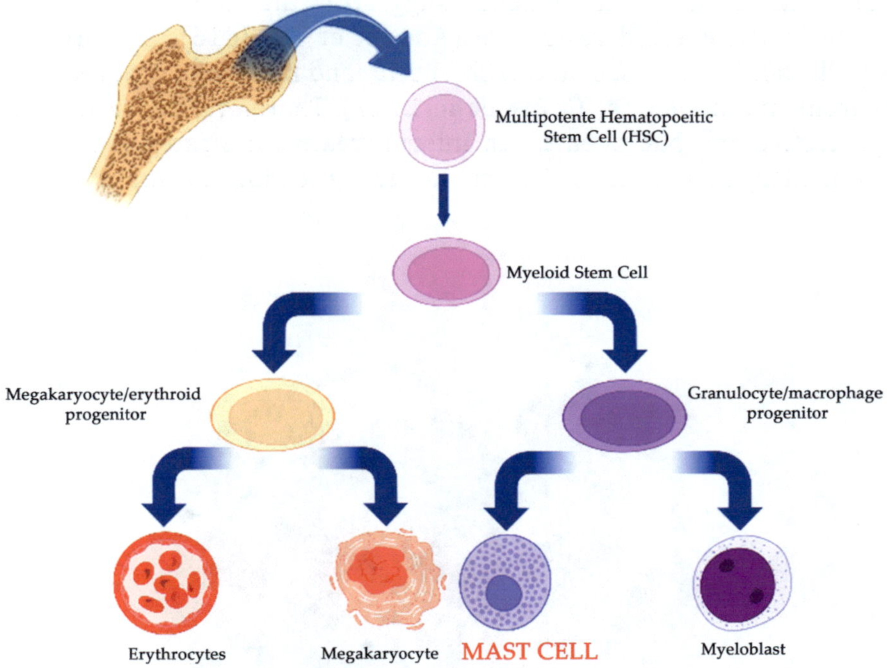

Figure 2.5. Mast cells play a critical role in the orchestration of inflammatory responses, particularly in the context of autoimmune diseases.

Source: https://www.mdpi.com/ijms/ijms-23-14004/article_deploy/html/images/ijms-23-14004-g001.png.

2.1.8. Neutrophils in Autoimmune Pathology

Among the various immune cells in the pathology of autoimmune diseases, the neutrophils have been implicated as major players in the disease process as well. Not only are these granulocyte components of the innate immune response, but they actively contribute to the pathogenesis of diseases , such as multiple sclerosis (MS) and rheumatoid arthritis. Increasing evidence suggests exacerbation of neuroinflammation and demyelination in MS models by neutrophils, particularly when they are recruited in response to chemokine signals , such as CXCL1. This signaling pathway has also been demonstrated to enhance neutrophil migration to the central nervous system, which leads to more demyelination and severity of disease (Doty et al., 2018). GM-CSF has additionally been identified as a factor for neutrophil activation and persistence within sites of inflammation, suggesting its role in many autoimmune diseases (Adorini et al., 2019). Thus, the targeting of neutrophils and their modulating pathways provides a good therapeutic approach to intervention in autoimmune diseases.

2.1.9. Eosinophils and Their Role in Specific Autoimmune Diseases

The eosinophil is a white blood cell with granular cytoplasm and has a multifaceted role in most autoimmune diseases, particularly those with an allergic and inflammatory etiology. These cells are most noted for their roles in fighting parasitic infections, but they also play an important role in tissue inflammation and destruction in autoimmune diseases. They play a role in sustaining airway inflammation in asthma, with evidence suggesting that their levels are associated with disease severity and corticosteroid resistance (Adcock et al., 2016). Also, research shows that increased eosinophilic activity is associated with obesity and metabolic syndrome, and thus reflects on their role in chronic inflammation (Crowe et al., 2017). Therefore, understanding the bipolarity of eosinophils, protective and pathogenic, can inform treatment strategies for the modulation of function in the context of autoimmune disease, hopefully leading to improved patient outcomes (Figure 2.6).

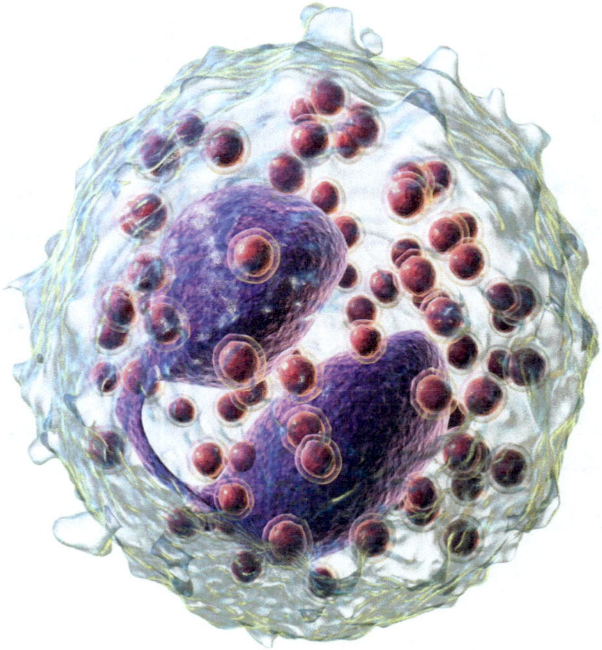

Figure 2.6. Eosinophils.

Source: https://upload.wikimedia.org/wikipedia/commons/1/19/Blausen_0352_Eosinophil_%28crop%29.png

Test Your Knowledge

1. Describe the functions of B-cells in autoimmunity and autoantibody production.
2. What is the function of regulatory T cells (Tregs) in self-tolerance?

2.2. Mechanisms of Autoimmunity

Learning Outcome

1. Explain molecular mimicry and its implications;
2. Recognize genetic predisposition for autoimmune disease;
3. Be aware of environmental triggers and their effects;
4. Emphasize dysregulation of immune tolerance;
5. Explain the role of cytokines in autoimmune response;
6. Understand the impact of gut microbiota on autoimmunity;
7. Recognize epigenetic factors influencing immune cells;
8. Recognize how hormones affect autoimmune diseases;
9. Explain the role of stress in provoking autoimmune diseases.

The autoimmunity pathogenesis is complex and multifactorial and encompasses genetic predispositions as well as environmental factors, which cumulatively overwhelm self-tolerance. The autoimmunity susceptibility can be determined by genetic factors, such as in autoimmune thyroid diseases (AITDs) , such as Graves' disease and *Hashimoto's thyroiditis*, which are even more prevalent in females due to the immune modulatory function of adipokines , such as leptin (Merrill & Mu, 2015). In the process, the environment can initiate or enhance autoimmune responses by mechanisms , such as molecular mimicry and bystander activation (Delogu et al., 2011). Such infections can induce the immune system by a cascade of inflammatory signals, which further upset the delicate balance of tolerance and lead to an attack on self-antigens. The interaction between these mechanisms highlights the contribution of intrinsic and extrinsic components towards the etiology of autoimmune diseases, and therefore the need for elaborate research in this area.

2.2.1. Molecular Mimicry and Its Implications

The phenomenon of molecular mimicry plays a crucial role in the etiology of most autoimmune diseases through blurring the distinction between self and non-self-antigens. This occurs when pathogen-derived epitopes share a similar structure with host tissues, where the immune system mistakenly attacks the body's own cells. Misrecognition here can lead to conditions like multiple sclerosis and type 1 diabetes, where viral infections are part of the disease process. As noted by new studies, the association between viral infections and autoimmune diseases needs further study in order to establish the mechanisms behind this mimicry (Piñeiro et al., 2017). In addition, this hypothesis has significant implications for the development of vaccines and public health. For instance, safety concerns over side effects from vaccines, such as the HPV vaccine, have been associated with the onset of autoimmune disorders in the context of widespread lack of trust in the safety of vaccines (Johnston, 2020). It is important to understand molecular mimicry in the formulation of strategies to mitigate such risks (Figure 2.7).

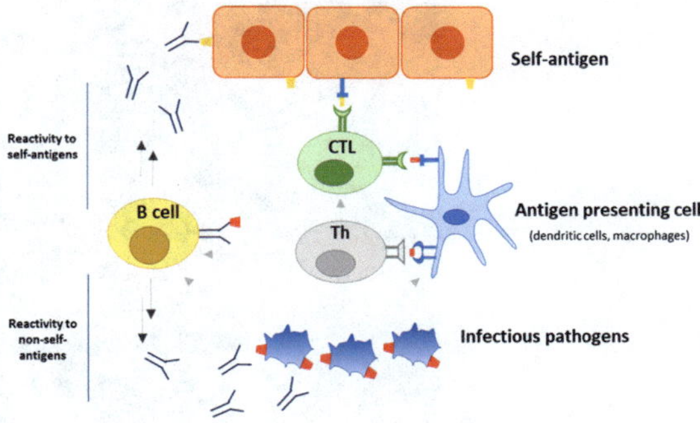

Figure 2.7. The phenomenon of molecular mimicry plays a crucial role in the development of various autoimmune diseases by blurring the lines between self and non-self-antigens.

Source: https://www.mdpi.com/ijms/ijms-24-13609/article_deploy/html/images/ijms-24-13609-g002.png.

2.2.2. Genetic Predisposition to Autoimmune Diseases

Genetic predisposition to autoimmune diseases is a significant area of research illustrating the complexity of immune system dysfunction. Various genes, including those found in the Human Leukocyte Antigen (HLA) system, are responsible for increasing the likelihood of acquiring such diseases as uveitis, ankylosing spondylitis, and Crohn's disease, particularly in individuals who are HLA-B27 positive (Cox et al., 2011). The genetic processes are synergized with environmental stimuli to suggest a multifactorial mode of disease development. According to recent studies, pathogens are able to trigger or exacerbate autoimmunity through mechanisms of molecular mimicry and bystander activation, supporting the idea that infectious agents tend to propel genetic predisposition (Delogu et al., 2011). These interactions need to be identified to establish targeted interventions and prevention measures, thus highlighting the significant role genetic markers play in population-at-risk identification and improved clinical outcomes of autoimmune disease.

2.2.3. Environmental Triggers and their Effects

Development of autoimmune diseases is largely most directly linked with environmental triggers, which have also been demonstrated as significant factors beyond inherited vulnerabilities. Infectious pathogens , such as viruses and bacteria, have been identified as major determinants that are capable of inducing or augmenting autoimmune responses, nearly breaking down immune tolerance that otherwise protects from self-antigens. The thyroid, for example, is extremely sensitive to such environmental factors, and adipokines like leptin and inflammatory cytokines like TNF-α and IL-6 play a role in triggering autoimmune thyroid diseases like Graves' disease and *Hashimoto's thyroiditis* (Merrill & Mu, 2015). Environmental triggers like infections utilize mechanisms like molecular mimicry, where microbial antigens resemble host tissues, to trigger autoimmunity (Delogu et al., 2011). Thus, understanding the interaction between such environmental factors and immune cells is the key to unraveling the complexities of autoimmune illness and inflammation (Figure 2.8).

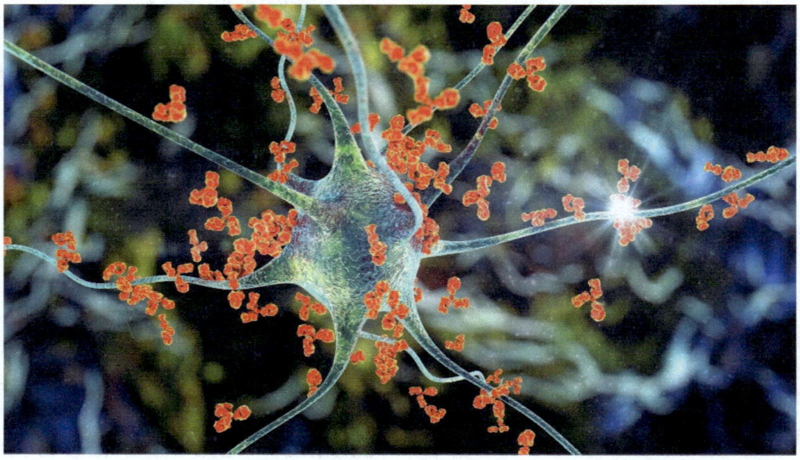

Figure 2.8. Pathogens , such as viruses and bacteria have been identified as critical factors that can initiate or exacerbate autoimmune responses, effectively breaking the immune tolerance that usually protects against self-antigens.

Source: https://www.news-medical.net/images/Article_Images/ImageForArticle_403_16619981729058147.jpg.

2.2.4. Dysregulation of Immune Tolerance

The dysregulation of immune tolerance is a fundamental process underlying autoimmune disorders in which the immune system mistakenly targets the body's own tissues. Loss of tolerance can lead to chronic inflammation and tissue destruction, such as in a variety of disorders like rheumatoid arthritis and multiple sclerosis. Key players in this process include immune cells , such as T and B-cells, which, upon inappropriate activation, contribute importantly to the autoimmune process. For instance, research has demonstrated that lipopolysaccharide (LPS) substances can trigger microglial activation, resulting in a neurotoxic environment that exacerbates neuroinflammation and interferes with immune homeostasis (Sfera et al., 2018). Additionally, the interaction between iron metabolism and immune processes can further amplify these abnormal pathways; increased cytosolic iron can engage deleterious inflammasomes, further impairing immune tolerance and driving autoimmune pathology (Dick et al., 2018). Thus, these processes are crucial for developing immunotherapeutic approaches to rebalance immune responses.

2.2.5. Role of Cytokines in Autoimmune Responses

Cytokines are the major players in autoimmune pathogenesis by mediating an inflammatory response that allows tissue damage and disease to continue. Among these, effector memory T (T-EM) cells are particularly noteworthy; they produce pro-inflammatory cytokines that promote activation and recruitment of many immune cells, including macrophages, neutrophils, and other T cells, thereby worsening inflammation of the tissues (Abdulahad et al., 2014).

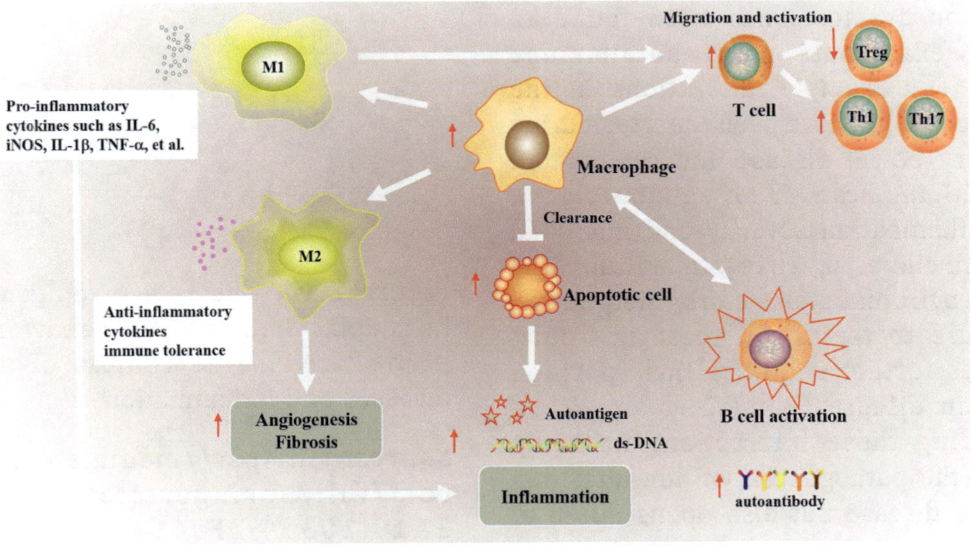

Figure 2.9. Cytokines play a pivotal role in the pathogenesis of autoimmune diseases by mediating inflammatory responses that drive tissue damage and disease progression.

Source: https://www.frontiersin.org/files/Articles/1080310/fimmu-14-1080310-HTML-r1/image_m/fimmu-14-1080310-g001.jpg.

Besides, GM-CSF is a representative of cytokine dual action in such diseases. While myeloid cell survival and activation by GM-CSF are guaranteed in chronic inflammatory conditions like rheumatoid arthritis and multiple sclerosis, GM-CSF may even exhibit protective actions in autoimmune conditions with humoral immunity like lupus and myasthenia gravis (Adorini et al., 2019). This complex interaction between cytokines reinforces their pivotal position in driving the inflammatory environment and therapeutic intervention in autoimmune disease (Figure 2.9).

2.2.6. Impact of Gut Microbiota on Autoimmunity

The intricate relationship between gut microbiota and autoimmunity has been of great interest in recent research, with the potential of being identified as an immune response modulator. Gut microbiota plays a major role in the attainment of immune homeostasis as it maintains control over the function of many immune cells, like Tregs and effector T cells, which are central to autoimmunity. Microbial imbalance or dysbiosis has been found to cause and exacerbate many autoimmune conditions. For example, alterations in the microbiota of the gut have been reported during inflammatory bowel disease and rheumatoid arthritis, with implications for an interrelation between inflammation severity and microbial change (D'Amelio et al., 2016). In addition, the impact of environmental factors, diet, stress, and exposure to toxins, on these microbial communities further solidifies their position as drivers in disease (Bonifaz et al., 2018). Understanding these interactions not only illuminates the pathogenesis of non-intestinal autoimmune disease but also opens doors to future therapeutic targeting of gut well-being.

2.2.7. Epigenetic Factors Influencing Immune Cells

The role of epigenetic elements in regulating the behavior of immune cells is pivotal, particularly in autoimmune diseases and inflammation. They are epigenetic changes like DNA methylation and histone modification that can potentially enormously influence the genes' expression in immune cells, hence influencing their function. For instance, microRNAs , such as miR-155 are key regulators of immune responses; their dysregulation is linked with inflammatory disease and autoimmunity (Alivernini et al., 2018). In addition, CD4 T cell differentiation and memory are largely dependent on epigenetic modification that regulates their activation and effector function. These memory CD4 T cells can respond rapidly to previously encountered antigens, illustrating how epigenetic modifications enable rapid immune reactions, which, when inappropriately executed, can lead to pathologic outcomes in autoimmune disorders (Jaigirdar & MacLeod, 2015). Hence, it is important to elucidate these epigenetic mechanisms for the identification of new therapeutic avenues for the treatment of autoimmune disorders (Figure 2.10).

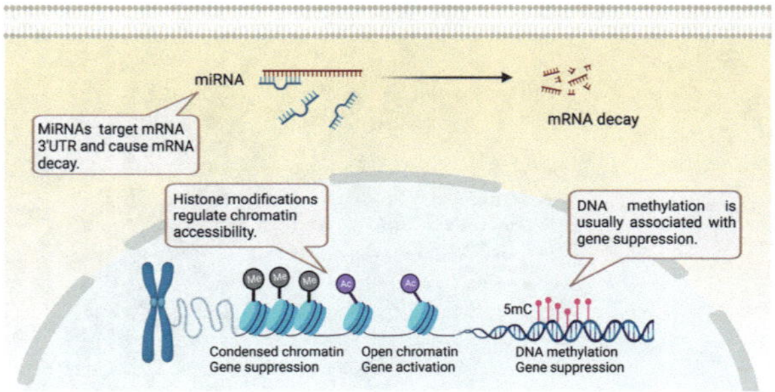

Figure 2.10. The role of epigenetic factors in shaping immune cell behavior is pivotal, particularly in the context of autoimmune diseases and inflammation.

Source: https://media.springernature.com/full/springer-static/image/art%3A10.1038%2Fs41423-022-00933-7/MediaObjects/41423_2022_933_Fig1_HTML.png.

2.2.8. Hormonal Influences on Autoimmune Diseases

The intricate hormone-autoimmune disease relationship reveals some of the fundamental features of the pathogenesis of the disease, particularly in females who have a higher prevalence of autoimmune diseases. Hormonal actions, most notably estrogen and androgens, play crucial roles in immune modulation, being the basis for the gender divide so apparent in autoimmune disease. AITDs , such as Graves' disease and *Hashimoto's thyroiditis*, for instance, are highly prevalent in women, suggesting that elevated estrogen levels enhance thyroid susceptibility to autoimmunity by means of inflammatory cytokine mediators , such as leptin and TNF-α, so central to immune modulation (Merrill & Mu, 2015). Similarly, Sjögren syndrome studies emphasize the bimodal role of androgens in regulating immune gene expression, highlighting strain-specific responses that can exacerbate or moderate inflammation in glandular tissues (Kam et al., 2019). Such hormonal balances are significant in designing focused therapeutic regimens in autoimmune conditions.

2.2.9. The Role of Stress in Exacerbating Autoimmune Conditions

The relationship between stress and autoimmune disease is more and more recognized as the central mediator in the pathogenesis of disease exacerbations. Stress activates a chain of physiological responses that derange immune homeostasis, elevating inflammation and vulnerability to autoimmune exacerbations. Specifically, chronic stress may influence the activity of critical immune cells , such as iNKT cells, which participate in disease pathogenesis in pSS (Barbera et al., 2019). These cells can initiate abnormal immune activity by the generation of an inflammatory cytokine profile. Besides, the psychological burden of chronic stress has been found to lead to maladaptive coping mechanisms, which in turn would be expected to weaken immune regulation and exacerbate underlying autoimmune diseases. Given the harmful influence of stress on immune homeostasis, it is requisite to study the therapeutic methods for decreasing stress as a method of improving the prognosis of the sufferers of such disorders (Rosa et al., 2015) (Figure 2.11).

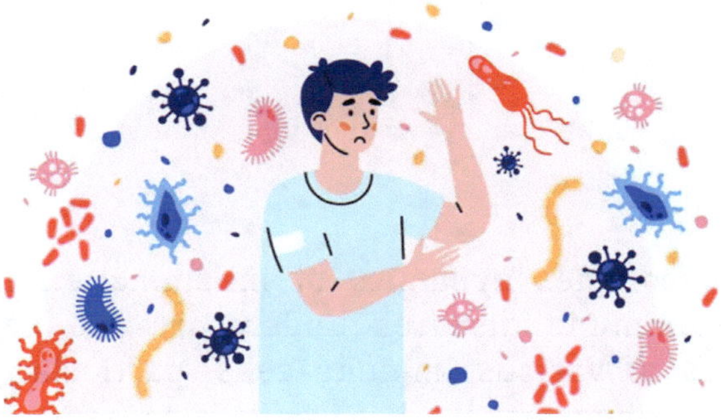

Figure 2.11. The interplay between stress and autoimmune conditions is increasingly recognized as a significant factor in disease exacerbation.

Source: https://thumbnails.icloudhospital.com/tr:w-1536,f-webp,q-75/1-autoimmune-1-b524de18-8ebb-47a0-b41b-0595bcd8f5b7.webp

Test Your Knowledge

1. How does epitope spreading exacerbate autoimmune responses?
2. What is the role of environmental triggers (e.g., infections, toxins) in autoimmunity?

2.3. Inflammation in Autoimmune Diseases

Learning Outcome

1. Know the definition and types of inflammation;
2. Discuss acute vs. chronic inflammation;
3. Focus on cytokine storms and their implications;
4. Know the role of inflammation in tissue damage;
5. Define inflammatory mediators and their sources;
6. Highlight the connection between inflammation and autoimmunity;
7. Understand clinical manifestations of inflammation in autoimmune diseases;
8. Learn therapeutic targets in inflammatory processes;
9. Discuss the role of inflammation in the disease process.

The complex dynamics of inflammation in autoimmune diseases underscore the key roles of various immune cells, particularly T lymphocytes, in disease development. In disorders , such as systemic autoimmune diseases, T-EM cells become significant players, causing tissue damage through their release of pro-inflammatory cytokines that are well known to recruit macrophages, neutrophils, and other leukocytes into areas of inflammation (Abdulahad et al., 2014).

This heightened activity is reflected in autoimmune thyroid disease, where a surge in inflammatory mediators like adipokines , such as leptin and cytokines , such as TNF-α and IL-6, tilts the balance of the immune response and prevents tolerance to thyroid antigens (Merrill & Mu, 2015). The convergence of these immune responses not only accounts for the pathophysiology of autoimmunity but also identifies putative therapeutic targets aiming at modulating the inflammatory responses and thereby relieving tissue damage and re-establishing homeostasis in injured organs.

2.3.1. Definition and Types of Inflammation

Inflammation is an essential biological reaction to damaging stimuli, and it can be classified into two broad types: acute and chronic inflammation. Acute inflammation is usually an acute and reversible process that consists of a sudden immigration of immune cells into the injured or infected area, which results in signs , such as redness, heat, swelling, and pain.

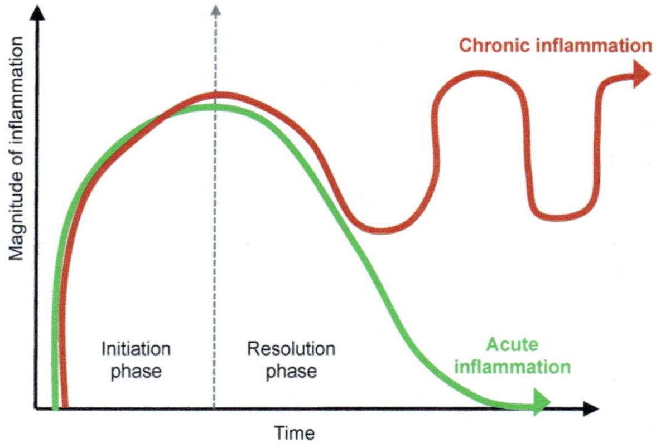

Figure 2.12. Inflammation serves as a critical biological response to harmful stimuli, and it can be classified into two primary types: acute and chronic inflammation.

Source: https://www.mdpi.com/ijms/ijms-23-14905/article_deploy/html/images/ijms-23-14905-g001.png.

Chronic inflammation is a prolonged and dysregulated inflammatory response that can be caused by persistent infections, autoimmune diseases, or chronic exposure to irritants. This type of inflammation will most often activate a complex interaction of various immune cells , such as macrophages and T cells, which, in attempting to rid the body of disease-causing pathogens, end up promoting tissue destruction and perpetuating disease. It is essential to grasp these inflammatory processes because they leave doors open for therapeutic intervention that can regulate immune reactions in diseases , such as multiple sclerosis, where certain gene expression patterns in astrocytes offer strong clues into the disease pathology (Staunton et al., 2013) (Figure 2.12).

2.3.2. Acute vs. Chronic Inflammation

The distinction between acute and chronic inflammation is critical in the understanding of immune response, particularly autoimmune diseases. Acute inflammation is characterized by the rapid development of signs , such as redness, swelling, and pain, typically as an adaptive response to infection or injury. Acute inflammation entails the activation of innate immune cells, such as neutrophils and macrophages, which respond to eliminate pathogens and initiate repair (Bluestone et al., 2005). Chronic inflammation, however, is a sustained inflammatory reaction that can potentially lead to tissue damage and the causation of various autoimmune conditions. In such a scenario, Tregs responsible for immune tolerance can be impaired or depleted, encouraging the inflammation and leading to disease (Ballardini et al., 1988). Therefore, knowing the balance and interaction between these two forms of inflammation is crucial in the development of targeted therapeutic interventions for autoimmune disorders.

2.3.3. Cytokine Storms and Their Consequences

Cytokine storms are an extreme dysregulation of the immune system, usually resulting in extreme inflammatory effects that cause autoimmune diseases to worsen to an extent that could be catastrophic.

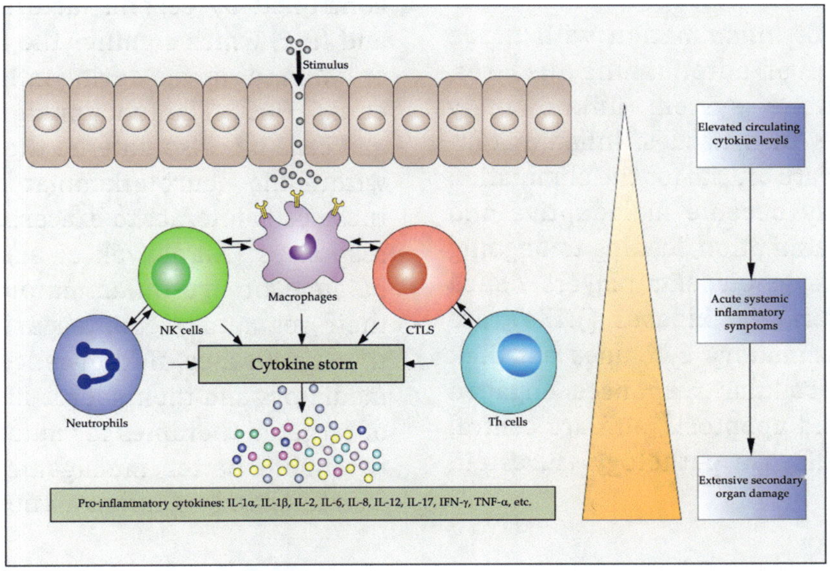

Figure 2.13. During a cytokine storm, an overproduction of cytokines occurs, driven primarily by an influx of white blood cells responding to infection or inflammation.

Source: https://www.mdpi.com/ijms/ijms-22-13009/article_deploy/html/images/ijms-22-13009-g001.png.

There is excessive production of cytokines during a cytokine storm, powered predominantly by a surfeit of white blood cells responding to infection or inflammation. The immense release of cytokines can cause widespread tissue damage and systemic effects, including acute respiratory distress syndrome and multi-organ failure, both of which are typically observed in conditions like COVID-19. The NLRP3 inflammasome plays a role in the amplification of this process, as it regulates the activation of pro-inflammatory cytokines , such as IL-1 beta and is crucial in the pathogenesis of many inflammatory diseases (Basile et al., 2023). Again, the increasing incidence of cytokine storms, particularly during viral pandemics, has served as an indicator of the urgent need for effective therapeutic interventions to help control their negative effects (Aldoori et al., 2022) (Figure 2.13).

2.3.4. The Role of Inflammation in Tissue Damage

The cooperation of inflammation with tissue damage is a part of autoimmune diseases, where the immune system unknowingly attacks the body's own tissues. Inflammatory responses, as they are crucial for the elimination of pathogens, may become maladaptive and cause chronic inflammation, leading to ongoing tissue damage. Key molecular players , such as the c-Jun N-terminal kinases (JNKs), are activated by inflammatory cytokines and link inflammation to cellular responses engaged in proliferation and apoptosis, and are central to autoimmune disease pathology (Firestein et al., 2012). In addition, hypoxia also often cycles inflammatory processes because chronic hypoxic states trigger the proinflammatory pathways to be activated, causing further tissue remodeling and injury (Carnevale et al., 2015). Such complex interaction evidently demands certain therapeutic interventions capable of modulating the inflammatory process in a way that it is unable to cause tissue injury, which is a major feature in the comprehension and treatment of autoimmune diseases effectively.

2.3.5. Inflammatory Mediators and their Sources

Inflammatory mediators play a key role in the pathophysiology of autoimmune disorders and their responses can potentially lead to tissue damage when not regulated appropriately. Among these mediators, cytokines , such as interleukin-17 (IL-17) and transforming growth factor-beta (TGF-β) are particularly notable. The Th17 cell differentiation, along with their production of pro-inflammatory cytokines, is controlled by certain factors , such as IL-1β and IL-6, which signifies the inter-relationship of immune signals during inflammation (Brand et al., 2009). The functioning of mast cells and glia cells has also entered the scene, especially within the neuroinflammatory milieu, where these cells interact to exacerbate inflammatory responses (Alhouayek et al., 2017). The fine balance of pro-inflammatory cytokines and their regulatory counterparts thus points to the significance of knowledge regarding these mediators and their source in the development of targeted therapies for autoimmune illnesses to enable better management of conditions characterized by inflammation (Figure 2.14).

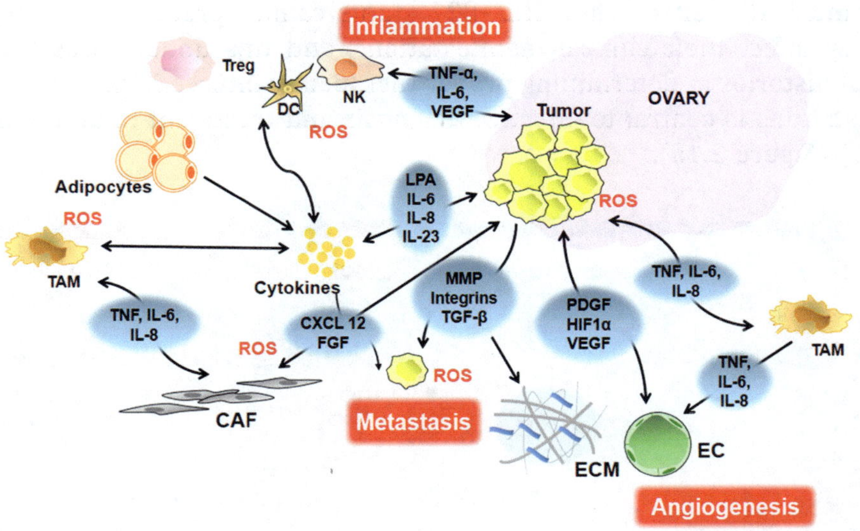

Figure 2.14. Inflammatory mediators play a crucial role in the pathophysiology of autoimmune diseases, orchestrating responses that can lead to tissue damage if dysregulated.

Source: https://www.mdpi.com/cancers/cancers-10-00251/article_deploy/html/images/cancers-10-00251-g002.png.

2.3.6. The Interplay between Inflammation and Autoimmunity

The interplay between inflammation and autoimmunity is intertwined in the pathophysiologic processes of most autoimmune conditions to the point that inflammatory mediators have a central role. In AITDs , such as Graves' disease and *Hashimoto's thyroiditis*, for instance, the balance of inflammatory cytokines like TNF-α and IL-6 triggered by stimuli , such as adipokines of adipose tissue illustrates how inflammation can favor the generation of autoantibodies and break self-tolerance (Merrill & Mu, 2015). Similarly, within RA, mucosal interactions and environmental insults , such as smoking and microbiome dysbiosis, trigger immune responses that have the potential to result in autoimmune expression (Conti et al., 2019). These cases illustrate that not only does inflammation fuel existing autoimmunity, but it can also be a key inciting factor for its onset, in showing a multi-faceted dialogue among immune system dysregulation and inflammatory processes in such diseases.

2.3.7. Clinical Manifestations of Inflammation in Autoimmune Diseases

Clinical features of autoimmune diseases typically comprise an ever-changing list, primarily characterized by inflammation that may involve multiple organ systems. A common example would be the presentation of sensorineural hearing loss in systemic autoimmune diseases, which would either be sudden or gradual and would most commonly affect both ears. This diagnosis, however often mistaken, points towards the need for comprehensive clinical watchfulness since prompt corticosteroid treatment will comparatively easily restore hearing function (Ralli et al., 2018). Furthermore, HLA-B27 positivity in patients could make them susceptible to some autoimmune diseases like ankylosing spondylitis and Crohn's disease, with secondary complications being likely , such as internal uveitis. While HLA-B27 status cannot predate the occurrence of these conditions, it may affect their clinical manifestations, and this underscores the importance of thorough medical histories in determining proper therapeutic interventions. Thus, the information on these manifestations is central to effective diagnosis and treatment in autoimmune conditions (Cox et al., 2011) (Figure 2.15).

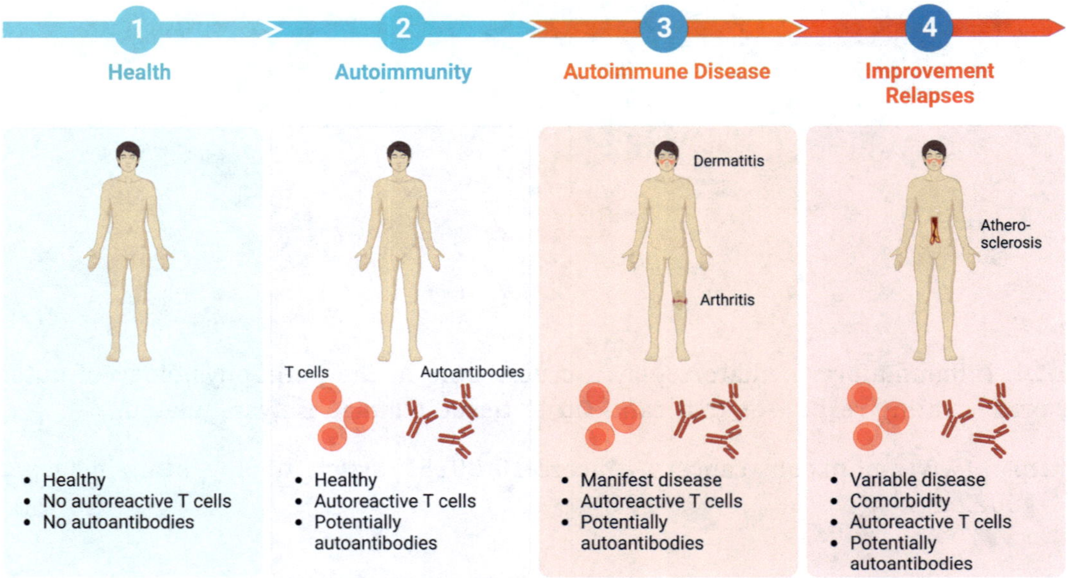

Figure 2.15. Autoimmune diseases often present with a complex array of clinical manifestations, primarily characterized by inflammation that can affect multiple organ systems.

Source: https://www.frontiersin.org/files/Articles/1159396/fimmu-14-1159396-HTML/image_m/fimmu-14-1159396-g001.jpg.

2.3.8. Therapeutic Targets in Inflammatory Pathways

The multifaceted interaction between inflammation and a number of disease states highlights the likely therapeutic targets in inflammatory pathways. It has been discovered through studies that extended hypoxia is a key inducer of pro-inflammatory responses, which may induce widespread cellular injury and chronic disease states, including autoimmune diseases (Carnevale et al., 2015). Most significant among these pathways are transcription factors , such as nuclear factor κB (NF-κB) and nuclear factor of activated T-cells (NFAT), which mediate the regulation of critical pro-inflammatory cytokines and other immune response factors.

The bifunctionality of the factors is what renders them so attractive as therapeutic targets; they can modulate tissue repair and are also able to mediate inflammatory damage. NF-κB and NFAT as specific targets may modulate immune processes in dermatomyositis and polymyositis and thus admit the possibility of a more nuanced control of inflammation and permitting recuperation (Paepe et al., 2017). Consequently, the evolution of our understanding of such signaling pathways may bring new hope for the therapy of autoimmune disorders.

2.3.9. The Role of Inflammation in Disease Progression

The involvement of inflammation in disease progression is best observed in autoimmune conditions, where the body's immune response becomes abnormal, often leading to injury of tissues and persistent inflammation. When inflammatory cells release reactive oxygen species (ROS) and reactive nitrogen species (RNS), they initiate processes that cause DNA damage, leading to gene mutations and genomic instability in target cells (Chen et al., 2018). This genomic upset is crucial, not only for maintaining disease but also for initiating the onset of autoimmune disorders. Besides, the inflammatory character of the disease takes on various forms , such as major oral manifestations, which can serve as prodromal symptoms of autoimmune conditions. This makes dentists very instrumental in the detection of these manifestations, which can facilitate better diagnosis and treatment procedures and consequently contribute to the overall quality of life of victims (Bossù et al., 2018). The intricate interplay of inflammation and exacerbation of disease underscores the need for a thorough understanding and regulation of autoimmune diseases (Figure 2.16).

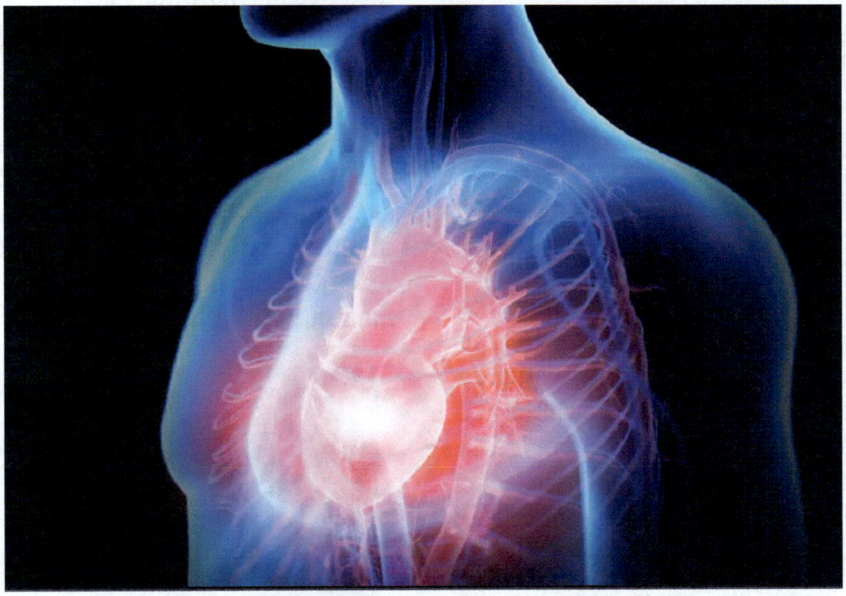

Figure 2.16. The role of inflammation in disease progression is particularly evident in autoimmune diseases, where the body's immune response becomes dysregulated, often leading to tissue damage and chronic inflammation.

Source: https://www.asterhospitals.in/sites/default/files/styles/optimize_images/public/2024-10/CHRONIC%20INFLAMATION.jpg.webp?itok=tDU5ZjT8

Test Your Knowledge

1. Explain the role of chronic inflammation in causing tissue damage and fibrosis in autoimmune diseases.
2. How do chemokines regulate immune cell migration to inflamed tissues in autoimmunity?

2.4. Current Research and Therapeutic Approaches

Learning Outcome

1. Understand new progress in immunotherapy for autoimmune diseases;
2. Identify biological agents acting upon specific immune cells;
3. Explain small-molecule inhibitors in the therapy;
4. Discuss the role of stem cell therapy;
5. Understand personalized medicine for the treatment of autoimmune disease;
6. Highlight clinical trials and why they are crucial;
7. Discuss challenges faced in the development of useful therapies;
8. Explain future approaches in autoimmune disease research.

Recent research has significantly advanced the cellular mechanisms of autoimmune diseases and inflammation and has subsequently introduced new therapeutic approaches. Targeted therapies attacking the specific immune cells involved in rheumatoid arthritis and immune-mediated inner ear disease are emphasized in recent research. For instance, mechanistic mathematical models are currently being developed to describe the biological mechanisms that underlie disease onset and to optimize therapeutic interventions for rheumatoid arthritis, a chronic autoimmune disease presenting formidable health threats (Chaplain et al., 2019).

Similarly, in autoimmune inner ear disease, timely corticosteroid therapy has yielded excellent outcomes in hearing loss reversal, highlighting the necessity of early diagnosis and treatment to alleviate symptoms of systemic autoimmune diseases (Ralli et al., 2018). Overall, the advancement of research is necessary in enhancing the effectiveness of treatments and patient outcomes in autoimmune diseases characterized by inflammatory reactions.

2.4.1. Advances in Immunotherapy for Autoimmune Diseases

As researchers continue to explore newer treatment modalities, immunotherapy has been a new beacon of hope for the treatment of autoimmune diseases, which are characterized by dysregulated immune responses. Among the latest advances is the development of monoclonal antibodies that selectively target pathogenic cells, thereby suppressing the inflammatory processes responsible for these conditions. The precision of these therapies relies on the ability to selectively find and follow disease indicators, so a requirement for advanced diagnostic devices. Radiolabeled antibodies, for instance, can be utilized in assessing the antigenic surroundings in inflammatory tissue to enable individualized treatment strategies to optimize patient outcomes and eliminate harmful side effects (Auletta et al., 2016).

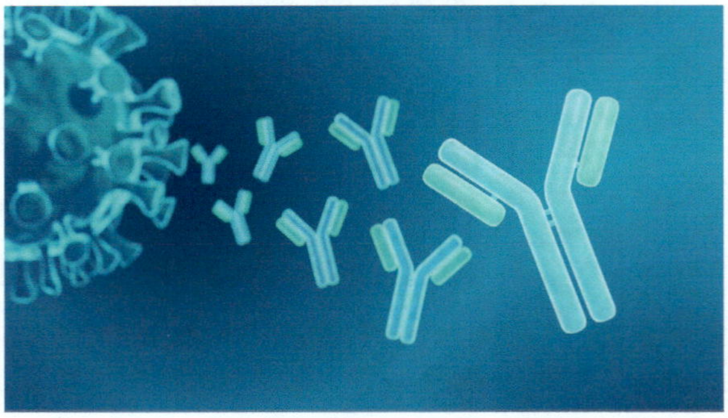

Figure 2.17. Immunotherapy for autoimmune diseases.

Source: https://ysm-res.cloudinary.com/image/upload/c_limit,f_auto,h_810,q_auto,w_1440/v1/yms/prod/32020180-8925-4ee4-bd2f-6db99112577e.

Additionally, the involvement of exosomes in immunomodulation is another breakthrough as extracellular vesicles facilitate cross-talk among immune cells and may serve as carriers for drugs, thereby maximizing the efficacy of immunotherapies (Cacalano et al., 2019). All these advancements pave the way for more effective interventions in treating autoimmune diseases (Figure 2.17).

2.4.2. Biological Agents Targeting Specific Immune Cells

The identification of biological agents that target specific immune cells represents a promising frontier for the treatment of autoimmune diseases and inflammation. These medications, intended to control the immune system, can effectively suppress augmented inflammatory processes characteristic of diseases , such as idiopathic inflammatory myopathies (IIM). In IIM, for instance, the intricate cytokine network is pivotal in maintaining muscle inflammation by various mediators, including Tumor Necrosis Factors (TNF) and Interleukins (IL-1 and IL-6) (Paepe et al., 2015). Furthermore, chronic hypoxia, a state frequently induced during inflammatory attacks, has been shown to activate NK cells, pro-inflammatory pathways that result in additional dissemination of tissue damage and fibrosis (Carnevale et al., 2015). Therefore, the biological agents with selective targeting of these immune cells and their associated pathways not only show therapeutic potential but bring on the horizon additional personalized therapeutic strategies, ultimately maximizing patient benefit in autoimmune diseases and inflammatory diseases.

2.4.3. Small Molecule Inhibitors in Treatment

The treatment landscape of autoimmune diseases has undergone a striking transformation with the introduction of small-molecule inhibitors that interfere with selected intracellular pathways of signaling, which are responsible for controlling immune cell function. Such inhibitory drugs, particularly Janus kinase (JAK) inhibitors, have succeeded in diseases , such as rheumatoid arthritis by interrupting the cytokine signal that results in inflammation and tissue damage. Research indicates that cytokine inhibitors have played a crucial role in determining the position of tumor necrosis factor α and interleukin 6 in autoimmune disease pathogenesis, hence opening the gateway for effective treatments (McInnes & Schett, 2017). Additionally, small molecule inhibitors might also act on the complex interaction between hypoxia and inflammation, a correlation that is linked to chronic autoimmune reactions and tissue remodeling (Carnevale et al., 2015). Thus, the design and deployment of such inhibitors not only underscore their therapeutic potential but also point to key pathways essential for effective modulation of autoimmune inflammation (Figure 2.18).

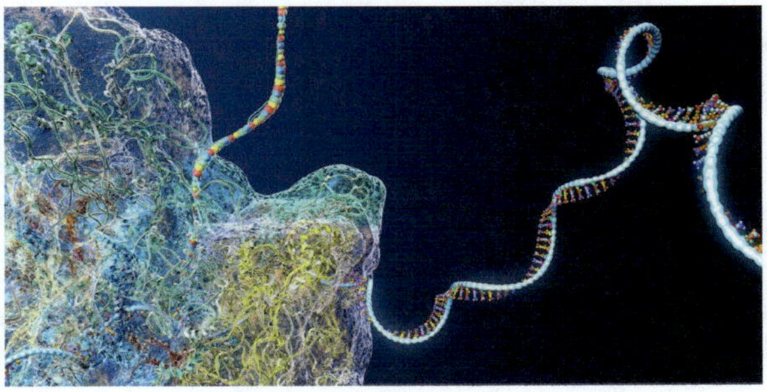

Figure 2.18. Small molecule inhibitors.

Source: https://www.activemotif.com/uploads/images/web_site/resources-page/blog/fto-inhibitors-target-rna-modifications/rna-molecule.jpg.

2.4.4. The Role of Stem Cell Therapy

The use of stem cell therapy has been a major area of research in the management of autoimmune diseases and inflammation, particularly in view of the limitations of conventional therapies. Stem cells possess unique properties for self-renewal and differentiation and are therefore a promising source for regenerative medicine. In disorders , such as MS, where inflammation causes extensive neurodegeneration, transplantation of neural and mesenchymal stem cells has been found to be promising as a result of their immunomodulatory effects as well as tissue repair-promoting capability. Studies have found that these stem cells are capable of inducing remyelination as well as functional mobility in affected individuals, and thus are of therapeutic interest (Guan et al., 2016). Besides, the interaction between inflammation and hypoxia complicates the course of disease, since inflammatory responses can be amplified by the hypoxic environment and lead to long-term tissue injury (Carnevale et al., 2015). Stem cell therapy, thus, not only offers a novel model of treatment but also opens new insights into the complex cell-cell interactions in autoimmune diseases and inflammation.

2.4.5. Personalized Medicine in Autoimmune Disease Management

The establishment of personalized medicine has greatly changed autoimmune disease treatment so that more individualized therapy is given with respect to patient-specific profiles. By using advanced diagnostic machinery, it is now possible for clinicians to detect more precise autoantigens and immune responses located in a patient's individual biological environment. For instance, the availability of biologic therapy necessitates highly precise diagnostic methods capable of measuring noninvasively disease mechanisms to optimize treatment. Radiopharmaceuticals used for SPECT or PET imaging, and radiolabeled monoclonal antibodies directed to specific antigens, allow accurate measurements of inflammatory disease and therapeutic response, maximizing treatment options available to the patient. Furthermore, these newer modalities not only aid in initial treatment selection but also provide very valuable information for ongoing adaptation of the therapy, so treatments are as effective as possible for individual patients (Auletta et al., 2016). This shift towards personalized medicine ultimately points towards the complex interdependence between cellular processes and therapeutic precision in the treatment of autoimmune diseases (Staunton et al., 2013) (Figure 2.19).

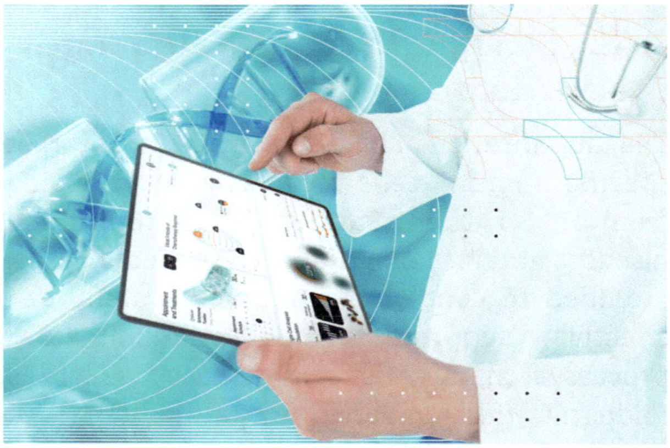

Figure 2.19. The evolution of personalized medicine has profoundly transformed the management of autoimmune diseases, enabling more tailored therapeutic approaches that consider individual patient profiles.

Source: https://www.bgosoftware.com/blog/wp-content/uploads/2024/01/bgo-software-blog_post-size-%E2%80%93-Personalized-Medicine_no_title.png.

2.4.6. Clinical Trials and Their Significance

The value of clinical trials to our build-up of knowledge and treatment of autoimmune diseases is that they can objectively evaluate the safety and efficacy of new treatments. The trials are generally investigating cellular mechanisms of these diseases and, as part of it, providing useful information about the complex immune system processes. For instance, studies on populations with MS have adopted cell-specific approaches to identify astrocyte gene expression variation across various neuroanatomical areas during inflammatory attacks, emphasizing the need for targeted therapeutic intervention (Ao et al., 2017). Besides, clinical studies of disorders like dry eye syndrome highlight the need to understand concealed cellular inflammation in testing the efficacy of new treatment strategies to restore ocular surface homeostasis (Albietz et al., 2017). Thus, by way of scrupulously designed research, clinical trials help bridge benchside results with bedside interventions, ultimately culminating in improved patient outcomes in the treatment of autoimmune diseases.

2.4.7. Challenges in Developing Effective Treatments

The development of successful treatments for autoimmune disorders remains an intimidating challenge, primarily due to the intricacy of immune system dysregulation and the diversity of such diseases. Autoimmune disorders generally entail a broad spectrum of cellular interactions and inflammatory responses; hence, it is not simple to identify shared therapeutic targets. For example, corticosteroid treatments can radically alleviate symptoms in some instances, but their effectiveness is frequently unreliable, and side effects can restrict long-term treatment. Additionally, misdiagnosis often makes treatment regimens difficult, since presentation can be exceptionally varied and mimic other conditions, which highlights the importance of accurate diagnostic protocols. The challenge of separating individual frameworks of immunopathology, combined with a dearth of strong evidence depicting diverse clinical outcomes, is part of the broader issue of therapy efficacy. Emphasis on the need for personalized interventions, identification of systemic involvement, and refinement in diagnostic accuracy is essential to enhance the effectiveness of treatment, especially in complex cases involving conditions like sensorineural hearing loss in association with autoimmune processes, where therapy may be very effective if given cautiously (Staunton et al., 2013; Ralli et al., 2018) (Figure 2.20).

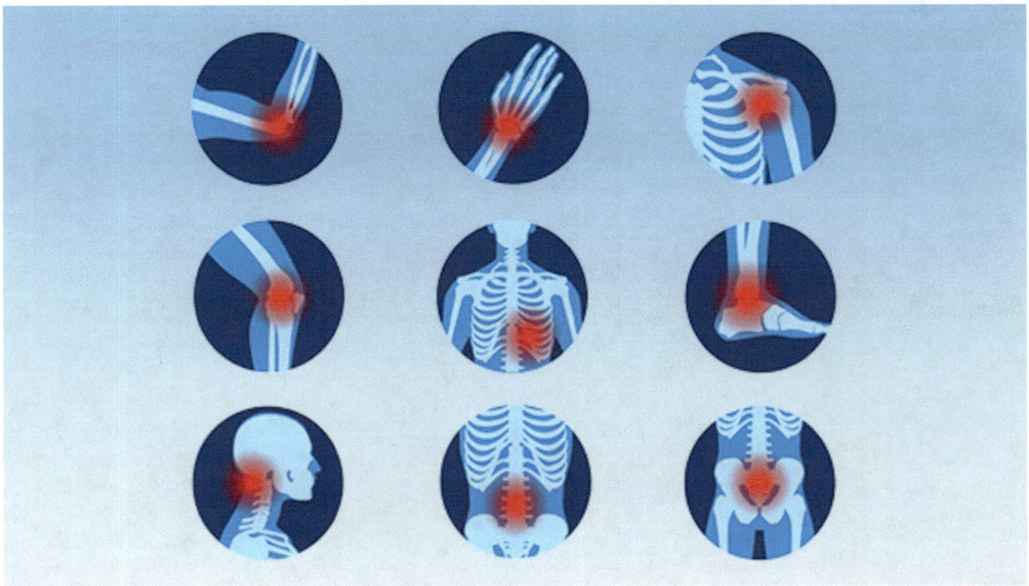

Figure 2.20. Autoimmune diseases often involve a broad spectrum of cellular interactions and inflammatory responses, making it difficult to identify universal therapeutic targets.

Source: https://www.autoimmuneinstitute.org/wp-content/uploads/2024/02/Inflammation-A-Driving-Force-of-Autoimmune-Disease-1.jpg.

2.4.8. Future Directions in Autoimmune Disease Research

The future of autoimmune disease research is promising, with directions that have the potential to change our understanding of disease mechanisms and therapeutic strategies. Refinement of cellular and molecular techniques adds to the improved understanding of autoimmune disease pathophysiology. For instance, advanced genomic technologies can decode the roles of single immune cells, thereby opening new therapeutic targets. Beyond this, understanding environmental factors that interact with gene predispositions is crucial in the development of personalized medicine approaches. Another emerging interest lies in the role of the gut microbiota in shaping immune function, and possibly new therapeutic horizons. In addition, research into biological drugs, such as those for tumor necrosis factor-alpha, and extensive studies of rare conditions like Cogan's syndrome, all indicate future potential for tailored therapy. Increased research into the pathophysiology of autoimmunity will undoubtedly improve diagnostic and therapeutic outcomes (Staunton et al., 2013; D'Aguanno et al., 2017).

Test Your Knowledge

1. How may microbiome modulation be applied to treating autoimmune disease?
2. What are some of the new treatments or clinical trials in autoimmune disease studies?

Summary

The intricate interaction between various immune cells plays a pivotal role in the pathogenesis of autoimmunity and inflammation, emphasizing the necessity of an intelligent appreciation of these processes for effective therapeutic strategies. Studies have unraveled the role of Tregs in tolerance but their relative scarcity in peripheral blood questions their therapeutic utility in treating autoimmune diseases (Bluestone et al., 2005). In addition, chronic inflammation, exemplified by uveitis, is typically the result of homeostasis breakdown and attempts at regulation that have failed, and this underscores the complexity of immune regulation in organs , such as the eye (Amadi-Obi et al., 2014). As we continue to untangle these multifaceted interactions, it more clearly emerges that targeted methods of enhancing Treg function and immune homeostasis are of potential value for the treatment of autoimmune disease and suppression of inflammatory responses within the involved tissue.

The multifaceted interaction among numerous cell types lies at the core of the understanding of autoimmune disease and inflammation. Central among them are immune cells that respond to aberrant signals, leading to chronic inflammatory disease. For instance, recent research has placed in the spotlight the role of mixed lineage kinase domain-like protein (MLKL) in programmed necrosis during autoimmune hepatitis, demonstrating its upregulation and activation by activation with inflammatory cytokines like IFN-gamma, suggesting it is involved in the etiology of the disease (Kremer et al., 2016). Moreover, the impact of mitochondria in cellular stress response cannot be overlooked; they are presently recognized as principal regulators of cellular aging and inflammation, thereby defining the course of autoimmune disorders (Haas, 2019). Overall, these findings emphasize that both mitochondrial necrosis and dynamics have a pivotal function in understanding the cellular pathogenesis of autoimmune disorders, which is moving towards future therapeutic intervention.

KEY TERMS FROM THIS CHAPTER

- Immune system
- Autoimmune thyroid diseases (AITDs)
- Hashimotos thyroiditis
- Infectious agents
- Viruses
- Bystander activation
- Immune cells
- Inflammation
- Autoimmunity
- Graves' disease
- Hormones
- Bacteria
- Molecular mimicry
- Autoimmune diseases
- Cytokines
- Pathogen

Critical Thinking Questions

1. Which immune cell is most accountable for autoantibody generation in autoimmune diseases?

a. T helper cells
b. Cytotoxic T cells
c. B-cells
d. Natural killer (NK) cells

2. Which subset of T cells plays a critical role in suppressing immune responses and preventing autoimmunity?

a. Th1 cells
b. Th2 cells
c. Cytotoxic T cells
d. Regulatory T cells (Tregs)

3. Which of the following cells is known to release histamine and contribute to the inflammatory response?

a. Neutrophils
b. Eosinophils
c. Mast cells
d. Macrophages

4. Which innate immune cell is often the first responder during inflammation and acts by phagocytosis?

a. B lymphocytes
b. Neutrophils
c. T lymphocytes
d. Basophils

5. Which cytokine is primarily produced by activated macrophages and plays a major role in systemic inflammation?

a. IL-4
b. IL-10
c. TNF-α
d. IFN-γ

Short Answer Questions

1. What is the role of T helper cells ($CD4^+$) in the development of autoimmune responses?
2. In autoimmune disease, how do cytotoxic T cells ($CD8^+$) cause tissue damage?
3. Define central tolerance and peripheral tolerance, and explain how their failure leads to autoimmunity.
4. What is molecular mimicry, and how does it contribute to the development of autoimmune diseases?
5. What are the main pro-inflammatory cytokines that are involved in autoimmune inflammation?
6. How do intrinsic immune responses initiate and maintain inflammation in autoimmune diseases?
7. What are the currently available biologic drugs utilized to treat autoimmune diseases (e.g., TNF inhibitors, IL-6 antagonists)?
8. How do JAK inhibitors work, and which autoimmune diseases are they approved to treat?

Answers to Critical Thinking Questions

1. (c); 2. (d); 3. (c); 4. (b); 5. (c)

References

1. Abdulahad, A., Abdulahad, A., Abdulahad, A., Abdulahad, A., Abdulahad, A., Abdulahad, A., Ait-Oufella, H., et al. (2014). T cells in vascular inflammatory diseases. https://core.ac.uk/download/pdf/82869901.pdf (accessed on 17th June 2025).

2. Alivernini, S., Tolusso, B., Ferraccioli, G., Gremese, E., Kurowska-Stolarska, M., & McInnes, I. B. (2018). Driving chronicity in rheumatoid arthritis: perpetuating role of myeloid cells. *Clinical and experimental immunology, 193*(1), 13–23. https://doi.org/10.1111/cei.13098 (accessed on 17th June 2025).

3. Adcock, I. M., Auffray, C., Baribaud, F., Chanez, P., et al. (2016). A transcriptome-driven analysis of epithelial brushings and bronchial biopsies to define asthma phenotypes in U-BIOPRED. https://core.ac.uk/download/77018710.pdf (accessed on 17th June 2025).

4. Ralli, M., D'Aguanno, V., Di Stadio, A., De Virgilio, A., Croce, A., Longo, L., Greco, A., & de Vincentiis, M. (2018). Audiovestibular Symptoms in Systemic Autoimmune Diseases. *Journal of immunology research, 2018*, 5798103. https://doi.org/10.1155/2018/5798103 (accessed on 17th June 2025).

5. Adorini, L., Ahn, J., Alnek, K., Ananthakrishnan, R., Aram, J., Aricha, R., Basdeo, S., et al. (2019). Roles of GM-CSF in the pathogenesis of autoimmune diseases: An update. https://core.ac.uk/download/225130666.pdf (accessed on 17th June 2025).

6. Albietz, J., Alio, J. L., Ambrosio, R., Djalilian, A. R., Dogru, M., Li, D. Q., Nebbioso, M., et al. (2017). Analysis of the pathogenic factors and management of dry eye in ocular surface disorders. https://core.ac.uk/download/127587951.pdf (accessed on 17th June 2025).

7. Aldoori, Z. A. A., & Hameed, N. I. A. (2022). Article review: The phenomenon of cytokine storm. https://core.ac.uk/download/597862228.pdf (accessed on 17th June 2025).

8. Alhouayek, M., Amor, S., Amor, S., Appel, S. H., Bankston, A. N., Biber, K., Biran, V., et al. (2017). Neuroinflammation, mast cells, and glia: Dangerous liaisons. https://core.ac.uk/download/129593018.pdf (accessed on 17th June 2025).

9. Al-Riyami, L., Al-Riyammi, A., Aoyama, T., Baev, D., Bashir, R., Bogoyevitch, M., Borghouts, C., et al. (2010). The therapeutic potential of the filarial nematode-derived immunodulator, ES-62 in inflammatory disease. https://core.ac.uk/download/9028724.pdf (accessed on 17th June 2025).

10. Al-Riyami, L., Harnett, M. M., Harnett, W., Pineda, M. A., et al. (2014). Lessons from helminth infections: ES-62 highlights new interventional approaches in rheumatoid arthritis. https://core.ac.uk/download/42352576.pdf (accessed on 17th June 2025).

11. Amadi-Obi, A., Arida, A., Cortes, A., Fox, A., Jager, A., Peters, A., Rothova, A., et al. (2014). Autoimmune and autoinflammatory mechanisms in uveitis. https://core.ac.uk/download/29416272.pdf (accessed on 17th June 2025).

12. Ao, Y., Burda, J., Farkhondeh, V., Itoh, N., et al. (2017). Cell-specific and region-specific transcriptomics in the multiple sclerosis model: Focus on astrocytes. https://core.ac.uk/download/323076468.pdf (accessed on 17th June 2025).

13. Auletta, S., Carideo, L., Galli, F., Lauri, C., et al. (2016). Immunoscintigraphic for therapy decision making and follow-up of biological therapies. https://core.ac.uk/download/153364883.pdf (accessed on 17th June 2025).

14. Ballardini, G., Baum, H., Berg, T., Bernuau, J., Demetris, A. J., et al. (1988). Pathologic analysis of liver transplantation for primary biliary cirrhosis. https://core.ac.uk/download/12204240.pdf (accessed on 17th June 2025).

15. Barbera, L. L., Ciccia, F., Guggino, G., Pizzo, M. L., Rizzo, C., & Sireci, G. (2019). Invariant NKT cells and rheumatic disease: Focus on primary Sjögren syndrome. https://core.ac.uk/download/287859163.pdf (accessed on 17th June 2025).

16. Basile, U., Marino, M., Napodano, C., & Pocino, K. (2023). NLRP3 inflammasome involvement in heart, liver, and lung diseases—A lesson from cytokine storm syndrome. https://core.ac.uk/download/597594059.pdf (accessed on 17th June 2025).

17. Bluestone, J. A., Bonyhadi, M. L., Earle, K. E., Liu, Y., et al. (2005). *In vitro* expanded human CD4+CD25+ regulatory T cells suppress effector T cell proliferation. https://core.ac.uk/download/323073865.pdf (accessed on 17th June 2025).

18. Bonifaz, L. C., Boudin, H., Bueno, S. M., Coronado-Arrázola, I., et al. (2018). Intestinal microbiota influences non-intestinal related autoimmune diseases. https://core.ac.uk/download/288897809.pdf (accessed on 17th June 2025).

19. Bossù, M., Di Carlo, G., Giovarruscio, F., Polimeni, A., et al. (2018). Autoimmune diseases and their manifestations on oral cavity: Diagnosis and clinical management. https://core.ac.uk/download/159635803.pdf (accessed on 17th June 2025).

20. Brand, S. (2009). Crohn's disease: Th1, Th17 or both? The change of a paradigm: New immunological and genetic insights implicate Th17 cells in the pathogenesis of Crohn's disease. https://core.ac.uk/download/12175178.pdf (accessed on 17th June 2025).

21. Simakou, T., Butcher, J. P., Reid, S., & Henriquez, F. L. (2019). Alopecia areata: A multifactorial autoimmune condition. *Journal of autoimmunity*, *98*, 74–85. https://doi.org/10.1016/j.jaut.2018.12.001(accessed on 17th June 2025).

22. Cacalano, N. A., Huyan, T., Li, Q., Peng, X., et al. (2019). Exosomes: Versatile nano mediators of immune regulation. https://core.ac.uk/download/323078768.pdf (accessed on 17th June 2025).

23. Carnevale, I., De Santis, E., Limana, F., Perrone, A., et al. (2015). One special question to start with: Can HIF/NFkB be a target in inflammation? https://core.ac.uk/download/54248898.pdf (accessed on 17th June 2025).

24. Chaplain, M. A. J., Eftimie, R., & Macfarlane, F. R. (2019). Quantitative predictive modelling approaches to understanding rheumatoid arthritis: A brief review. https://core.ac.uk/download/286356117.pdf (accessed on 17th June 2025).

25. Chen, H., Choi, E. T., Cueto, R., Drosatos, K., et al. (2018). DNA checkpoint and repair factors are nuclear sensors for intracellular organelle stresses—inflammations and cancers can have high genomic risks. https://core.ac.uk/download/213438588.pdf (accessed on 17th June 2025).

26. Conti, F., Di Franco, M., Guzzo, M. P., Iannuccelli, C., et al. (2019). Mucosa-environment interactions in the pathogenesis of rheumatoid arthritis. https://core.ac.uk/download/231748449.pdf (accessed on 17th June 2025).

EFFECTOR MECHANISMS IN AUTOIMMUNITY AND INFLAMMATION

3

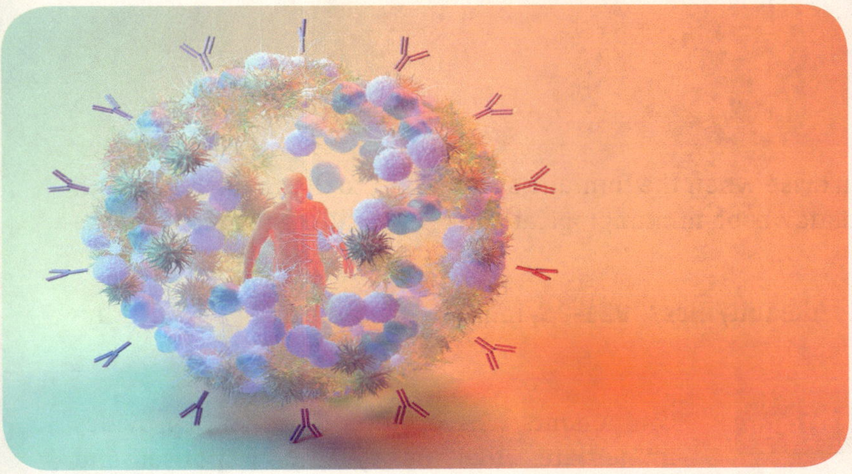

LEARNING OBJECTIVES

After studying this chapter, you will be able to:

1. Define immune system overview;
2. Describe effector T cells in autoimmunity;
3. Explain B-cells and antibody production;
4. Remember inflammatory mediators and pathways.

Introduction

The interface between effector mechanisms of autoimmunity and inflammation is central to understanding the pathophysiology of most autoimmune diseases. Autoimmune diseases often arise when the immune system is incapable of differentiating between self and non-self, and the immunological tolerance fails, leading to tissue injury. As in diseases like Rheumatoid Arthritis (RA), recurrent inflammation occurs due to the improper activation of myeloid cells and ongoing inflammatory pathways, eventually causing irreversible disability and tissue injury (Alivernini et al., 2018). Also, co-stimulatory receptors , such as CD28, play a role in the activation of T-cells and regulatory T-cell function, which affects the balance between immune activation and tolerance (Aruffo et al., 2018). The identification of these effector mechanisms is crucial for creating targeted therapy that will restore immune homeostasis and impede the pathogenic consequences of autoimmunity and chronic inflammation, leaving room to explore further in this chapter (Figure 3.1).

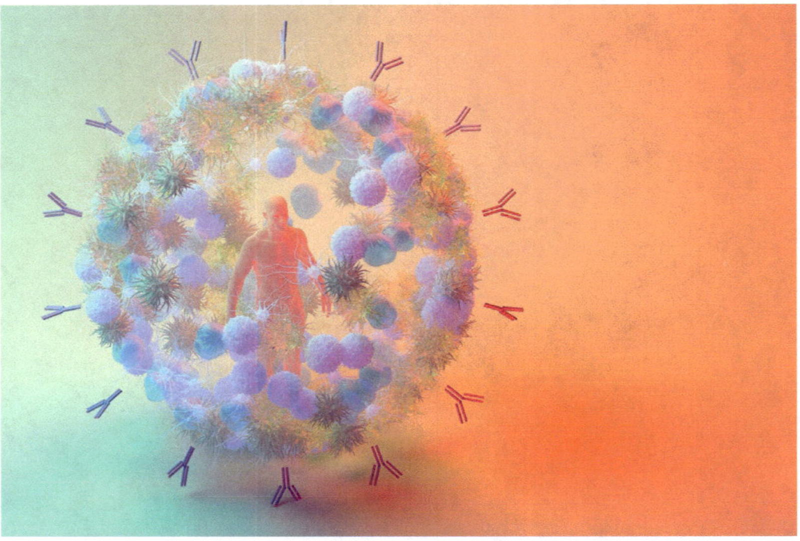

Figure 3.1. Autoimmune diseases often arise when the immune system fails to distinguish between self and non-self, leading to the breakdown of immunological tolerance and subsequent tissue damage.

Source: https://magazine.ucsf.edu/sites/default/files/2021-05/immune-system-turn-covid-deadly-featured.jpg.

3.1. Immune System Overview

Learning Outcome

1. Identify components of the immune system;
2. Describe the function of innate immunity;
3. Discuss the function of adaptive immunity;
4. Learn the mechanism of the immune response;
5. Discuss the interaction between innate and adaptive immunity;
6. Know the importance of immune regulation;
7. Understand an overview of immune tolerance;
8. Learn the consequence of immune dysregulation;
9. Explain the key players in the immune response.

The immune system is the body's primary defense system, elegantly coordinating attacks against a huge diversity of pathogens and maintaining homeostasis. It is comprised of a delicate balance of innate and adaptive components, wherein innate immunity provides immediate, albeit nonspecific, responses and adaptive immunity plans a highly sophisticated defense against individualized antigens over time. One of the characteristic aspects of this mechanism is regulatory processes that prevent overreaction to non-detrimental stimuli. Overactivation of such regulatory processes, on the other hand, results in autoimmunity, immunity that targets self-tissues as a result of misidentification, for example, alopecia areata, wherein there is lymphocytic invasion and antibody targeting against hair follicular cells (Simakou et al., 2019).

Additionally, the eye is a unique immune microenvironment, employing some immunoregulatory mechanisms in resisting inflammation, such as uveitis (Amadi-Obi et al., 2014). Understanding such specificity is vital for the development of correct therapy for autoimmune diseases and inflammation.

3.1.1. Components of the Immune System

The immune system comprises various components that work together to protect the body from infection and provide homeostasis. The key elements are the natural immune cells, such as macrophages and dendritic cells, that initiate infection responses, and adaptive immune cells, such as T and B lymphocytes, that initiate long-term immunity. Molecules like cytokines and chemokines also facilitate communication among the cells to be more competent at responding to threats. Notably, microRNAs (miRNAs) , such as miR-155 are critical controllers of immune responses; dysregulated, they have the ability to cause autoimmunity and chronic inflammation, their therapeutic potential being highlighted for use as a target in diseases , such as Rheumatoid Arthritis (Alivernini et al., 2018). Also, natural killer (NK) cells are an important component, with active behaviors driven by the local microenvironment, capable of modulating their capacity to induce inflammatory effects at the site of injury or infection (Shi et al., 2011). All these components are the best example of the fine balance required for effective immune function and the consequent effects of dysregulation (Figure 3.2).

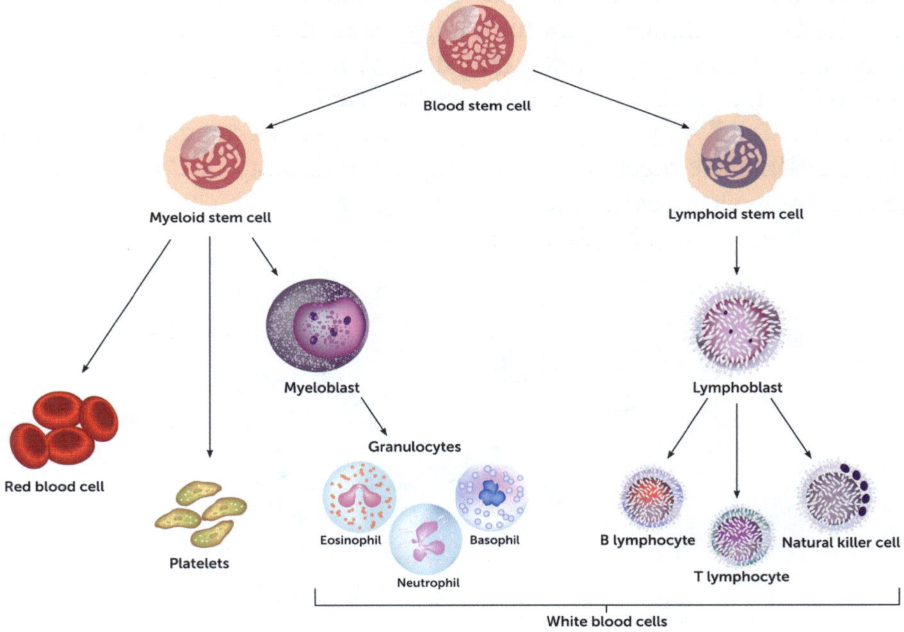

Figure 3.2. Components of the immune system.

Source: https://m2.healio.com/~/media/images/education-lab/learning-sites/learn-immuno-oncology/the-immune-system/learnimmunoblood.jpg.

3.1.2. Role of Innate Immunity

Natural immunity is behind initiating and regulating inflammatory reactions that are normally present in autoimmune disease. Natural immunity is the initial defense and consists of diverse cellular and molecular mechanisms that respond to infection or tissue damage. In rheumatoid arthritis, for instance, studies highlight the role of immune-mediated pathogenesis and its link with dysregulation of stromal tissue that causes chronic inflammation and joint destruction (Firestein &

McInnes, 2017). The dysregulation that is seen can partly be explained by the interplay between innate immune cells, such as macrophages and dendritic cells, that release pro-inflammatory cytokines. Interestingly enough, parasitic infection, particularly from helminths, has been found to modify the cytokine environment and induce anti-inflammatory responses, thereby informing therapeutic strategies for managing autoimmune disease (Fleming et al., 2017). These interactions attest to the two-faced role of innate immunity as both a protector against infection and an inducer of autoimmune disease.

3.1.3. Role of Adaptive Immunity

The adaptive immunity has a key role in understanding the complex interaction between autoimmunity and chronic inflammation, particularly in conditions , such as rheumatoid arthritis (RA). Unlike the innate immune response, which acts to offer immediate but non-specific mechanisms of protection, adaptive immunity offers an individualized action through T-cell and B-cell activation. This specificity, although necessary to defend effectively against pathogens, can also be held accountable for self-directed phenomena that lead to autoimmune diseases. The pre-RA phase generally offers a lead-in to clinical symptomatology and is characterized by the emergence of autoantibodies and inflammatory cytokines that disrupt immunological homeostasis. In addition, the microRNA miR-155 has also been shown to be crucial in the modulation of the immune response and, therefore, following deregulation, plays a role in chronic inflammation (Alivernini et al., 2018). Thus, unraveling the mechanisms of adaptive immunity not only sheds light on disease pathogenesis but also reveals potential therapeutic targets with which to re-establish immunologic balance (Firestein & McInnes, 2017) (Figure 3.3).

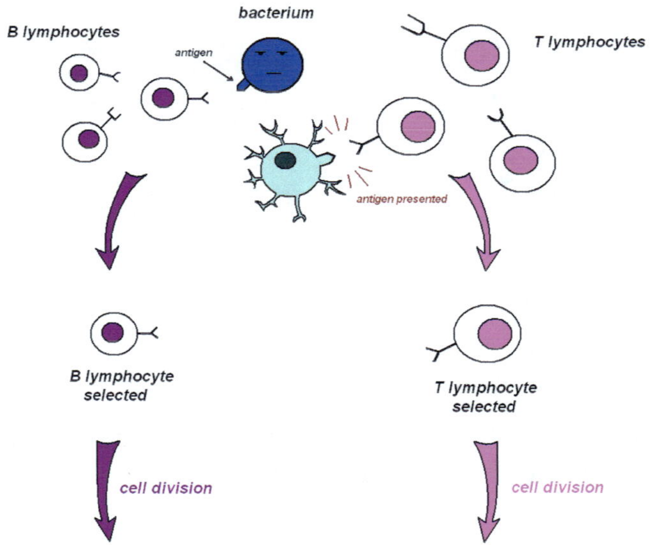

Figure 3.3. The role of adaptive immunity is fundamental in understanding the complex interplay between autoimmunity and chronic inflammation, particularly within conditions , such as rheumatoid arthritis (RA).

Source: https://www.ucl.ac.uk/~zchabg4/pics/selection1.gif.

3.1.4. Mechanisms of Immune Response

Understanding immune response mechanisms is most important in the disclosure of the complexities involved in autoimmunity and inflammation, particularly in diseases , such as RA. Immune dysregulation triggers a series of inflammatory events that are linked with the presence of autoantibodies and elevated inflammatory cytokines and chemokines, which cause chronic inflammation and tissue injury. Certain molecular players, such as microRNAs, have emerged to be of interest; e.g., miR-155 is crucial for immune function but, when deregulated, can exacerbate chronic inflammation and autoimmunity, such as in RA (Alivernini et al., 2018). This pro-inflammatory state is not merely a coincidence of immune stimulation but a central component propelling articular degradation. Therapeutic intervention targeting immune strategies aiming to restore immunologic homeostasis holds a promising prospect, as aligned with the ultimate aim of drug-free remission and redefining success in the treatment of autoimmunity (Firestein & McInnes, 2017). These reports further clarify the immune mechanisms underlying disease onset.

3.1.5. Interaction between Innate and Adaptive Immunity

The interaction between innate and adaptive immunity is a dynamic and complex process that is responsible for the pathogenesis of autoimmune conditions and inflammation. Innate immune cells, such as NK cells, are among the first to respond to signals of danger and trigger inflammatory cascades that drive adaptive immune responses. These natural cells not only contribute to the immediate defense but also participate in the development and activation of adaptive T and B lymphocytes, thus creating a connection between the two branches of immunity. For instance, in diseases , such as rheumatoid arthritis, innate immune activation leads to cytokine and chemokine generation that coordinates the inflammatory environment to create a milieu for generating autoreactive T cells as well as the generation of autoantibodies (Firestein & McInnes, 2017). Besides, organ-specific characteristics of innate immunity highlight the manner in which local microenvironments can modulate such interactions, once more making the autoimmunity and inflammation landscape intricate (Shi et al., 2011) (Figure 3.4).

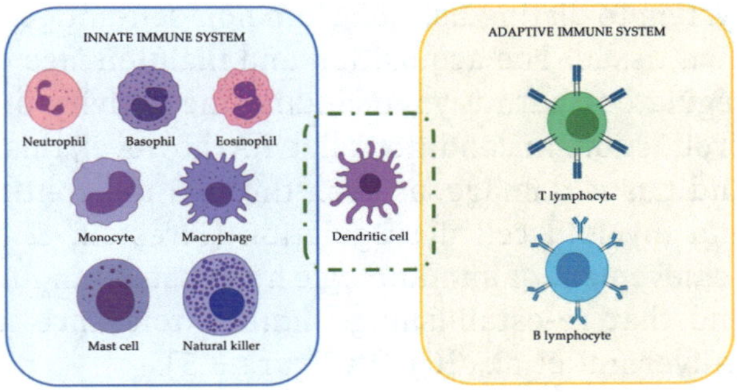

Figure 3.4. The interaction between innate and adaptive immunity is a complex and dynamic process that plays a crucial role in the pathogenesis of autoimmune diseases and inflammatory responses.

Source: https://www.mdpi.com/nanomaterials/nanomaterials-11-02991/article_deploy/html/images/nanomaterials-11-02991-g001.png.

3.1.6. Importance of Immune Regulation

The significance of immune regulation must not be exaggerated while thinking in terms of the mechanisms of effector functions that cause autoimmunity and inflammation. Without good immune regulatory mechanisms, the body would be susceptible to inflammatory diseases, as seen in rheumatoid arthritis and uveitis. For instance, in rheumatoid arthritis, immune-mediated pathogenesis demonstrates how dysregulation of stromal tissue leads to autoimmune aggression, characterized by circulating autoantibodies and heightened inflammatory cytokines, leading to joint destruction (Firestein & McInnes, 2017). Similarly, in uveitis, ocular tissues under normal conditions employ unique immunoregulatory mechanisms to maintain homeostasis despite immune aggression. Interference with these processes causes chronic inflammation, fueled by mechanisms , such as imbalanced myeloid cell function and T cell deregulation (Amadi-Obi et al., 2014). Thus, comprehension and promotion of immune regulatory processes are essential for creating effective therapies to achieve balance and control in autoimmune disease, which will lead to better patient outcomes.

3.1.7. Overview of Immune Tolerance

Immune tolerance is a critical mechanism that prevents autoimmune disease by maintaining a balance between immune activation and suppression. This physiological state enables the immune system to distinguish self from non-self-antigens and prevent unwanted reactions against the body's own tissue. The acquisition and maintenance of immune tolerance are multiple cell processes and regulatory pathways, including the activity of regulatory T cells and anti-inflammatory cytokine production. In conditions like RA, however, this tolerance is broken, leading to chronic inflammation and tissue damage, as seen through the continued activation of inflammatory signaling pathways and myeloid cell dysregulation (Firestein & McInnes, 2017). Recent research suggests that the achievement of immunologic homeostasis in RA patients may be the doorway to drug-free remission and that re-establishing immune tolerance may be a paradigm shift in treatment approaches (Alivernini et al., 2018) (Figure 3.5).

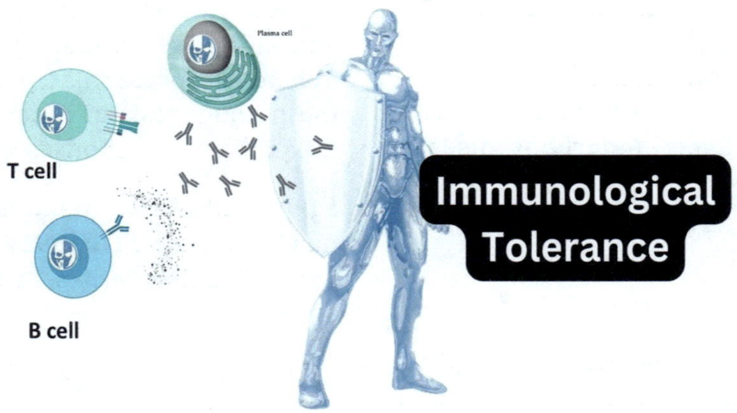

Figure 3.5. Immune tolerance is a critical mechanism that prevents autoimmune diseases by maintaining a balance between immune activation and suppression.

Source: https://biologynotesonline.com/wp-content/uploads/2022/10/Immunological-Tolerance.jpg.

3.1.8. Consequences of Immune Dysregulation

The consequences of immune dysregulation are observed in various pathological conditions, particularly autoimmune diseases, where the immune system mistakenly targets the self-tissues. RA is a classic example where inflammation due to chronicity causes joint damage and systemic comorbidities like cardiovascular and metabolic diseases. Studies indicate that the pre-RA period can involve increasing autoantibodies and inflammatory cytokines, with mention of a subtle interaction among immune mediators and tissue environments (Firestein & McInnes, 2017). Besides, epithelial cells play a crucial role in maintaining immune homeostasis; dysregulation results in the overstimulation of immune responses and can drive type 2 immunity under stress, which further aggravates the pathological landscape (Agrawal et al., 2014). This multicomponent immune response can exacerbate tissue damage and hinder healing, demonstrating that immune dysregulation is not only capable of compromising local tissue integrity but can also have distant consequences on overall well-being and disease causation.

3.1.9. Key Players in Immune Response

The immune response is regulated by an array of cellular participants, each of which has a significant role to play in maintaining homeostasis and combating disease. Among these, Treg are of particular interest due to their capacity to impose peripheral immune tolerance and consequently prevent autoimmune phenomena. In disease states like Multiple Sclerosis (MS), however, Treg frequency or function defects lead to self-tolerance loss and result in unbridled immune attack and inflammatory consequences (Carbone, 2011). In addition, immune checkpoint molecules , such as PD-1 and CTLA-4, play critical roles in the regulation of the immune response; the mechanisms are responsive to therapeutic interference for augmenting anti-tumor immunity in cancer treatment (Mai et al., 2017). Clarity of the Treg cell-immune checkpoint factor interaction is key to understanding the complexity of autoimmunity and inflammation since it opens doors to new therapeutic strategies aimed at the restoration of immune homeostasis (Figure 3.6).

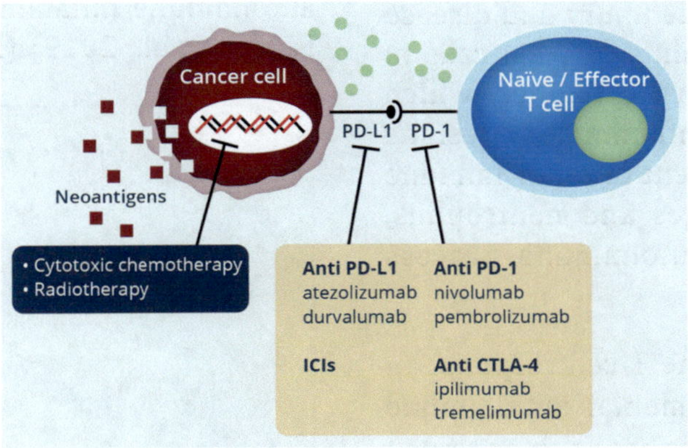

Figure 3.6. Immune checkpoint molecules , such as PD-1 and CTLA-4 are crucial in modulating the immune response; these pathways can be manipulated therapeutically to enhance anti-tumor immunity in cancer treatment.

Source: https://www.oatext.com/img/CRT-8-370-g002.gif.

Test Your Knowledge

1. What is the role of the thymus and bone marrow in immune development?
2. Explain the differences between humoral and cell-mediated immunity.

3.2. Effector T Cells in Autoimmunity

Learning Outcome

1. Recognize types of effector T cells;
2. Describe mechanisms of T cell activation;
3. Discuss CD4+ T helper cell role;
4. Describe the CD8+ Cytotoxic T cell role;
5. Recognize contribution to tissue damage;
6. Emphasize cytokine production by T Cells;
7. Learn about memory T cells and autoimmunity;
8. Recognize therapeutic targeting of T cells.

The function of effector T cells in autoimmunity is also found to play a significant role as an essential part in the pathogenesis of different autoimmune diseases. These lymphocytes, specifically the effector memory T (T-EM) cells, are known to play an essential role in the inflammatory reactions that lead to tissue injury and disease development. Evidence points to T-EM cells in releasing pro-inflammatory cytokines, which are frequently seen in inflammatory lesions and enhance the recruitment of other immune cells, such as macrophages and neutrophils, thus perpetuating the autoimmune process (Abdulahad et al., 2014).

Also, modulation of the T cell response in some models, like experimental autoimmune encephalomyelitis (EAE), has been demonstrated in some studies to have a significant effect on the outcome of the disease. For instance, administration of kirenol was shown to inhibit the proliferation and activation of autoreactive T cells, suggesting a new therapeutic pathway in autoimmune disease (Xiao et al., 2015). This is an indicator of the therapeutic potential of targeting effector T cells as a means of limiting detrimental inflammatory reactions.

3.2.1. Types of Effector T Cells

Diversification of effector $CD4^+$ T cells is a key mediator of immunity and may play a role in the pathogenesis of autoimmunity. The major subsets include the $CD4^+$ helper T cells and $CD8^+$ cytotoxic *T lymphocytes*, both with specialized functional capabilities evolved to react to different pathologies. $CD4^+$ T cells further differentiate into several lineages, including Th1, Th2, and Th17 cells, that secrete cytokines that steer the immune response towards inflammation or healing of tissues. The $CD8^+$ T cells, however, are predominantly responsible for killing infected or tumor cells directly. In autoimmune disorders, like type 1 diabetes, β-cell-specific effector T cell proliferation can perpetuate islet inflammatory processes, as has been highlighted in recent research. The balance between these populations of effector T cells and immune regulatory mechanisms illustrates the fine line necessary for maintaining immune homeostasis and preventing chronic autoimmune inflammation (Clark et al., 2017; Fahmy et al., 2019) (Figure 3.7).

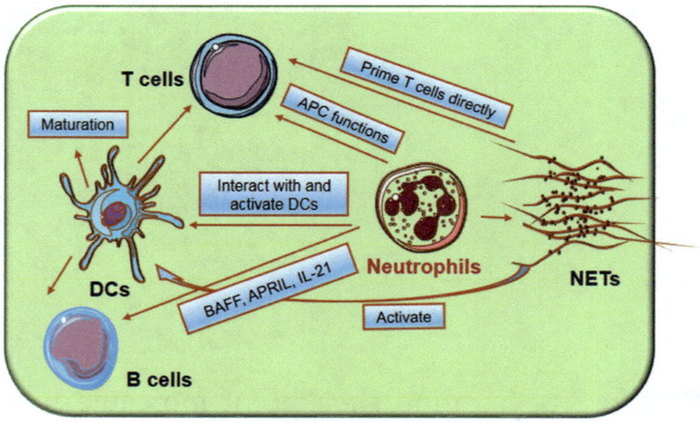

Figure 3.7. The diversification of effector T cells plays a crucial role in mediating immune responses and can contribute to the pathogenesis of autoimmune diseases.

Source: https://media.springernature.com/lw1200/springer-static/image/art%3A10.1186%2Fs12964-019-0471-y/MediaObjects/12964_2019_471_Fig1_HTML.png.

3.2.2. Mechanisms of T Cell Activation

T cell activation is a fundamental process in orchestrating immune responses, especially in autoimmunity and inflammation. This intricate process initiates with the recognition of antigen-presenting cells (APCs) presenting specific peptides on major histocompatibility complex (MHC) molecules. Upon engagement of these antigens, T cells undergo a series of signal transductions that lead to their proliferation and differentiation into effector cells for mediating immune responses. In autoimmune conditions like rheumatoid arthritis, the inappropriate activation of T cells can cause repeated inflammation characterized by the infiltration of immune cells into the affected tissues, sustaining the disease cycle of tissue damage (Firestein & McInnes, 2017). Furthermore, the role of regulatory cells and local microenvironment is a significant function in the T cell response modulation, indicating the subtle balance between tolerance and activation, which is often disrupted in inflammatory diseases (Shi et al., 2011). Clarification of these processes is essential for the development of specific therapies in order to restore immunological homeostasis.

3.2.3. Role of CD4⁺ T Helper Cells

CD4⁺ T helper cells are pivotal in controlling immune responses, particularly in the contexts of autoimmunity and inflammation. They do not respond; they directly influence the behavior of other immune cells by producing specific cytokines, which can induce or resolve inflammation. In multiple sclerosis pathology, for example, induction of self-reactive CD4⁺ T cells into the central nervous system increases inflammation, particularly by compromising the integrity of the blood-brain barrier and thereby inducing neuroinflammation (Kunkl et al., 2020). In addition, the reservoir of memory CD4⁺ T cells harbors important information about previous immune encounters to enable rapid responses upon reactivation, a function that can serve well in disease protection but is harmful in autoimmunity (Jaigirdar & MacLeod, 2015). Understanding the nuances of CD4⁺ T cell activation and differentiation will be key in developing targeted treatments that might offset their pathological effects while augmenting protective immunity (Figure 3.8).

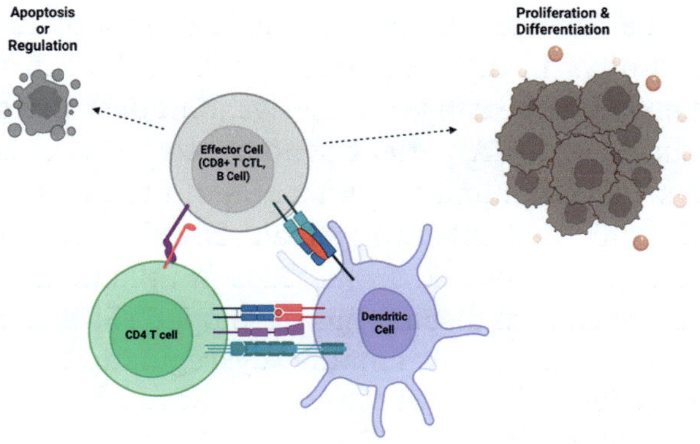

Figure 3.8. CD4⁺ T helper cells play a pivotal role in orchestrating immune responses, particularly in the contexts of autoimmunity and inflammation.

Source: Crater JM, Dunn DC, Nixon DF, Furler O'Brien RL. A History and Atlas of the Human CD4⁺ T Helper Cell. *Biomedicines*. 2023; 11(10):2608. https://doi.org/10.3390/biomedicines11102608

3.2.4. Role of CD8⁺ Cytotoxic T Cells

The role of CD8⁺ cytotoxic T cells during autoimmune diseases and inflammatory responses is important, as these effector T cells are largely accountable for direct cytotoxicity against infected or diseased cells. In autoimmune diseases, such as alopecia areata, CD8⁺ T cells have been identified to attack healthy tissues by mistake in targeting, leading to pathological conditions of tissue inflammation and destruction. Lymphocytic infiltration around hair follicles in alopecia areata is an example, since CD8⁺ T cells orchestrate the local immunity and strengthen the secretion of inflammatory cytokines like IFN-γ, thereby fueling the autoimmunity (Simakou et al., 2019). Moreover, $CD8^+$ T cells demonstrate a complex interaction with other immune mediators like TRAIL, indicating their dual role in destroying tumor cells and controlling the immune environment, which could dampen or amplify inflammation (Baukloh et al., 2019). This complex balance reflects the function of $CD8^+$ T cells in shaping the trajectories of autoimmune and inflammatory diseases.

3.2.5. Contribution to Tissue Damage

Chronic inflammation, like that which occurs in diseases of RA, is an organizing mechanism of tissue damage and loss of function common to autoimmunity. Prolonged activation of inflammatory pathways in myeloid cells sets a context in which repair of the tissue is secondary to ongoing damage, increasing progressive joint destruction and disability. It has been demonstrated in current studies that RA patient synovial tissue is constantly exposed to inflammatory stimuli, leading to dysregulation and amplification of the inflammatory response, thus playing a crucial role in tissue destruction (Alivernini et al., 2018). The pre-RA period also demonstrates how a build-up of autoantibodies and an increase in inflammatory mediators sets the stage for chronic damage long before clinical disease has developed (Firestein & McInnes, 2017). This complex interplay between tissue damage and immune dysregulation underscores the imperative requirement for particular therapeutic interventions aimed at reestablishing immunologic equilibrium to halt autoimmunity's development (Figure 3.9).

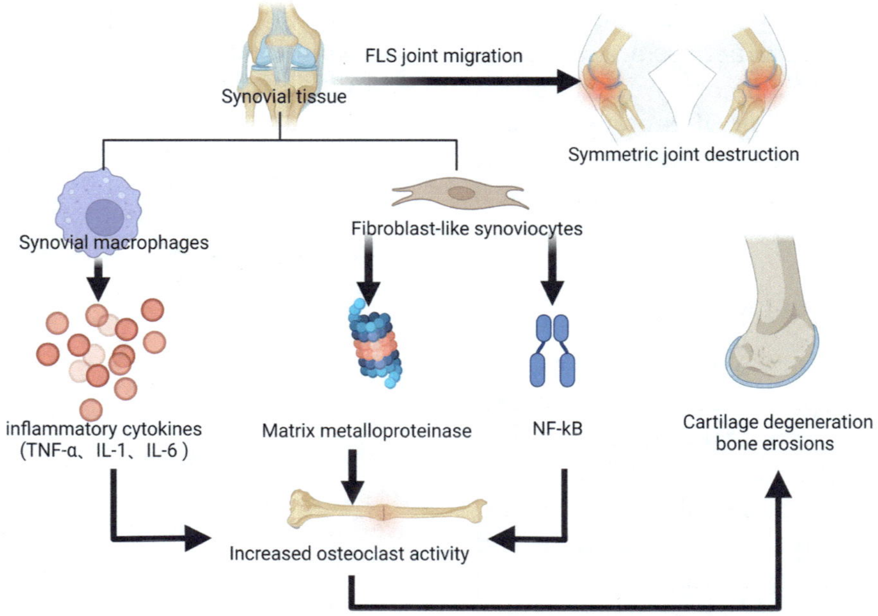

Figure 3.9. Chronic inflammation, particularly evident in conditions like rheumatoid arthritis (RA), plays a pivotal role in tissue damage and the subsequent loss of function characteristic of autoimmunity.

Source: https://www.frontiersin.org/files/Articles/1051082/fimmu-13-1051082-HTML-r1/image_m/fimmu-13-1051082-g001.jpg.

3.2.6. Cytokine Production by T Cells

The role of T cell cytokine secretion is important in the context of autoimmunity and inflammation, as it is primarily responsible for forming the pathological environment of most diseases, including RA. Activated T cells become differentiated into various subsets that produce a variety of cytokines, some of which can increase inflammation or contribute to tissue homeostasis. In RA, dysregulation of cytokine production leads to chronic inflammation and joint damage, with proof of an early phase of elevated levels of inflammatory cytokines and autoantibodies prior to clinical symptoms (Firestein & McInnes, 2017). In addition, miR-155, an important microRNA in T cell biology, has been shown to control cytokine expression, linking its deregulation with the chronic inflammatory state observed in autoimmune diseases (Alivernini et al., 2018). The complexity in the production of cytokines by T cells must hence be appreciated for the development of focal therapeutic approaches that seek to target immunologic balance in infected patients.

3.2.7. Memory T Cells and Autoimmunity

The role of autoimmunity by memory T cells has been of great interest in recent times because they can sustain chronic inflammatory responses characteristic of most autoimmune diseases. Such cells, having been generated subsequent to initial antigenic encounter, can be re-stimulated upon secondary exposure to certain antigens and hence contribute to the pathology of such diseases as rheumatoid arthritis and multiple sclerosis. Their dysregulation can lead to hyperactivation of the immune system and tissue damage, and such highlights the fine-tuning involved in immune homeostasis. Dysregulation of microRNAs, like miR-155, for instance, is known to control the activation and differentiation of memory T cells, and subsequently induce chronic inflammation and autoimmunity (Alivernini et al., 2018). Similarly, EAE research emphasizes autoreactive T cells' pathogenic role in demyelination, demonstrating how therapeutic approaches that control the activity of T cells, such as kirenol, decrease autoimmune activity (Xiao et al., 2015) (Figure 3.10).

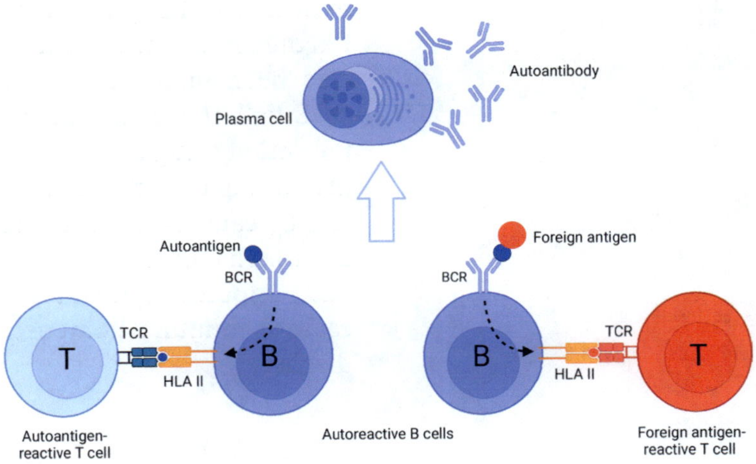

Figure 3.10. The role of memory T cells in autoimmunity has garnered significant attention due to their ability to sustain chronic inflammatory responses that are characteristic of various autoimmune diseases.

Source: https://www.pnas.org/cms/10.1073/pnas.2401337121/asset/e2d8dd11-918b-4d23-b4f6-a6de1a35b713/assets/images/large/pnas.2401337121fig01.jpg.

3.2.8. Therapeutic Targeting of T Cells

Therapeutic targeting of T cells has been a promising field in autoimmune disease treatment, particularly RA, characterized by chronic inflammation and immune dysregulation. Development in the understanding of the pathogenic function of some T cell subsets has paved the way for the creation of targeted immunotherapies for the re-establishment of immune homeostasis. For instance, microRNAs , such as miR-155 have been implicated as major regulators of T cell activation and modulation; when abnormally controlled, they are responsible for chronic inflammation in conditions like RA (Alivernini et al., 2018). The dynamic shifts of immune responses, particularly in the pre-RA stage marked by autoantibody induction and inflammatory cytokine induction, highlight the likelihood of interventions restoring tolerance with no compromise on needed immune functions (Firestein & McInnes, 2017). These therapeutic modalities ultimately lead to disease remission and improved patient outcomes, and highlight the precarious balance between therapeutic and immune homeostasis.

Test Your Knowledge

1. What mechanisms usually prevent autoreactive T cells from activation?
2. How do cytotoxic $CD8^+$ T cells induce tissue damage in autoimmune disease?

3.3. B-cells and Antibody Production

Learning Outcome

1. Discuss the function of B-cells in immune response;
2. Understand mechanisms of B-cell activation;
3. Emphasize antibody classes and functions;
4. Explain autoantibody production in autoimmunity;
5. Explain B-cell memory and what it is;
6. Learn B-cell-T cell interaction;
7. Discuss B-cell differentiation and role of cytokines;
8. Define therapeutic strategies against B-cells;
9. Provide examples of diseases that are B-cell-driven.

B-cells are responsible for playing a key role in the immune response, largely by the production of antibodies that are directed against antigens. When autoimmunity and inflammation are at issue, dysregulation of B-cell function can result in the production of autoantibodies, which inadvertently attack the body's own tissues. Such a dysregulated immune response is particularly observed in conditions , such as RA, where the presence of autoantibodies is a significant marker of the disease condition, reflecting the transition from a pre-RA phase of inflammatory cytokines to full synovitis and systemic manifestations (Firestein & McInnes, 2017). Furthermore, microRNAs like miR-155 have also been implicated as significant regulators of B-cell function; their overexpression can potentially augment chronic inflammation by promoting the activation of autoreactive B-cells and by causing tissue damage (Alivernini et al., 2018). The understanding of these mechanisms adds impetus to targeted therapy that aims to restore immune homeostasis in autoimmune disease.

3.3.1. Role of B-cells in the Immune Response

The role of B-cells in immunity is central, especially in autoimmunity and inflammation. The role of the cells is primarily the secretion of antibodies that neutralize pathogens and modulate immune responses. Dysregulation of B-cell function can lead to chronic autoimmune disease conditions, including RA, in which ongoing inflammation causes tissue damage. It has been proven through studies that microRNAs, particularly miR-155, play an important part in the dysregulation of the activation of B-cells, which propels the inflammatory condition observed in diseases like RA. This microRNA is extremely present in immune cells and, when deregulated, can strengthen immune responses, leading to long-term inflammation, as supported by recent studies (Alivernini et al., 2018). How the intricate processes of B-cell activation and their role in autoimmunity are conceived is paramount to the development of targeted therapies, particularly considering the fact that there is no known cure available currently for RA (Firestein & McInnes, 2017) (Figure 3.11).

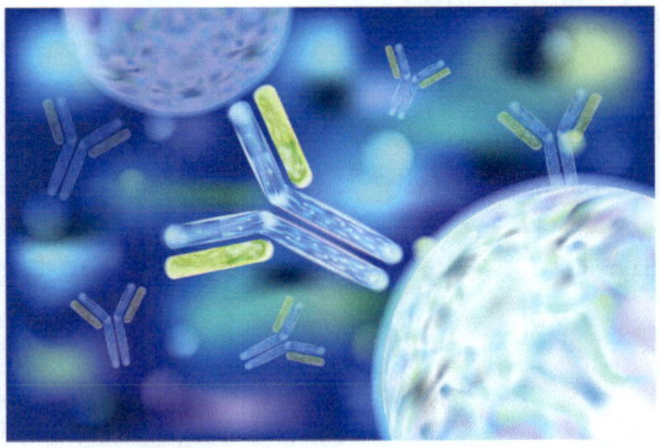

Figure 3.11. The role of B-cells in the immune response is critical, especially in the context of autoimmunity and inflammation.

Source: https://criver.widen.net/content/yehyl9tphw/jpeg/110068852_xl.jpg.

3.3.2. Mechanisms of B-cell Activation

Under autoimmunity and inflammation conditions, understanding the mechanisms of B-cell activation is essential, as such cells are at the center of unregulated immune responses common in such conditions. T cell-dependent and T cell-independent mechanisms are usually the forms in that B-cell activation occurs.. The former is the recognition of individual antigens presented by antigen-presenting cells together with the co-stimulatory signals needed from T helper cells, while the latter can be directly induced by polysaccharide or other structural antigens. In RA, as shown in recent studies, chronic activation of B-cells has been linked to chronic inflammation through the production of autoantibodies and pro-inflammatory cytokines, enhancing tissue damage and disease progression (Firestein & McInnes, 2017). Moreover, dysregulated B-cell signaling may also enhance inflammatory processes in myeloid cells to create a positive feedback loop, and it fuels the pathology of autoimmune diseases (Alivernini et al., 2018). Detection of such mechanisms is vital in the creation of targeted treatments that aim to reinstate immune homeostasis.

3.3.3. Antibody Classes and Functions

The immune system utilizes various classes of antibodies, or immunoglobulins, each with distinct functions that are critical in the battle against pathogens and inflammation. The five principal antibody classes, IgG, IgA, IgM, IgE, and IgD, are each tailored for an activity; for instance, IgG prevails in secondary immune response and long-term immunity, while IgA is essential on mucosal surfaces to avert attack by pathogens at entry points. In autoimmunity, dysregulation of the antibodies leads to pathologies, such as in rheumatoid arthritis, where autoantibodies contribute significantly to inflammation and destruction of joints (Firestein & McInnes, 2017).

Furthermore, the role of antibodies during antibody-mediated rejection demonstrates the intricacy of their interaction, where both HLA and non-HLA antibodies are capable of inducing graft rejection, thereby affecting the outcome of transplants (Butler et al., 2017). Understanding these classes and how they operate is key to the formulation of immunotherapeutic interventions in treating autoimmune conditions as well as in ensuring graft survival (Figure 3.12).

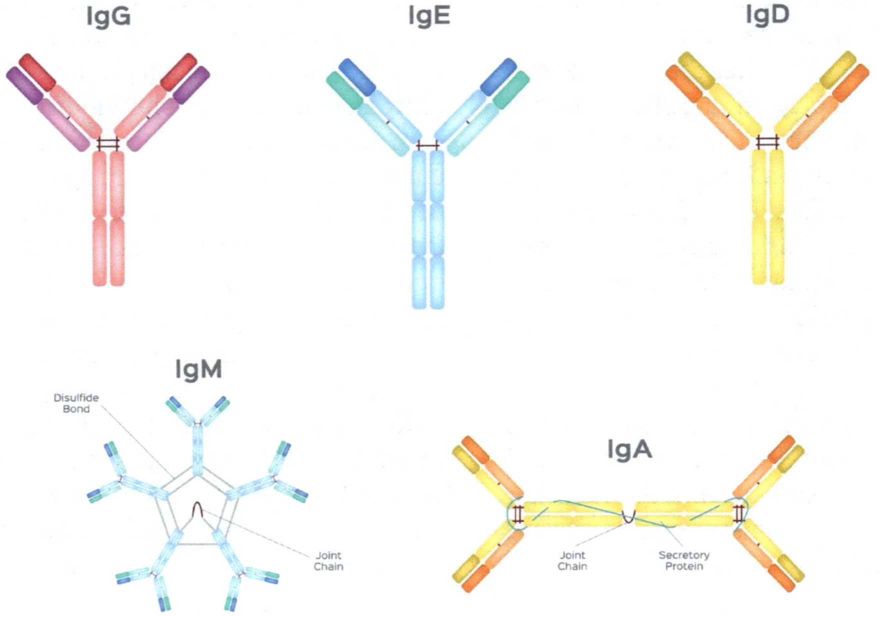

Figure 3.12. The immune system utilizes various classes of antibodies, or immunoglobulins, each serving distinct functions crucial to combating pathogens and mediating inflammatory responses.

Source: https://www.news-medical.net/images/Article_Images/ImageForArticle_16427_17386092428414821.jpg.

3.3.4. Autoantibody Production in Autoimmunity

Production of autoantibodies is characteristic of autoimmune diseases and a significant effector mechanism in the pathogenesis of inflammation. These autoantibodies, which target self-antigens, are responsible for tissue injury and chronic inflammatory responses. There is evidence to indicate that in conditions , such as RA, autoantibodies typically precede clinical onset, and there consequently exists a pre-RA period during which there is an increase in circulating autoantibodies and inflammatory mediators. This chronic immune activation not only facilitates synovitis but also results in systemic comorbidities and highlights the intricacy of autoimmunity (Firestein & McInnes, 2017; McInnes & Schett, 2017). Furthermore, treatments of such autoimmune responses have been shown to restore tolerance in the immune system and reduce inflammatory burden. Understanding autoantibodies thus provides insight not only into mechanisms of disease but also into therapeutic approaches of restoring immunologic balance, a crucial goal in managing autoimmune conditions like RA.

3.3.5. B-cell Memory and its Implications

The role of B-cell memory in autoimmune disease and inflammation has significant implications for the pathogenesis of chronic autoimmune disease. In rheumatoid arthritis, for instance, evidence suggests that autoantibody persistence, derived from memory B-cells, plays a crucial role in maintaining inflammatory processes and tissue damage to cause chronic synovitis and systemic comorbidities (Firestein & McInnes, 2017). Furthermore, experimental models , such as experimental autoimmune encephalomyelitis demonstrate how autoreactive B-cells and the cytokine microenvironment, such as pro-inflammatory cytokines , such as IFN-γ and IL-17A, contribute to the maintenance and activation of these memory responses (Xiao et al., 2015). Dysregulation of B-cell memory not only underscores the complexities of autoimmune pathologies but also suggests potential therapeutic strategies towards re-establishing immune tolerance with implications for new treatment paradigms aimed at these effector mechanisms in inflammation and autoimmunity (Figure 3.13).

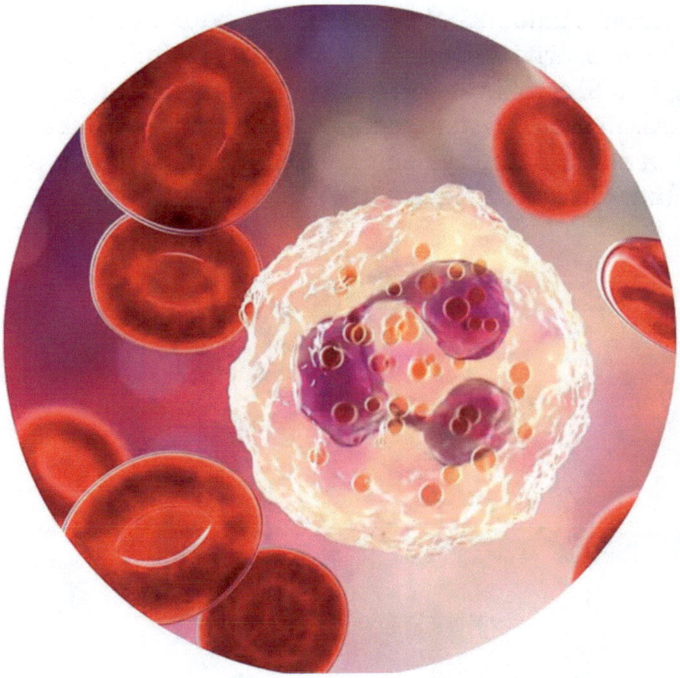

Figure 3.13. The role of B-cell memory in autoimmune responses and inflammation presents significant implications for understanding the pathogenesis of chronic autoimmune conditions.

Source: https://www.autoimmuneinstitute.org/wp-content/smush-webp/2024/02/Inflammation-A-Driving-Force-of-Autoimmune-Disease-graphics-1024x683.jpg.webp.

3.3.6. Interaction between B-cells and T Cells

B-cell-T cell interaction is quite crucial in the modulation of immune responses, particularly autoimmunity and inflammation. B-cells are associated with antibody production, something that is typically triggered by their interaction with T cells. Specifically, $CD4^+$ T helper cells, through various cytokines and costimulatory stimuli, facilitate the proliferation and differentiation of B-cells to yield high-affinity antibodies. This cooperative process, when dysregulated, has been involved in autoimmune disease pathogenesis , such as RA, wherein an immune-mediated pathogenesis is the cause of tissue destruction and chronic inflammation (Firestein & McInnes, 2017). Moreover, the disruption of immunological tolerance, which is caused most often by regulatory T cell failure as a result of interactions between B and T cells, plays a pivotal role in autoimmunity (Aruffo et al., 2018). Understanding such interactions gives insight into potential therapeutic strategies to restore immune homeostasis and establish tolerance to autoimmune illnesses.

3.3.7. Role of Cytokines in B-cell Differentiation

Cytokines also play a critical role in the differentiation of B-cells, an occurrence that is crucial for generating effective humoral immune responses. Various cytokines, such as interleukin-4 (IL-4) and interleukin-21 (IL-21), are critical in regulating B-cell lineage commitment and development, which affects their ability to produce antibodies. In diseases like autoimmune RA and MS, deregulation of these cytokines can lead to disturbed B-cell function, leading to more inflammation and tissue damage. For instance, excessive amounts of inflammatory cytokines associated with RA increase the survival of autoreactive B-cells, driving chronic inflammation within the joints (Firestein & McInnes, 2017). Correspondingly, in MS, cytokines derived from T helper cells augment B-cell activation and migration into the central nervous system, enhancing processes of neuroinflammation (Kunkl et al., 2020). Clarification of these pathways emphasizes the importance of cytokine modulation in the therapy of autoimmune diseases (Figure 3.14).

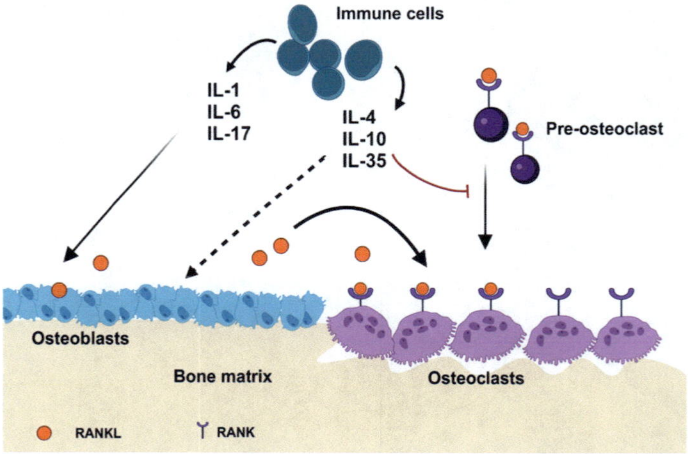

Figure 3.14. Various cytokines, such as interleukin-4 (IL-4) and interleukin-21 (IL-21), are fundamental in guiding B-cell lineage commitment and maturation, influencing their ability to produce antibodies.

Source: https://www.mdpi.com/ijms/ijms-25-08163/article_deploy/html/images/ijms-25-08163-g001.png.

3.3.8. Therapeutic Strategies Targeting B-cells

In the case of autoimmune diseases, therapeutic strategies targeting B-cells have been the object of intervention, particularly in RA cases. These treatments aim to modify the pathogenic activities of B-cells while they engage in the chronic inflammation and tissue damage of these diseases. Evidence suggests that B-cells contribute to the production of autoantibodies and increase inflammatory responses through cytokine release, perpetuating the disease cycle. Advances in the area of targeted immunotherapies, such as monoclonal antibodies depleting or inhibiting B-cells, have shown promise in restoring immune homeostasis in patients with RA and may potentially induce sustainable remission and improved quality of life. The ongoing challenge lies in modulating B-cell function properly without compromising general immune competence, balancing the need to dampen inflammation without losing protective immunity to pathogens (Alivernini et al., 2018; Firestein & McInnes, 2017).

3.3.9. Examples of Diseases Driven by B-cell Activity

B-cell function contributes to many autoimmune diseases, where aberrant immune responses induce widespread pathology. For instance, RA is characterized by an autoimmunity process where B-cells produce autoantibodies that contribute to long-term inflammation and joint damage. The condition often begins with a pre-clinical course characterized by circulating autoantibodies and elevated inflammatory cytokines with synovitis and extracellular complications, as noted in recent studies (Firestein & McInnes, 2017). Similarly, uveitis demonstrates that B-cell activation can result in inflammation of ocular tissues, typically by inducing latent infection. Uveitis underscores the tightrope walked between host-protective and pathogenic functions of B-cells, where failure to restore mechanisms results in chronic inflammation and tissue damage (Amadi-Obi et al., 2014). These pathophysiologic mechanisms inform therapeutic strategies for restoring immune homeostasis in such patients (Figure 3.15).

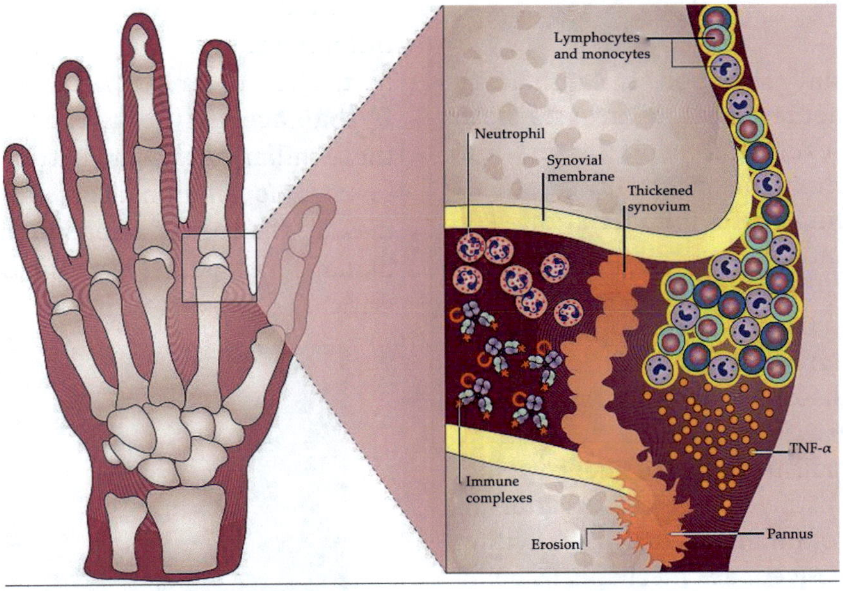

Figure 3.15. Rheumatoid arthritis (RA) is characterized by an autoimmune process where B-cells produce autoantibodies that contribute to chronic inflammation and joint destruction.

Source: https://www.immunopaedia.org.za/wp-content/uploads/2016/02/Figure-21.jpg.

Test Your Knowledge

1. What is the role of plasma cells and memory B-cells in long-term immunity?
2. How do autoantibodies contribute to autoimmune disease pathology?

3.4. Inflammatory Mediators and Pathways

Learning Outcome

1. Give an overview of inflammatory mediators;
2. Explain the role of cytokines in inflammation;
3. Comprehend chemokines and their functions;
4. Emphasize prostaglandins and leukotrienes;
5. Understand the role of the complement system;
6. Explain inflammatory pathways in tissue damage;
7. Emphasize chronic inflammation and autoimmunity;
8. Explain mechanisms of resolution of inflammation;
9. Learn therapeutic interventions against inflammation.

The fine interplay between inflammatory pathways and mediators is central to both initiation and resolution of inflammation, particularly autoimmune disorders , such as RA. During health, acute inflammation is a protective mechanism, enabling leukocytes to migrate into damaged or infected tissue for effective destruction of pathogens. When these pathways are dysregulated, as in the case of chronic disease, chronic inflammatory responses can lead to massive tissue damage and functional impairment. New evidence points toward the role of myeloid cell activation in the maintenance of inflammation in RA, with a network of positive-feedback mechanisms being identified as maintaining the disease (Alivernini et al., 2018). In addition, microRNAs, namely miR-155, emerge as major controllers of immune responses; their deregulation contributes to chronic inflammation and autoimmunity and are thus potentially feasible therapeutic targets for dampening the progression of disease (Alivernini et al., 2018). Understanding these mediators offers crucial information on possible interventions against autoimmunity.

3.4.1. Overview of Inflammatory Mediators

Their role in autoimmunity and chronic inflammation is pivotal, as inflammatory mediators control the complex interactions that underlie the immune process. Cytokines, chemokines, and growth factors are a few of the mediators released by immune cells and are engaged in both anti-inflammatory and pro-inflammatory processes. For instance, granulocyte-macrophage colony-stimulating factor (GM-CSF) has been shown to initiate the activation and migration of myeloid cells to sites of inflammation, thereby enhancing the inflammatory response and disease pathogenesis of autoimmune diseases like RA and MS (Adorini et al., 2019).

In contrast, mediators of resolution of inflammation also play an important role in tissue repair as well as in homeostasis. Dysbalance in the production or action of these inflammatory mediators most often leads to chronic inflammation and tissue damage, making the role of selective therapies that can manage the pathways effectively even more critical (Alivernini et al., 2018) (Figure 3.16).

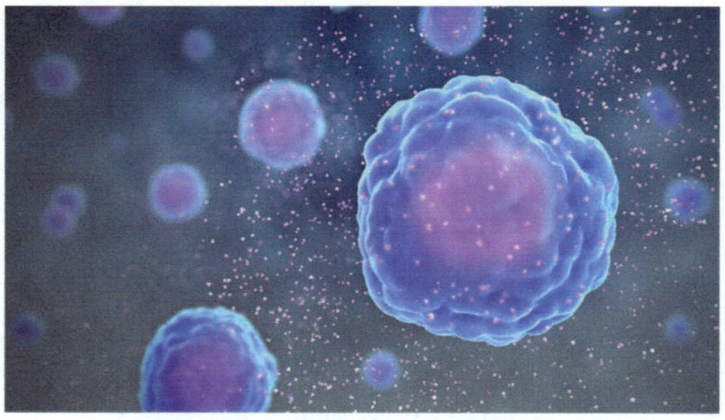

Figure 3.16. Cytokines play a pivotal role in mediating inflammation, particularly in autoimmune disorders , such as multiple sclerosis (MS).

Source: https://upload.wikimedia.org/wikipedia/commons/f/fa/Cytokine_release.jpg.

3.4.2. Role of Cytokines in Inflammation

Cytokines are also a key mediator of inflammation, particularly in autoimmune diseases , such as MS. These cytokine signal proteins are primarily produced by immune cells and have dramatic effects on the host's inflammatory response in terms of nature and magnitude. In MS, autoreactive T cell invasion into the CNS prompts the resident cells to produce a variety of pro-inflammatory cytokines, further amplifying the inflammatory milieu. Specifically, T helper cell-derived cytokines like Th1 and Th17 have been implicated in the breakdown of the blood-brain barrier and augmentation of neuroinflammation, reinforcing their pivotal role in disease pathogenesis. In addition, B-cell involvement in inflammation has been accentuated by their ability to secrete cytokines, express autoantigens and ectopic lymphoid structures within the CNS, which are associated with poorer clinical outcomes in MS patients (Mitsdoerffer & Peters, 2016; Kunkl et al., 2020). Understanding such intricate interactions is important in order to develop target therapeutic interventions.

3.4.3. Chemokines and Their Functions

Chemokines also play a role in the regulation of immune responses, particularly those that are autoimmunity or inflammation-related. They are short signaling proteins that manage leukocyte populations' migration into sites of injury or infection to cause an instantaneous and effective immune response. In conditions , such as RA, dysregulation of the chemokine signal plays a significant role in the pathophysiology of chronic inflammation and tissue damage. As highlighted in recent studies, continuous myeloid cell activation sustains this inflammatory process, with chemokines playing key roles that recruit more immune cells into the synovial tissue and contribute further to joint destruction (Firestein & McInnes, 2017). Moreover, the promise of targeted therapeutics that adjust chemokine function holds potential for re-establishing immunologic homeostasis and inducing drug-free remission among RA patients, underscoring the role of chemokines not only in disease pathophysiology but also in therapeutic intervention (Alivernini et al., 2018) (Figure 3.17).

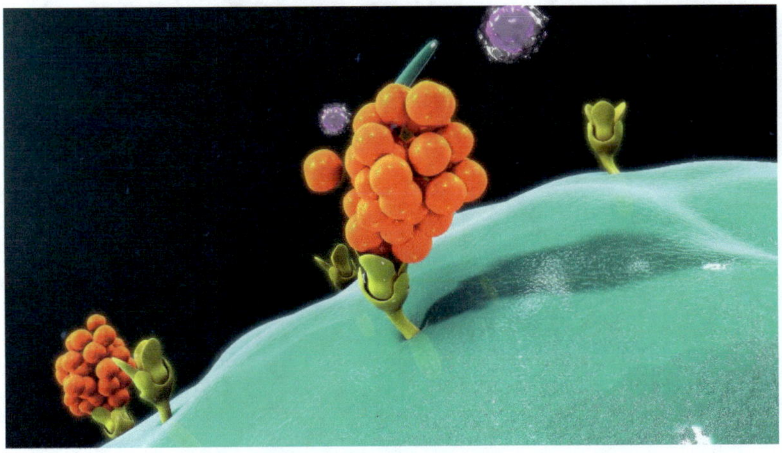

Figure 3.17. Chemokines play a crucial role in the regulation of immune responses, particularly in the context of autoimmunity and inflammation.

Source: https://www.news-medical.net/images/Article_Images/ImageForArticle_3844_16620956280404150.jpg.

3.4.4. Prostaglandins and Leukotrienes

Of the intricate landscape of immune responses, prostaglandins and leukotrienes are key players as eicosanoids that control inflammation and govern autoimmunity. Lipid mediators that are derived from arachidonic acid are pivotal for the regulation of heterogeneous physiological processes, including vasodilation and mobilization of immune cells. Prostaglandins, and particularly PGE2, have been reported to elevate vascular permeability and produce fever, both in the acute and chronic phases of inflammatory diseases. Similarly, leukotrienes, and particularly leukotriene B4, are equally responsible for the mobilization of neutrophils to sites of infection or injury, thus heightening inflammatory reactions. Latest research has indicated that dysregulation of these mediators is not only able to lead to autoimmune disease, but that treatments targeting modulating their pathways are potentially therapeutic for them. Such mechanisms must be targeted, as the intricate interaction between these mediators dictates the trajectory of the resultant overall immune response in autoimmune disease (Al-Riyami et al., 2014; Jutel et al., 2023).

3.4.5. Role of the Complement System

The complement system plays a multifunctional role in the maintenance of homeostasis and modulation of inflammatory responses. Being a component of the innate immunity system, it participates in pathogen destruction, inflammation, and clearance of apoptotic cells.

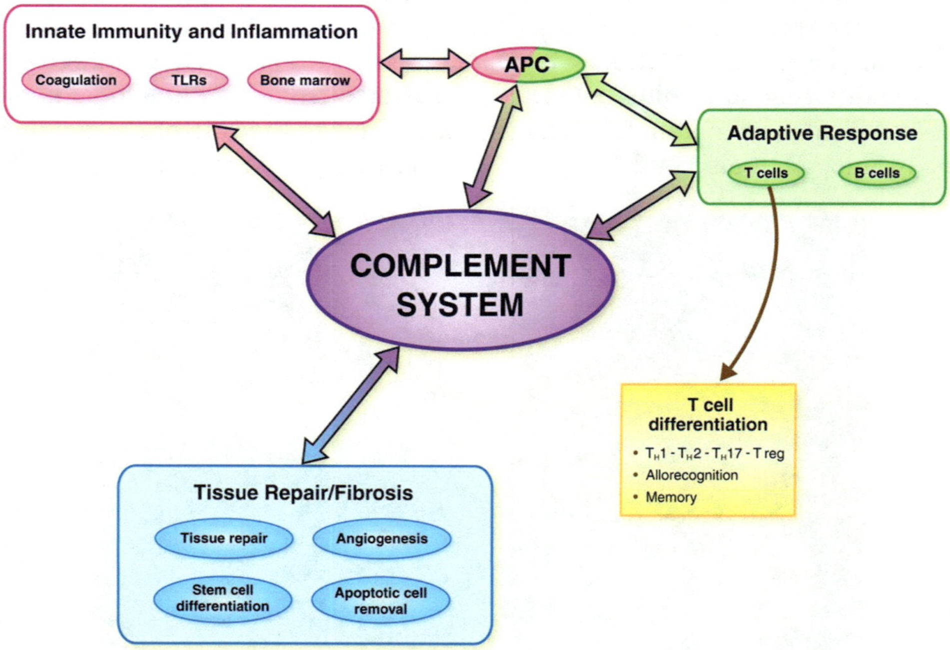

Figure 3.18. The complement system plays a multifaceted role in the maintenance of homeostasis and the modulation of inflammatory responses.

Source: https://media.springernature.com/lw1200/springer-static/image/art%3A10.1186%2F1755-1536-7-16/MediaObjects/13069_2014_Article_154_Fig2_HTML.jpg.

Activation of the complement cascade is particularly of interest in autoimmune diseases, where its activity can lead to tissue damage and contribute to chronic inflammation. For instance, enhanced complement activation was linked with neuroinflammation in neurodegenerative diseases , such as Alzheimer's disease, where inflammatory mediators can enhance further neuronal damage and cognitive impairment, as recently demonstrated, where microglial activation and iron pathology occurred upon exposure to inflammatory stimuli (Sfera et al., 2018). Besides, obesity-induced chronic inflammation illustrates how a dysregulation of complement activity can promote macrophage infiltration, thereby worsening metabolic syndrome (Crowe et al., 2017). These observations are indicative of the role of this system in autoimmunity and inflammation (Figure 3.18).

3.4.6. Inflammatory Pathways in Tissue Damage

The intricate dance between inflammatory pathways and tissue injury is exemplified by autoimmune diseases , such as RA. Chronic inflammation, a product of an uncontrolled immune response, is the cause of ongoing tissue damage and disability. In RA, cytokines and chemokines are central to perpetuating inflammatory processes, which create a negative feedback loop that sustains tissue damage and suppresses healing mechanisms. The synovial tissue is turned into a war zone, with myeloid cell activation prolonging inflammation and continuing joint damage. Increasing research highlights the significance of clarifying these pathways, with therapeutic targets potentially lying in achieving normal immunologic homeostasis and moving toward a drug-free remission (Firestein & McInnes, 2017). Furthermore, the transition from acute to chronic inflammation underlines the need for a more specific course of therapy, pointing out anti-inflammatory mediators that can potentially reverse the degradative nature of inflammation and enable tissue repair (Alivernini et al., 2018).

3.4.7. Chronic Inflammation and Autoimmunity

It is a multifaceted phenomenon where the interaction between chronic inflammation and autoimmunity has a profound contribution to many diseases, and RA serves as a shining example. In RA, chronic inflammation is more than a reaction to injury and occurs as a consequence of dysregulated immune mechanisms, characterized by pathogenic autoantibodies and a network of inflammatory cytokines and chemokines that perpetuate tissue damage and systemic comorbidities (Firestein & McInnes, 2017).

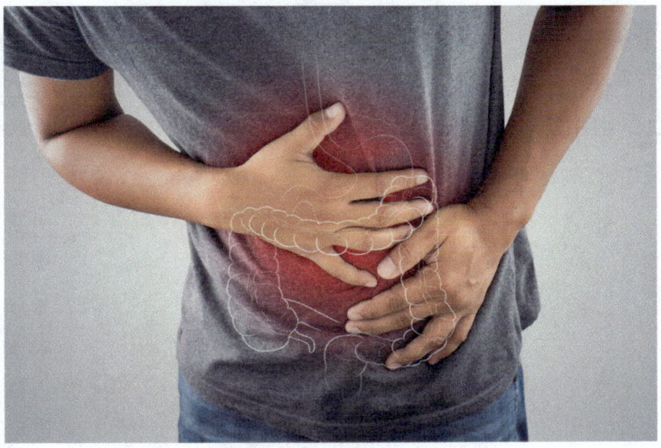

Figure 3.19. Chronic inflammation and autoimmunity.

Source: https://drmaggieyu.com/wp-content/uploads/2023/06/iStock-962782170-1184x789.jpg.

The chronically inflamed milieu creates a feedback mechanism that violates immune tolerance, which in turn leads to further autoreactive responses. Furthermore, microRNAs, particularly miR-155, play a critical role in regulating such immune mechanisms. Defects in miR-155 have been implicated in chronic inflammation and autoimmunity, and therefore represent a key target for modulating immune activation in conditions like RA (Alivernini et al., 2018). Elucidating such effector mechanisms is also relevant in the development of effective interventions that may restore immune balance and stem disease progression (Figure 3.19).

3.4.8. Mechanisms of Resolution of Inflammation

Although inflammation is crucial in defense by the host, the mechanisms of its resolution are equally crucial in maintaining homeostasis and preventing chronic pathology. Resolution of inflammation is regulated by a cascade of well-orchestrated events that involve apoptosis of neutrophils, macrophage clearance of apoptotic cells, and generation of anti-inflammatory mediators , such as resolvins and protectins. These processes stop inflammatory reactions from going on unchecked and prevent tissue injury and chronic dysfunction. When mechanisms of resolution are defective, as often in chronic inflammatory diseases like Rheumatoid Arthritis, the inflammatory reaction feeds on itself, leading to prolonged tissue damage and autoimmune activity (Alivernini et al., 2018). Furthermore, disturbances in inflammatory resolution could be linked to oral dysbiosis, which suggests significant implications in periodontitis disease, thus demonstrating the complex interplay between immune dysregulation and inflammation (Arboleda et al., 2020). Lastly, knowing these processes is crucial for developing targeted interventions to restore balance in autoimmune diseases.

3.4.9. Therapeutic Interventions Targeting Inflammation

The therapeutic panorama of anti-inflammatory treatments has radically evolved, particularly in the management of autoimmune diseases , such as RA.

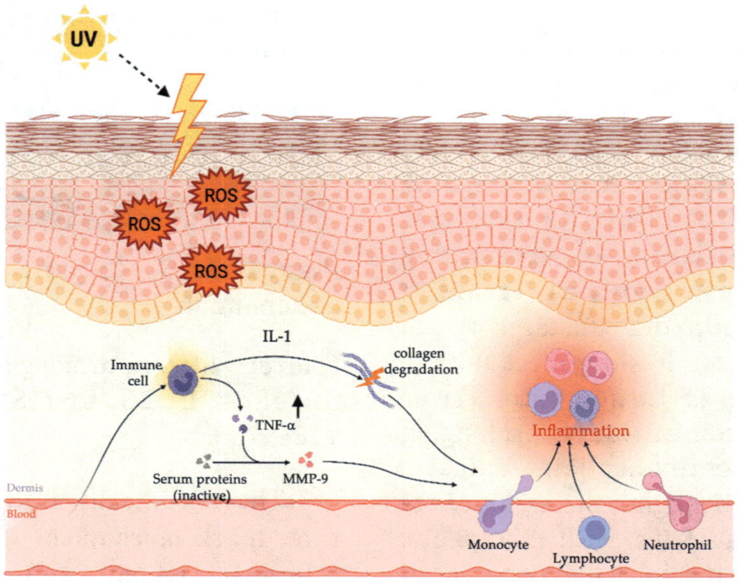

Figure 3.20. Agents that block tumor necrosis factor α and interleukin 6 have demonstrated notable efficacy in mitigating articular damage and restoring functional capacity.

Source: Pocino K, Carnazzo V, Stefanile A, Basile V, Guerriero C, Marino M, Rigante D, Basile U. Tumor Necrosis Factor-Alpha: Ally and Enemy in Protean Cutaneous Sceneries. International Journal of Molecular Sciences. 2024; 25(14):7762. https://doi.org/10.3390/ijms25147762

New understanding of RA's immunopathogenesis has prompted the development of targeted biologics and small-molecule drugs specifically inhibiting pro-inflammatory cytokines, transforming therapeutic paradigms. For instance, blockade agents of tumor necrosis factor α and interleukin 6 have been found to be significantly effective in alleviating articular damage and restoring functional capacity, highlighting their pivotal role in interrupting pathologic inflammatory cascades (Firestein & McInnes, 2017). Furthermore, with the emergence of Janus kinase (JAK) inhibitors, the importance of cytokine signaling pathways has come to the forefront, promising new therapeutic approaches towards drug-free remission and enhanced immunologic homeostasis (McInnes & Schett, 2017). Overall, these therapies represent a paradigm shift in the direction of personalized medicine in autoimmune disorders, underlining the necessity of unraveling complex inflammatory networks for effective intervention (Figure 3.20).

Test Your Knowledge

1. How do reactive oxygen species (ROS) contribute to inflammatory damage?
2. What are the major steps in the inflammatory cascade, and how are they controlled?

Summary

Study of effector mechanisms in autoimmunity and inflammation emphasizes the balance that controls immune reactions. Explaining the pathways involved, including Kirenol's role in controlling T cell activity, has promise in therapeutic intervention, particularly in diseases , such as multiple sclerosis, where autoinflammatory processes are prevalent (Xiao et al., 2015). Moreover, MALT1's role in regulating T cell homeostasis provides a critical area for treatment methods for autoimmune diseases. Because MALT1's proteolytic activity is crucial to maintaining the effector-to-regulator T cell ratio, modulation of therapies that enhance or inhibit such mechanisms can influence disease course and magnitude (Baens et al., 2019). These findings taken together encourage further research into these mechanisms in the hope that they can provide effective measures for managing, if not preventing, autoimmune diseases in order to ultimately affect patient outcomes.

The intricate interplay of effector mechanisms of autoimmunity and inflammation reveals some key aspects key to understanding disease progression. miR-155, the key inducer of chronic inflammation, is a microRNA essential in regulating immune response. Its deregulation could lead to aberrant immune activation, exacerbating diseases like RA and potentially acting as a biomarker and therapeutic target (Alivernini et al., 2018). Secondly, failure by RA to resolve inflammation is extremely key in initiating tissue damage and lasting disability. Research points out that chronic activation of positive-feedback regulatory loops between myeloid cells results in inflammation, which accentuates their pathogenic role (Alivernini et al., 2018). Combined, these findings illustrate the delicate balance demanded of immune system function, and the potential for targeted therapy, as well as the complexity involved in addressing chronic inflammatory disease. These results are integral to the design of efficacious treatment regimens in inflammation and autoimmunity.

KEY TERMS FROM THIS CHAPTER

- Rheumatoid Arthritis (RA)
- T-cells
- Homeostasis
- Stimuli
- Macrophages
- Innate immunity
- Natural killer (NK) cells
- Dendritic cells
- Co-stimulatory receptors
- Targeted therapy
- Chronic inflammation
- Alopecia areata
- B lymphocytes
- Chemokines
- Microenvironment
- Parasitic infection

Critical Thinking Questions

1. **Which one of the following is an effector mechanism most often responsible for tissue damage in autoimmune reactions?**
   a. Apoptosis of autoreactive T cells
   b. Complement activation
   c. Antigen sequestration
   d. Clonal deletion
2. **Which hypersensitivity reaction is most mediated by antibodies and complement, leading to cell lysis?**
   a. Type I (IgE-mediated)
   b. Type II (antibody-mediated cytotoxicity)
   c. Type III (immune complex-mediated)
   d. Type IV (delayed-type hypersensitivity)
3. **In systemic lupus erythematosus (SLE), immune complexes are deposited in tissues. This is what kind of immune mechanism?**
   a. Type I hypersensitivity
   b. Cell-mediated cytotoxicity
   c. Type III hypersensitivity
   d. Autoantibody neutralization
4. **Which cytokine is strongly associated with Th17 cell differentiation and chronic inflammation in autoimmune diseases?**
   a. IL-4
   b. IL-10
   c. IL-17
   d. TGF-β
5. **Cytotoxic T lymphocytes (CTLs) mediate tissue damage in autoimmunity by:**
   a. Releasing histamine
   b. Producing antibodies
   c. Inducing apoptosis via perforin and granzyme pathways
   d. Blocking cytokine production

Short Answer Questions

1. What are the major constituents of the innate and adaptive immune systems?
2. How do antigen-presenting cells initiate an adaptive immune response?
3. What are the primary functions of $CD4^{+}$ effector T cells during immune responses?
4. What are the functions of Th1 and Th17 cells in autoimmune pathogenesis?
5. How are B-cells activated and what do they require?
6. How is a T-dependent different from a T-independent B-cell response?
7. What are the primary pro-inflammatory cytokines, and what do they do?
8. How do chemokines function in the regulation of immune cell traffic to inflamed tissues?

Answers to Critical Thinking Questions

1. (b); 2. (b); 3. (c); 4. (c); 5. (c)

References

1. Abdulahad, A., Abdulahad, A., Abdulahad, A., Abdulahad, A., Abdulahad, A., Abdulahad, A., Ait-Oufella, H., et al. (2014). T cells in vascular inflammatory diseases. https://core.ac.uk/download/pdf/82869901.pdf (accessed on 17th June 2025).
2. Alivernini, S., Tolusso, B., Ferraccioli, G., Gremese, E., Kurowska-Stolarska, M., & McInnes, I. B. (2018). Driving chronicity in rheumatoid arthritis: perpetuating role of myeloid cells. *Clinical and experimental immunology*, *193*(1), 13–23. https://doi.org/10.1111/cei.13098(accessed on 17th June 2025).
3. Adorini, L., Ahn, J., Alnek, K., Ananthakrishnan, R., Aram, J., Aricha, R., Basdeo, S., et al. (2019). Roles of GM-CSF in the pathogenesis of autoimmune diseases: An update. https://core.ac.uk/download/225130666.pdf (accessed on 17th June 2025).
4. Jutel, M., Agache, I., Zemelka-Wiacek, M., Akdis, M., Chivato, T., Del Giacco, S., Gajdanowicz, P., Gracia, I. E., Klimek, L., Lauerma, A., Ollert, M., O'Mahony, L., Schwarze, J., Shamji, M. H., Skypala, I., Palomares, O., Pfaar, O., Torres, M. J., Bernstein, J. A., Cruz, A. A., ... Akdis, C. A. (2023). Nomenclature of allergic diseases and hypersensitivity reactions: Adapted to modern needs: An EAACI position paper. *Allergy*, *78*(11), 2851–2874. https://doi.org/10.1111/all.15889(accessed on 17th June 2025).
5. Agrawal, S., Aguado, B., Al-Shami, A., Allakhverdi, Z., Angkasekwinai, P., Arwert, E., Balkwill, F., et al. (2014). Beneficial autoimmunity at body surfaces–Immune surveillance and rapid type 2 immunity regulate tissue homeostasis and cancer. https://core.ac.uk/download/76991376.pdf (accessed on 17th June 2025).
6. Firestein, G. S., & McInnes, I. B. (2017). Immunopathogenesis of Rheumatoid Arthritis. *Immunity*, *46*(2), 183–196. https://doi.org/10.1016/j.immuni.2017.02.006(accessed on 17th June 2025).
7. Al-Riyami, L., Harnett, M. M., Harnett, W., Pineda, M. A., et al. (2014). Lessons from helminth infections: ES-62 highlights new interventional approaches in rheumatoid arthritis. https://core.ac.uk/download/42352576.pdf (accessed on 17th June 2025).
8. Amadi-Obi, A., Arida, A., Cortes, A., Fox, A., Jager, A., Peters, A., Rothova, A., et al. (2014). Autoimmune and autoinflammatory mechanisms in uveitis. https://core.ac.uk/download/29416272.pdf (accessed on 17th June 2025).
9. Kunkl, M., Frascolla, S., Amormino, C., Volpe, E., & Tuosto, L. (2020). T Helper Cells: The Modulators of Inflammation in Multiple Sclerosis. *Cells*, *9*(2), 482. https://doi.org/10.3390/cells9020482(accessed on 17th June 2025).
10. Arboleda, S., Garzón, H., Rodríguez, A., Suarez Londono, J., et al. (2020). Oral dysbiosis and autoimmunity: From local periodontal responses to an imbalanced systemic immunity. A review. https://core.ac.uk/download/487076676.pdf (accessed on 17th June 2025).
11. Aruffo, A., Levine, A., Paterson, A., Schneider, A., Salomon, B., Brunstein, C., Camperio, C., et al. (2018). CD28 between tolerance and autoimmunity: The side effects of animal models [version 1; referees: 2 approved]. https://core.ac.uk/download/158822581.pdf (accessed on 17th June 2025).
12. Baens, M., Beyaert, R., Demeyer, A., Driege, Y., et al. (2019). MALT1 proteolytic activity suppresses

autoimmunity in a T cell intrinsic manner. https://core.ac.uk/download/237010402.pdf (accessed on 17th June 2025).

13. Baukloh, A. K., Beyer, K., Kamphues, C., Kotsch, K., et al. (2019). Interactions of tumor necrosis factor–related apoptosis-inducing ligand (TRAIL) with the immune system: Implications for inflammation and cancer. https://core.ac.uk/download/288113975.pdf (accessed on 17th June 2025).
14. Simakou, T., Butcher, J. P., Reid, S., & Henriquez, F. L. (2019). Alopecia areata: A multifactorial autoimmune condition. *Journal of autoimmunity*, *98*, 74–85. https://doi.org/10.1016/j.jaut.2018.12.001 (accessed on 17th June 2025).
15. Butler, C. L., Reed, E. F., Thomas, K. A., Valenzuela, N. M., et al. (2017). Not all antibodies are created equal: Factors that influence antibody mediated rejection. https://core.ac.uk/download/323079645.pdf (accessed on 17th June 2025).
16. Carbone, F. (2011). Regulatory T cell proliferative potential as novel marker to investigate immune tolerance and clinical progression in multiple sclerosis. https://core.ac.uk/download/11918866.pdf (accessed on 17th June 2025).
17. Clark, M., Kroger, C. J., & Tisch, R. M. (2017). Type 1 diabetes: A chronic anti-self-inflammatory response. https://core.ac.uk/download/304663457.pdf (accessed on 17th June 2025).
18. Crowe, J., Harnett, M. M., Harnett, W., Lumb, F. E., et al. (2017). Parasite excretory-secretory products and their effects on metabolic syndrome. https://core.ac.uk/download/78908151.pdf (accessed on 17th June 2025).
19. Xiao, J., Yang, R., Yang, L., Fan, X., Liu, W., & Deng, W. (2015). Kirenol attenuates experimental autoimmune encephalomyelitis by inhibiting differentiation of Th1 and th17 cells and inducing apoptosis of effector T cells. *Scientific reports*, *5*, 9022. https://doi.org/10.1038/srep09022(accessed on 17th June 2025).
20. Fahmy, T. M., Horwitz, D. A., La Cava, A., Piccirillo, C. A., et al. (2019). Rebalancing immune homeostasis to treat autoimmune diseases. https://core.ac.uk/download/573405299.pdf (accessed on 17th June 2025).
21. Fleming, J. O., Maizels, R., & Varyani, F. (2017). Helminths in the gastrointestinal tract as modulators of immunity and pathology. https://core.ac.uk/download/80697189.pdf (accessed on 17th June 2025).
22. Jaigirdar, S. A., & MacLeod, M. K. (2015). Development and Function of Protective and Pathologic Memory CD4 T Cells. *Frontiers in immunology*, *6*, 456. https://doi.org/10.3389/fimmu.2015.00456(accessed on 17th June 2025).
23. Shi, F. D., Ljunggren, H. G., La Cava, A., & Van Kaer, L. (2011). Organ-specific features of natural killer cells. *Nature reviews. Immunology*, *11*(10), 658–671. https://doi.org/10.1038/nri3065(accessed on 17th June 2025).
24. Mai, A., Mazzone, R., Valente, S., Zwergel, C., et al. (2017). Epi-drugs in combination with immunotherapy: A new avenue to improve anticancer efficacy. https://core.ac.uk/download/98345233.pdf (accessed on 17th June 2025).
25. McInnes, I. B., & Schett, G. (2017). Pathogenetic insights from the treatment of rheumatoid arthritis. *Lancet (London, England)*, *389*(10086), 2328–2337. https://doi.org/10.1016/S0140-6736(17)31472-1(accessed on 17th June 2025).

26. Mitsdoerffer, M., & Peters, A. (2016). Tertiary Lymphoid Organs in Central Nervous System Autoimmunity. *Frontiers in immunology*, *7*, 451. https://doi.org/10.3389/fimmu.2016.00451 (accessed on 17th June 2025).

27. Sfera, A., Sfera, A., Price, A. I., Osorio, C., Diaz, E., Cummings, M., & Gradini, R. (2018). Rusty microglia: Trainers of innate immunity in Alzheimer's disease. https://core.ac.uk/download/195777199.pdf (accessed on 17th June 2025).

28. Alivernini, S., Gremese, E., McSharry, C., Tolusso, B., Ferraccioli, G., McInnes, I. B., & Kurowska-Stolarska, M. (2018). MicroRNA-155-at the Critical Interface of Innate and Adaptive Immunity in Arthritis. *Frontiers in immunology*, *8*, 1932. https://doi.org/10.3389/fimmu.2017.01932 (accessed on 17th June 2025).

CLINICAL PRESENTATIONS OF RHEUMATIC DISEASE IN DIFFERENT AGE GROUPS

4

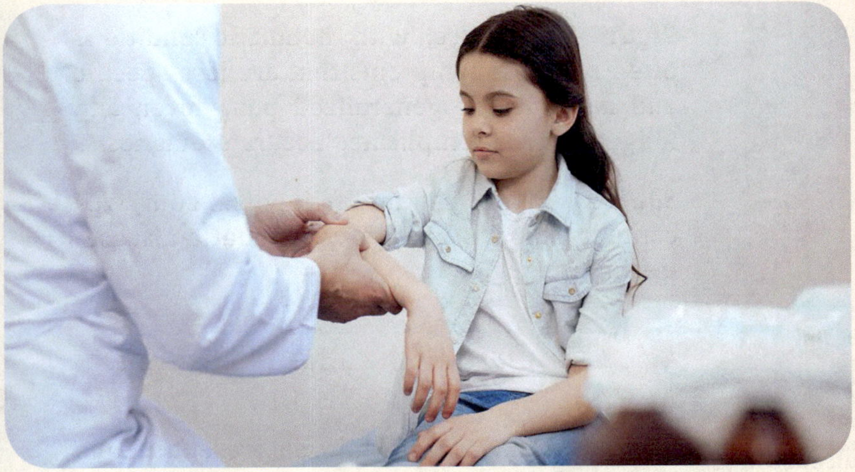

LEARNING OBJECTIVES

After studying this chapter, you will be able to:

1. Understand clinical presentations in pediatric population;
2. Explain clinical presentations in young adults;
3. Discuss clinical presentations in middle-aged adults;
4. Emphasize clinical presentations in the elderly.

Introduction

Rheumatic diseases are a heterogeneous group of disorders that present with inflammation and pain and can have a dramatic impact on the patient in any age category. Understanding the clinical presentations of these conditions is important because they manifest differently among children, adults, and the elderly and therefore necessitate particular diagnostic and treatment protocols. In youth, rheumatic fever and its complications, like rheumatic heart disease, are of primary concern, as indicated by studies that highlight specific HLA alleles that confer high risks on affected individuals (Eglite et al., 2003). Conversely, the elderly tend to present with comorbidities, their most common being cardiovascular diseases complicated by rheumatic diseases, making careful evaluation in this population very important (Kisenge, 2011). As their prevalence rises across the globe, an in-depth study of their manifestations across various age groups is necessary to enhance outcomes and guide proper clinical management.

4.1. Clinical Presentations in Pediatric Population

Learning Outcome

1. Describe common rheumatic diseases in children;
2. Learn symptoms and signs of juvenile idiopathic arthritis;
3. Understand the growth and development effect of rheumatic illnesses;
4. Describe diagnostic challenge in children;
5. Emphasize treatment technique and effectiveness;
6. Discuss long-term prognosis in children with rheumatologic diseases;
7. Understand the role of family history in pediatrics presentation;
8. Describe the psychological impact on children and families;
9. Understand early intervention and management significance.

The clinical presentation of rheumatoid disease in children is different and from that seen in adults. Rheumatic children present with nonspecific complaints that involve widespread pain, fever, and fatigue, and this poses challenges to proper diagnosis. Traditionally defined in the above study, the standard laboratory tests that have been used to evaluate rheumatologic conditions , such as antinuclear antibody (ANA) and rheumatoid factor (RF), have limited application in children and can lead to misdiagnosis and thus, require to have systematic evaluation methods (Eichenfield et al., 2008).

Additionally, conditions like Acute Rheumatic Fever (ARF) present unique challenges since the systemic inflammatory responses provoked by group A streptococcal infections overwhelmingly affect younger age groups with extreme variability in clinical presentations based on geographical and age factors (Fritzler et al., 2018). This necessitates nuanced pediatric presentation knowledge to refine diagnosis and treatment strategies (Figure 4.1).

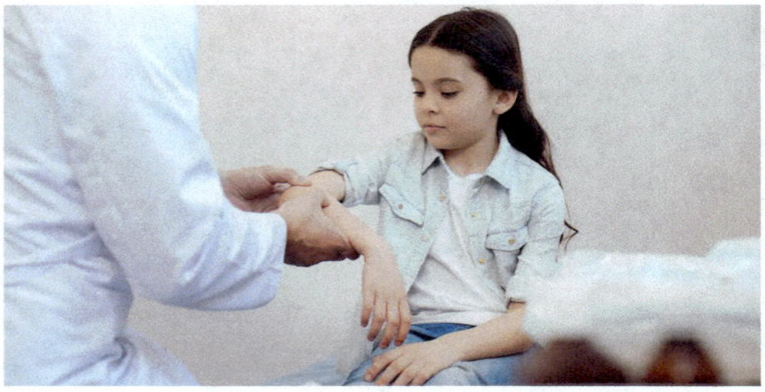

Figure 4.1. Children with rheumatic conditions often manifest symptoms that are less specific and may include generalized pain, fever, and fatigue, which complicates accurate diagnosis.

Source: https://inamdarhospital.com/wp-content/uploads/2024/04/rheumatic-disease-in-children.jpg.

4.1.1. Common Rheumatic Diseases in Children

Rheumatic diseases in children present unique clinical challenges that are very different from those of adults. One of the most prevalent conditions is juvenile idiopathic arthritis (JIA), which has many subtypes with chronic inflammation of the joint. The diagnostic approach to these conditions needs a careful examination of laboratory findings because findings , such as ANA and RF are not as useful diagnostically in children as in adults (Eichenfield et al., 2008). In addition, ARF is still rampant among children globally, particularly in the developing world, and highlights the need for timely detection and treatment of streptococcal infection to prevent long-term cardiac consequences (Fritzler et al., 2018). The understanding of these diseases' particular presentation and clinical implications is paramount to healthcare providers to foster successful treatment plans and improved overall health outcomes among the suffering children.

4.1.2. Symptoms and Signs of Juvenile Idiopathic Arthritis (JIA)

JIA, the most prevalent rheumatic disorder in children, presents a broad array of symptoms and signs that have a direct impact on a child's course of development. The illness usually manifests as pains, swelling, and stiffness in joints recurring repeatedly, largely in big weight-bearing joints , such as the knees and hips, but may be any joint (Hahn & Kim, 2010). In addition to these early indicators, additional extra-articular manifestations of chronic fever, rashes, and fatigue also occur relatively often, particularly in systemic-onset JIA with systemic inflammation. The variability of symptoms at times can also result in a delay in diagnosis, as parents may believe the initial presenting symptoms of fatigue or low-grade fever to be indicative of less severe disorders. Thus, the detection of these symptoms is critical for early treatment, since if left untreated, JIA can lead to permanent disability and joint deformity, affecting the quality of life and growth of a child (Chiang et al., 2015) (Figure 4.2).

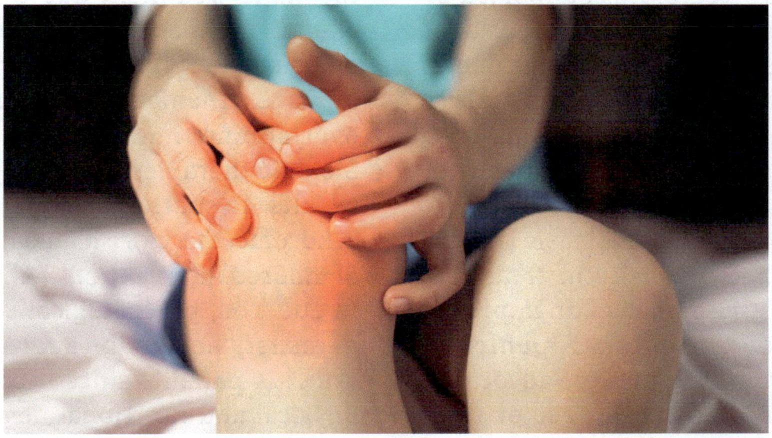

Figure 4.2. Juvenile idiopathic arthritis (JIA), classified as the most prevalent rheumatic disorder in children, presents with a diverse array of symptoms and signs that can significantly impact a child's developmental trajectory.

Source: https://d35oenyzp35321.cloudfront.net/Swelling_in_Minors_e77851b2d0.jpg.

4.1.3. Impact of Rheumatic Diseases on Growth and Development

Rheumatic diseases can severely impede growth and development at various phases of life, primarily in children and adolescents. JIA, for instance, may lead to chronic inflammation and pain, impacting negatively on physical activity and consequently on overall patterns of growth. These conditions are most likely to result in delayed puberty and osteopenia, compounded by therapies , such as corticosteroids, which induce further growth-related issues. Moreover, children with rheumatic diseases are also most likely to carry a higher prevalence of comorbidities, as evidenced in studies showing that 98% of rheumatoid arthritis patients have at least one comorbidity, adding to the complexity of issues they face. Additionally, as medical records observe, cardiovascular complications are prevalent among patients like them, and thus proper control and monitoring are essential to ensuring physical well-being as well as developmental potential (Kisenge, 2011). Effective management of these factors is key to ensuring better health results for this vulnerable population.

4.1.4. Diagnostic Challenges in Pediatric Patients

In pediatrics, the diagnosis of rheumatic conditions has unique challenges that require careful balancing of patient history and clinical presentation. Unlike in adults, where symptoms may more commonly align with established diagnostic criteria, children may present in an unusual fashion, making the clinical presentation complex. For instance, Sydenham's chorea (SC) presents as a central diagnostic symptom of acute rheumatic fever, and it is more common in children aged 5–15 years; it is supported by involuntary movements and neuropsychiatric presentations, whose aetiology may be due to other neurological disorders. The latest survey highlighted that clinicians chose hospitalization for SC suspects and recognized the need for careful diagnostics, including laboratory tests and brain MRI, to confirm the diagnosis (Battini et al., 2024). Also, heterogeneity in treatment approaches reflects the demand for improved clinical guidelines, as post-SC penicillin prophylaxis and steroid therapy were advocated, though opinions differed in respect of their duration (Battini et al., 2024) (Figure 4.3).

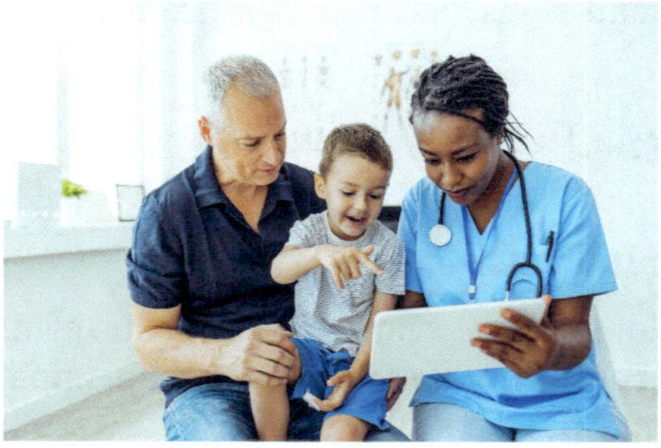

Figure 4.3. Diagnosing rheumatic diseases presents unique challenges that require careful consideration of clinical manifestations and patient history.

Source: https://images.ctfassets.net/yixw23k2v6vo/16pRWoAgzP2EPMIwYdh2oi/0f61887ac348f13fe949f4ce1f92b0ee/GettyImages-1415364203-3000x2000.jpg.

4.1.5. Treatment Options and Their Effectiveness

The treatment scenario in rheumatic diseases involves a complex interplay between age-related clinical presentation and therapeutic effectiveness. In the case of the young population, early treatment with biologics, especially in conditions , such as juvenile idiopathic arthritis, has been shown to be effective in managing inflammation and preventing long-term joint damage. But it has been demonstrated that older individuals may respond differently to the same treatment due to comorbidities and altered pharmacokinetics. For instance, a review of primary Sjögrens syndrome and systemic lupus erythematosus indicates that, despite overlapping immunologic features, current biologic therapies typically yield disappointing results in patients with primary Sjögrens syndrome, therefore highlighting the importance of tailored interventions (Ahwireng et al., 2021). In addition, psychological comorbidities , such as anxiety need to be addressed in rheumatoid arthritis patients since it correlate with worse physical and functional health, suggesting that integrative treatment models could enhance overall efficacy (Blaney, 2021). To this end, age-related nuances need to be grasped so that treatment paradigms can be optimized for rheumatic diseases.

4.1.6. Long-term Outcomes for Children with Rheumatic Diseases

Understanding long-term results for children who have rheumatic disorders is important to the development of intervention and treatment plans. Science shows that children who have diseases , such as JIA tend to have serious problems throughout their growth, such as an increased risk of infection because of immunosuppressive treatments. The Pharmachild registry indicates that in 15,284 patients, the most common adverse events were infections, which carry possible long-term health risks, and opportunistic infections were reported in many instances (Giancane, 2019). In addition, the importance of attending to the psychosocial aspects of rheumatic conditions should not be overemphasized, especially with regard to family planning and parenting, as seen in the patient needs survey of autoimmune rheumatic diseases (Phillips et al., 2018). Such considerations highlight the necessity of a holistic multidisciplinary provision of care and support to children with rheumatic conditions in such a way that their future health and well-being are of prime importance (Figure 4.4).

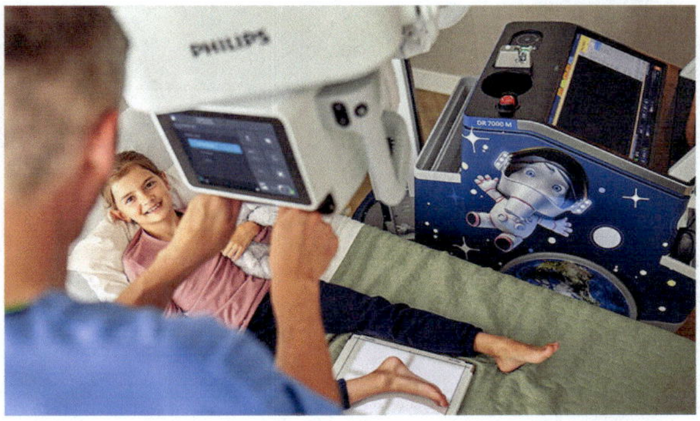

Figure 4.4. Understanding the long-term outcomes for children with rheumatic diseases is crucial for shaping interventions and treatment strategies.

Source: https://www.philips.com/c-dam/corporate/newscenter/global/standard/resources/healthcare/2024/q-and-a-with-atul-gupta-md/dr-7000-m-application-tech-pediatric-eth.jpg.

4.1.7. Role of Family History in Pediatric Presentations

Family history in pediatric presentation of rheumatic disease is crucial, as it can significantly impact diagnosis as well as management strategies. A detailed study of medical histories of the family helps clinicians recognize patterns that indicate hereditary diseases , such as JIA and rheumatic fever. For instance, the Pharmachild registry has confirmed the prevalence of autoimmune diseases in children with a family predisposition and demonstrated a genetic link for such occurrences (Giancane, 2019). In addition, recent findings indicate socioeconomic determinants of family background may influence disease severity, particularly in conditions like rheumatic heart disease, for which a higher degree of deprivation has been associated with adverse outcomes (de Loizaga et al., 2021). Thus, including family history in clinical assessment enhances predictive accuracy and allows for interventions to be specially focused, finally optimizing the treatment of children with rheumatic disease.

4.1.8. Psychological Impact on Children and Families

The psychological impact of rheumatic disorders on the children and families themselves is vast, oftentimes leading to profound emotional distress and disruption of daily life. Disorders like Juvenile Dermatomyositis not only have their physical symptoms like muscle weakness and skin rash, but also impose monumental psychosocial challenges, as alluded to in a study that used the metaphor of a rollercoaster to encapsulate the lived life of such afflicted children. Emotional distress in children under these circumstances can be linked to ambiguity regarding their health and the sense of being a burden to their families. Peer support that is limited and problems related to school can also cause psychological issues, and it is thus important for health professionals to prioritize psychosocial treatment alongside medical treatments (Murphy et al., 2010). Meanwhile, understanding the complexities of anxiety disorders like OCD, which might also coexist with rheumatic diseases, only serves to intensify the requirement for prolonged mental health treatment for such families (Murphy et al., 2010) (Figure 4.5).

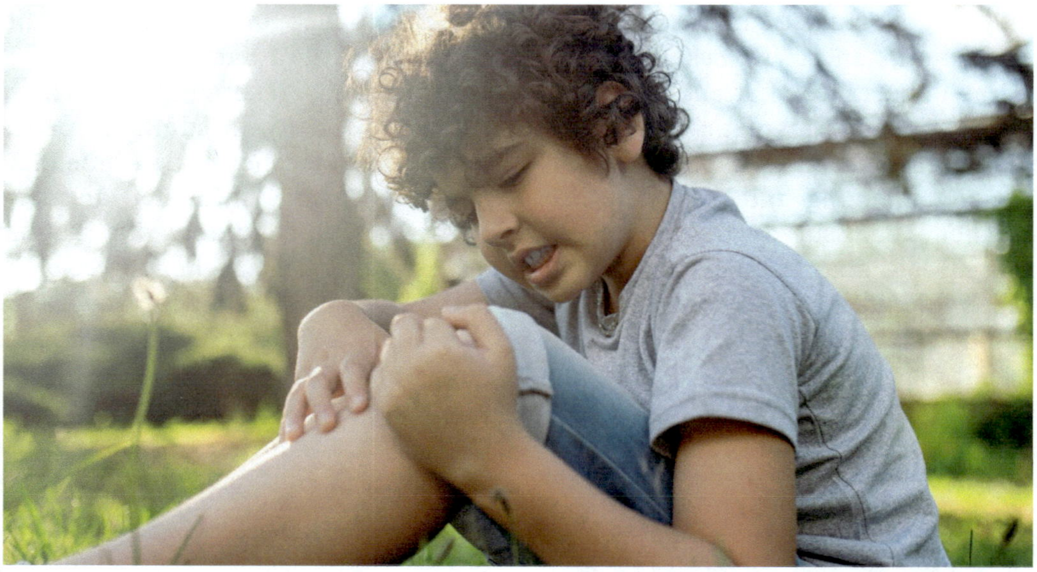

Figure 4.5. The psychological impact of rheumatic diseases on children and their families is profound, often leading to significant emotional distress and disruption in daily life.

Source: https://www.hindustantimes.com/ht-img/img/2024/04/24/1600x900/focused-dark-haired-boy-examining-his-damaged-knee_1713940850211_1713940884583.jpg.

4.1.9. Importance of Early Intervention and Management

The importance of early intervention and management of rheumatic diseases cannot be overstated, particularly in the context of their multifaceted clinical presentations among diverse age groups. Early diagnosis and appropriate management significantly lower the risk of severe complications, and this ultimately results in an overall improvement in the quality of life in patients. For instance, an early check-up for cardiovascular and hypertension diseases is necessary among the elderly because these diseases have been found to occur together and commonly in instances where hospitalization was caused by non-cardiovascular factors (Kisenge, 2011). Furthermore, for younger patients, control of the multifaceted needs of autoimmune rheumatic disease patients is essential to provide optimum clinical outcomes, especially in ontogenetic life periods , such as pregnancy and early parenthood (Phillips et al., 2018). By such targeted interventions, clinicians are able to facilitate better control of the disease and empower patients through shared decision-making, resulting in better clinical outcomes across all patient age groups.

Test Your Knowledge

1. How are rashes and fevers viewed in systemic rheumatic conditions of children?
2. What is the role of uveitis in pediatric rheumatologic conditions?

4.2. Clinical Presentations in Young Adults

Learning Outcome

1. Understand the prevalence in young adults of rheumatic conditions;
2. Describe age-related conditions prevalent in this group;
3. Discuss clinical features and symptoms;
4. Know the impact on daily activities and lifestyle;
5. Describe treatment strategy and compliance issues;
6. Highlight the physical therapy and rehabilitation role;
7. Describe psychological and social effects;
8. Discuss patient education and care importance.

The clinical presentations of rheumatic diseases in young adults indicate the unique challenges of this group. Young adults will often have a variety of symptoms that complicate diagnosis and treatment planning. For instance, diseases , such as JIA may persist into adulthood with joint pain, fatigue, and decreased mobility symptoms and lead to severe functional impairment. Additionally, the development of inflammatory bowel disease and spondylarthritis association in this group contributes to the complex clinical picture. Atypical presentation, such as systemic and extra-articular manifestations, may also present in young adults and necessitate a high suspicion and suspicion by physicians. Effective detection at the early stages is required to avoid long-term disability, and thus the need for specialized assessment tools like pGALSplus, which enable identification of severe musculoskeletal issues in young patients (Foster et al., 2024). Moreover, older presentations in this population, including cardiovascular sequelae, require overall management approaches (Kisenge, 2011).

4.2.1. Prevalence of Rheumatic Diseases in Young Adults

The prevalence of rheumatic disorders in young adults is a cause of serious public health concern, and further information regarding their clinical presentation is required in comparison with other age groups. Young adults, although having a generally milder presentation of these diseases, can nevertheless suffer from considerable morbidity that affects their quality of life and productivity. For instance, evidence indicates that conditions , such as rheumatoid arthritis and systemic lupus erythematosus are likely to have onset in this age group and cause symptoms that can be missed or misdiagnosed since they occur in an atypical manner. The evolving healthcare milieu calls for increased awareness and screening for these disorders in young adults, since they also have special psychosocial concerns that can affect control of the disease. This emphasis is critical because rheumatic diseases are susceptible to long-term implications, and as such, there is a necessity for early intervention and comprehensive models of care to capture their effect on this demographic (Kiseng, 2011) (Figure 4.6).

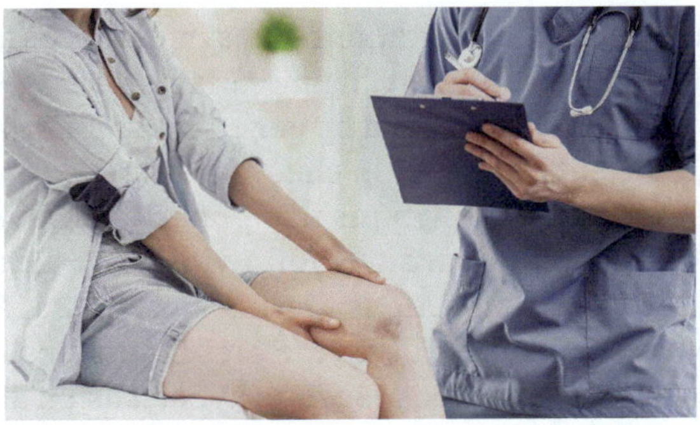

Figure 4.6. Young adults, who often experience a less severe manifestation of these conditions, may still suffer from considerable morbidity that affects both their quality of life and productivity.

Source: https://www.jointreplacementhawaii.com/wp-content/uploads/2021/04/Orthopedic-Surgeon-vs-Rheumatologist.jpg.

4.2.2. Specific Conditions affecting this Age Group

When investigating the special conditions affecting the elderly in the context of rheumatic diseases, one finds a notable overlap with cardiovascular disease. As an individual gets older, the prevalence of conditions , such as hypertension, congestive heart failure, and other forms of cardiovascular disease increases significantly. For instance, facts indicate that cardiovascular disease is the leading cause of death among individuals over 50 years and leads to high morbidity and disability among them (Kisenge, 2011). In addition, multisystemic presentation of autoimmune diseases can also manifest with audiovestibular symptoms like sensorineural hearing loss, thus complicating elderly systemic disease patients (Ralli et al., 2018). This is reinforced in the complexity that underscores the necessity of understanding the diverse clinical manifestations of the rheumatic diseases in the elderly because early intervention will improve patient outcomes and quality of life.

4.2.3. Symptoms and Clinical Manifestations

The clinical manifestations and symptoms of the rheumatic diseases are highly variable with age, a determinant influenced by genetic susceptibility and the environment. In children and teenagers, diseases like ARF typically present as fever, arthritis, and carditis following untreated streptococcal infections (Fritzler et al., 2018). Conversely, in the elderly, the presentation could be chronic conditions , such as hypertension and congestive heart failure, which could present as palpitations and shortness of breath (Kisenge, 2011). These differences not only indicate the age-related immune response and biological alterations but also the specific epidemiological patterns of the diverse rheumatic disorders. Besides, the occurrence of comorbidities, as with the case of obesity and anemia among elderly individuals, makes the clinical situation complicated and emphasizes the need for age-related risk factor-specific screening and intervention for the effective control of rheumatic illnesses (Figure 4.7).

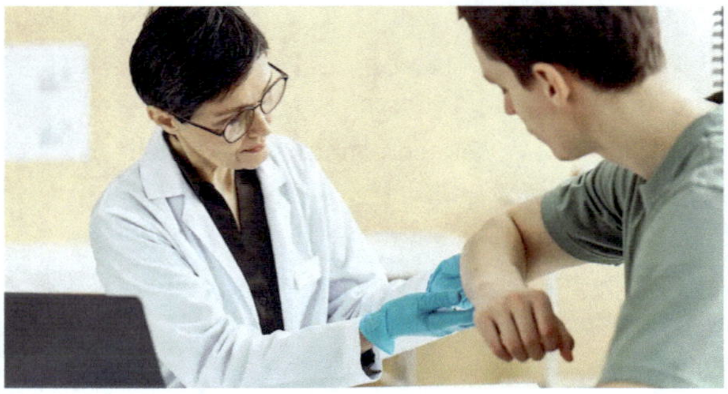

Figure 4.7. The symptoms and clinical manifestations of rheumatic diseases significantly vary across different age groups, influenced by both genetic predispositions and environmental factors.

Source: https://images.ctfassets.net/yixw23k2v6vo/f44YecGcVFnJAZWBoa4uf/3aba1f5b430151f613393b4104d917fb/large-GettyImages-1765430464-3000x2000.jpg?fm=webp&q=50&w=1200&h=600&fit=thumb.

4.2.4. Impact on Lifestyle and Daily Activities

The effect of rheumatic diseases on lifestyle and daily activities is sometimes significant, particularly because the manifestation of these diseases is age-dependent. For instance, pain and physical activity limitations are prevalent among the elderly; over three-quarters of knee osteoarthritis patients are below physical activity guidelines, which only aggravates mobility as well as overall health problems (Bramble et al., 2019). Therefore, such patients typically have highly disrupted daily activities that limit independence and socialization. On the contrary, adolescents would struggle with other issues, such as the psychological distress of long-term pain, which would adversely affect school performance and social relationships. The necessity for individualized preventive health interventions becomes apparent as health professionals navigate the complexities of differential influence on daily living and lifestyle, particularly among vulnerable populations. By addressing these multifaceted effects, physicians are able to significantly enhance the quality of life in individuals of any age.

4.2.5. Treatment Strategies and Adherence Issues

Strategies for the treatment of rheumatic conditions cannot simply address the clinical manifestations of the diseases but also the multifaceted issues of patient compliance with treatment. Research indicates that rheumatoid arthritis (RA) patients are often comorbid with depression and anxiety, which can significantly impair treatment adherence and general health outcomes, including functional disability and quality of life (Blaney, 2021).

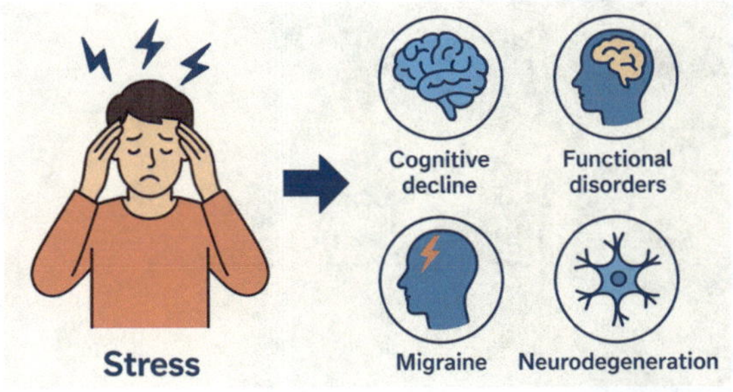

Figure 4.8. Patients with rheumatoid arthritis (RA) often experience comorbid anxiety and depression, which can significantly impair treatment adherence and overall health outcomes, including functional disability and quality of life.

Source: https://media.licdn.com/dms/image/v2/D5612AQFvY0RAXNh1SA/article-cover_image-shrink_720_1280/B56ZZanLyeHsAI-/0/1745276951040?e=2147483647&v=beta&t=40njbpsMdFj2_c_VxL0zHw5YzTee4_kYs3z5EPYLPBk.

Additionally, adherence to anticoagulation therapy is a major challenge in young adults with rheumatic heart disease (RHD), while ignorance and logistical issues are some of the determinants leading to poor compliance (Mangnall et al., 2017). Thus, an interdisciplinary team-based approach incorporating mental health counseling and patient education becomes imperative to ensure better compliance in various age groups. By solving these intricate adherence issues, physicians can improve therapeutic success and allow for easier control of rheumatic diseases across all age groups (Figure 4.8).

4.2.6. Role of Physical Therapy and Rehabilitation

Rehabilitation and physical therapy are part of the treatment of rheumatic diseases across the lifespan and play an important role in determining patients' quality of life and functional ability. Through the application of targeted therapeutic measures, physical therapists can diminish pain, optimize mobility, and improve overall physical function in patients with conditions , such as osteoarthritis and rheumatoid arthritis. Specifically, regional physical therapy networks, including continuing education for practitioners, have demonstrated positive results in enhancing clinical performance.

The evidence indicates that communication among physical therapists and rheumatologists improves through these networks, with better patient satisfaction and treatment adherence (Bakker et al., 2004). In addition, treatment of comorbidities , such as anxiety, frequent among rheumatic disease patients, can similarly be improved through customarily designed physical rehabilitation programs, hence providing comprehensive care with a holistic strategy to treat both physical and mental health aspects (Blaney, 2021). Generally, incorporation of physical therapy in the process of multidimensional treatment is essential for optimal patient management.

4.2.7. Psychological and Social Implications

Rheumatological conditions not only manifest physically, but also generate enormous psychological and social effects among different age groups. For instance, RA patients develop very high levels of anxiety, which exacerbate physical symptoms and lower well-being. Research indicates that increased anxiety is correlated with worse clinical outcomes, for example, increased functional disability, pain, and fatigue, and therefore augmenting the burden for the patients during the course of the day (Blaney, 2021). Additionally, the coexistence of anxiety along with other psychiatric disorders, for instance, obsessive-compulsive disorder (OCD), can contribute to the intricacy of the clinical presentation, leading to impaired social functioning and enhanced distress (Murphy et al., 2010). This interconnectedness of mental illness issues underscores the necessity of biopsychosocial therapy treatment of rheumatism, pointing out that an appropriate solution approach should not only address the physical but must also incorporate psychological counseling to enhance patient welfare and social integration (Figure 4.9).

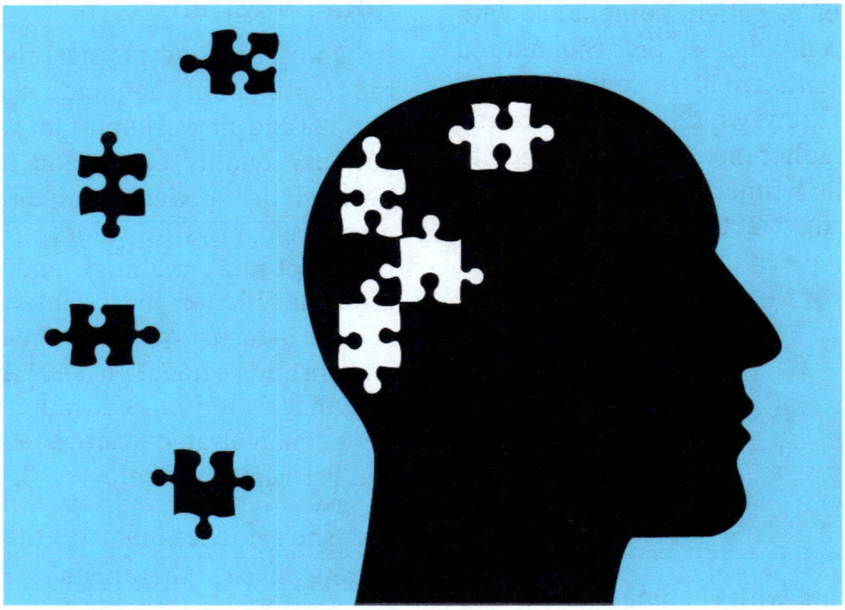

Figure 4.9. Rheumatic diseases not only manifest physically but also engender significant psychological and social implications across different age groups.

Source: https://scx2.b-cdn.net/gfx/news/hires/2018/mentalillness.jpg.

4.2.8. Importance of Patient Education and Support

Effective patient education and support are significant factors that come into play when treating rheumatic diseases among different age groups, particularly with regard to the complexities involved in such diseases. RA patients, for instance, tend to develop co-morbid mental disorders , such as anxiety, which may exacerbate physical symptoms as well as overall quality of life. Research has indicated that patients with more severe levels of anxiety yield less functional outcomes, and this highlights the necessity for mass educational interventions focused on physical and psychological aspects of care (Blaney, 2021). Furthermore, autoimmune rheumatic disease patients also often struggle to gain access to family planning, pregnancy, and integrative care information, highlighting a crucial shortfall in services (Phillips et al., 2018). By making patient education and multi-disciplinary support systems a priority, healthcare providers are able to empower patients, enhance treatment compliance, and ultimately improve outcomes and quality of life in persons suffering from rheumatic disease.

Test Your Knowledge

1. What is the clinical presentation of reactive arthritis following an infection?
2. How does psoriatic arthritis develop in young adults, and how does it differ from RA?

4.3. Clinical Presentations in Middle-Aged Adults

Learning Outcome

1. Identify the typical rheumatic diseases of middle-aged adults;
2. Highlight gender variations in disease presentation;
3. Identify clinical and symptom features;
4. Outline the comorbidities of rheumatic conditions;
5. Outline diagnostic challenges among middle-aged adults;
6. Highlight treatment options and their effectiveness;
7. Be familiar with the effect on work and productivity;
8. Understand the importance of lifestyle modification;
9. Implement long-term management strategies.

Middle-aged patients will have a complex range of clinical presentations of rheumatic disease that are an expression of the aging process and the cumulative effect of lifestyle factors. Joint pain, stiffness, and generalized symptoms like fatigue may be presenting features and can lead to conditions , such as rheumatoid arthritis or ankylosing spondylitis. Most prominently, cardiovascular complications are now higher in this group, and hypertension and heart failure commonly occur with rheumatic presentations. In one study of patients between, hypertension has been found to be present in over 67% of patients, as congestive heart failure was also a problem, pointing to the intersection of cardiovascular and rheumatic disease in this group (Kisenge, 2011). The management of such diseases needs an integrative approach that addresses not only musculoskeletal presentations but also comorbidities, as evidenced by reports of public health, which have demonstrated changes in demand for health among middle-aged individuals.

4.3.1. Common Rheumatic Diseases in Middle-aged Adults

Middle-aged adults frequently present with a range of common rheumatic diseases that significantly impact their quality of life. Among these, RA is especially common, with chronic inflammation and joint damage often leading to disability if untreated. Osteoarthritis (OA) also occurs as degenerative joint disease, interfering with mobility and activities of daily living due to cartilage loss. Systemic lupus erythematosus (SLE) also occurs in this population, causing systemic involvement as it impacts multiple organ systems. The burden of these conditions is then added to by co-morbid conditions , such as cardiovascular disease, which, as stated, is prevalent among the elderly and makes it more difficult to treat. Specifically, in studies , such as those carried out at Muhimbili National

Hospital, hypertension and congestive heart failure were listed as frequent complications, thus further supporting the need for holistic approaches to tackle middle-aged adults' health with rheumatic diseases (Kisenge, 2011) (Figure 4.10).

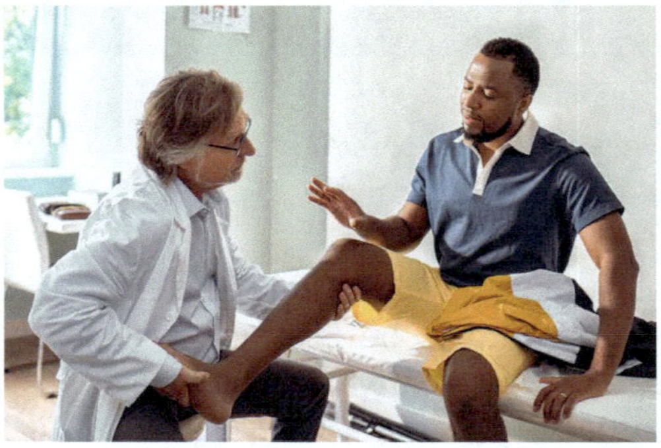

Figure 4.10. Middle-aged adults frequently encounter a range of common rheumatic diseases that significantly impact their quality of life.

Source: https://img.lb.wbmdstatic.com/vim/live/webmd/consumer_assets/site_images/article_thumbnails/other/doctor_examining_mans_leg_other/1800x1200_doctor_examining_mans_leg_other.jpg?resize=750px:*&output-quality=75.

4.3.2. Gender Differences in Disease Presentation

The research on gender differences in disease presentation depicts extensive gaps in the expression and progression of rheumatologic diseases between age groups. Specifically, studies have demonstrated that SLE is predominantly found in women, with a remarkable 94.9% of patients presenting with female characteristics in a study on the Pakistani population (Adil et al., 2024).

This gender difference is compatible with a broader understanding that autoimmune illnesses are more prevalent in women, according to hormonal and genetic factors. In contrast, cardiovascular disease, which is more responsible for morbidity among the elderly, fails to show significant gender variation in incidence among the elderly; both men and women suffer from equal rates of hypertension and cardiovascular complications (Kisenge, 2011). These differing findings emphasize the relevance of gender consideration when evaluating clinical presentations of rheumatic illnesses, since these differences may eventually affect diagnosis, therapy, and patient outcomes within various age groups.

4.3.3. Symptoms and Clinical Features

An evaluation of symptoms and clinical features of rheumatic diseases shows considerable differences at different ages, affecting diagnosis and treatment plans. In older adults, for instance, hypertension and congestive heart failure are also often present with rheumatic diseases, emphasizing the importance of comprehensive cardiovascular assessment in older adults (Kisenge, 2011).

The clinical presentations may involve frequent onset of symptoms , such as palpitations, dyspnea, and fatigue, and these pose challenges in making the diagnosis of underlying rheumatic diseases. In contrast, younger age groups present with more acute symptoms, with rapid onset of swelling and pain in joints that allows for rapid diagnosis of disorders like rheumatoid arthritis or juvenile idiopathic arthritis. Further, systemic manifestations , such as sensorineural hearing loss may be indicative of autoimmune involvement and can present similarly to other conditions and need careful evaluation (Ralli et al., 2018).

This underscores the need for age-specific diagnostic models to adequately address the complexity of rheumatic diseases (Figure 4.11).

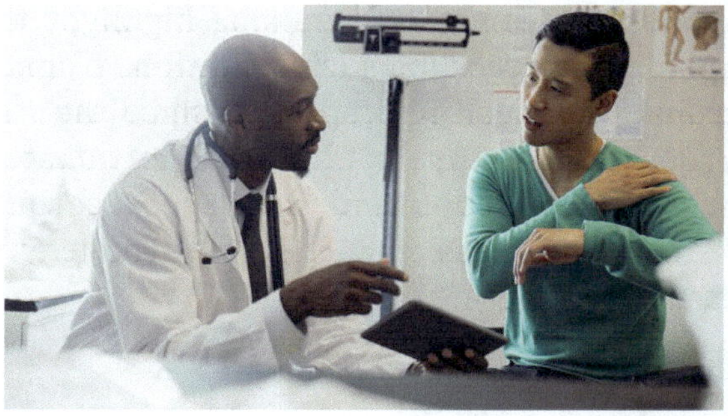

Figure 4.11. Examining the symptoms and clinical features of rheumatic diseases reveals notable variances across different age groups, impacting diagnosis and management strategies.

Source: https://dims.healthgrades.com/dims3/MMH/db456a2/2147483647/strip/true/crop/2121x1185+0+114/resize/800x447!/quality/75/?url=https%3A%2F%2Fucmscdn.healthgrades.com%2F8b%2F5c%2F707d7af749fe90f8b227cf801f6c%2Fimage-null.jpg.

4.3.4. Comorbidities Associated with Rheumatic Diseases

The prevalence of comorbidities among individuals with rheumatic diseases, and most notably RA, demonstrates the intricate nature of these diseases and overall wellness. Literature indicates that nearly all RA patients have one or more comorbidities, and, in a study on black South African patients with RA, the number of comorbidities per patient was a median of three. Amongst stated comorbidities are hypertension, osteoporosis, and diabetes mellitus, which are prevalent and complicate management and influence outcomes in patients (Lala, 1996). The rising expenditure of comorbidities is especially true in older adults, as aging remains a high-risk factor for the onset of rheumatic diseases as well as resultant comorbid conditions. For this reason, clinicians are required to embrace an integrative approach to treat not just the underlying rheumatic disease but also the gamut of comorbidities capable of worsening the clinical presentations reported in different age groups.

4.3.5. Diagnostic Challenges in this Age Group

In the field of rheumatic diseases, diagnostic challenges are usually encountered, particularly in older age groups, in which the complex presentation of clinical conditions hinders accurate diagnosis. With progressive aging, comorbid conditions become much more common, contributing to complicating the clinical picture and leading to potential misdiagnosis. For instance, studies on black South African RA patients revealed that an astonishing 98% of the patients had one or more comorbidities, and the median was three comorbidities in a population of 500 patients (Lala, 1996). Not only do these comorbidities aggravate rheumatic condition symptoms, but also mask usual clinical features, thus slowing down appropriate treatment steps. Furthermore, the interrelated nature of conditions like hypertension and diabetes mellitus, common in the elderly population, again indicates the necessity for greater sensitivity and longer diagnostic methods suited to the unique challenges in this scenario (Lala, 1996) (Figure 4.12).

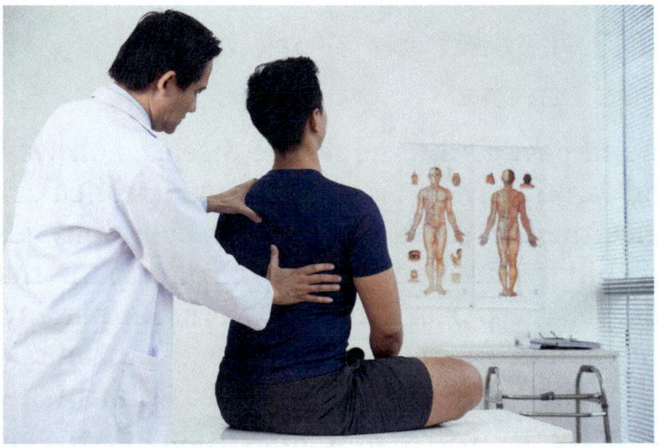

Figure 4.12. As individuals age, the prevalence of comorbidities significantly increases, often complicating the clinical picture and leading to potential misdiagnosis.

Source: https://www.rheum-care.com/wp-content/uploads/2021/01/annual-medical-examination-VNLVSRK-scaled.jpg.

4.3.6. Treatment Options and Their Effectiveness

The treatment modalities for rheumatoid diseases vary significantly between age groups, a reflection of the distinct patterns of presentation that occur in these patient groups. The most commonly employed traditional treatments in adults are non-steroidal anti-inflammatory drugs (NSAIDs) and Disease-Modifying Antirheumatic Drugs (DMARDs), but their effectiveness is undermined by comorbid conditions like anxiety, which is frequently observed in RA patients (Blaney, 2021). In contrast, children with JIA will react differently to the same regimen because their bodies are immature and their immune systems will differ. New analysis indicates that biologic therapies may provide differential interventions, particularly if they stratify patients by immunological profile, as seen in studies of primary Sjögrens syndrome and systemic lupus erythematosus (Ahwireng et al., 2021). This stratification regimen can maximize the effectiveness of therapy, and age- and individual-specific therapies are indicated in the management of rheumatic diseases.

4.3.7. Impact on Work and Productivity

The impact of the rheumatic diseases on work and productivity is tremendous, particularly since the disorders can lead to severe physical disability and debilitating chronic pain that hamper the performance of work. RA patients, for instance, may experience symptoms of different severity, leading to diminished capacity to work and absenteeism. In one study that analyzed administrative health care data, the variation in the number of RA cases detected merits careful observation when one is looking at the effects on productivity among the population as a whole, a sign of the loss in workforce performance brought about by such health conditions (Hanly et al., 2015). Moreover, health disparities between Indigenous and non-Indigenous Australians highlight the importance of tackling such conditions from an occupational health perspective since the risk of rheumatic disease could disproportionately affect some groups and further exacerbate existing disparities in workforce productivity and use (Figure 4.13).

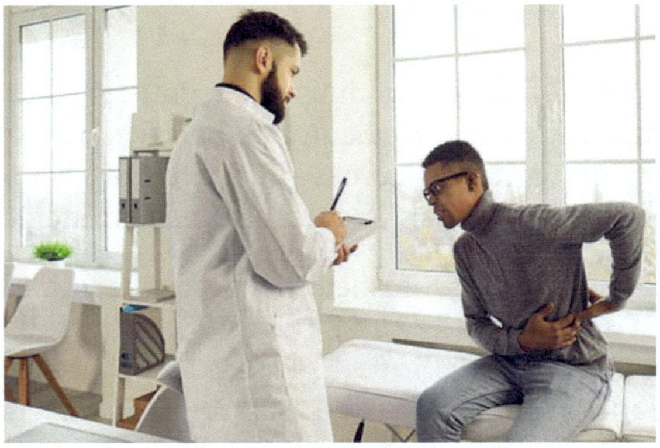

Figure 4.13. Individuals diagnosed with rheumatoid arthritis (RA), for instance, may experience varying degrees of severity in their symptoms, which can lead to decreased work capacity and increased absenteeism.

Source: https://media.assettype.com/healthday-en%2F2024-09-03%2Fipvtguej%2F408297821.jpeg?w=480&auto=format%2Ccompress&fit=max.

4.3.8. Importance of Lifestyle Modifications

The contribution of lifestyle changes in managing rheumatic disorders, particularly across various ages, cannot be overstated. These adjustments can include diet, increased exercise, and weight management, all of which are key parts of symptom relief and improved clinical outcomes. In the young patient population, early education about healthy habits can reduce the long-term morbidity from these chronic conditions. Older patients may find that adjustments consistent with their limitations, e.g., low-impact exercise or anti-inflammatory diets, are an important component of enhancing their quality of life.

In addition, there is a recent study that indicates chronic disease management is significantly improved when patients are encouraged regularly, particularly by health workers knowledgeable about their requirements (Balanescu et al., 2022). Last but not least, embracing these lifestyle modifications not only improves disease management but also stimulates more patient-oriented care, i.e., for the different experiences of rheumatic patients by age group (Jordá et al., 2019).

4.3.9. Long-term Management Strategies

Long-term care for rheumatic diseases must be adjusted to the different clinical presentations observed in different age groups. From recent studies, the reality is evident that elderly populations with disorders like knee OA do not attain recommended levels of exercise activity, impacting their functional outcomes and increasing the risk of disability (Bramble et al., 2019). Multidimensional intervention is required with a focus on the recognition of individualized clinical phenotypes to guide individualized interventions. For instance, the understanding of the various influences on physical activity, e.g., age, body mass index, comorbidities, enables clinicians to use interventions that support mobility and overall health in older patients (Bramble et al., 2019). In younger adults as well, early detection and treatment of immune-related adverse events caused by therapies, e.g., immune checkpoint inhibitors, underscore the need for ongoing monitoring and multidisciplinary care to reach optimal patient outcomes. These general plans are key to improving the quality of life for rheumatic disease patients throughout their lifespan (Figure 4.14).

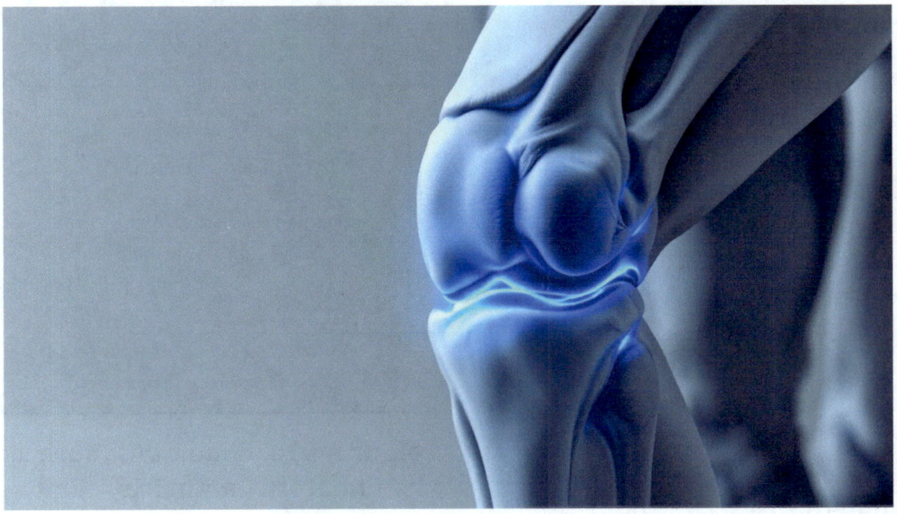

Figure 4.14. Older adults with conditions like knee osteoarthritis (OA) often do not meet recommended physical activity levels, impacting their functional outcomes and increasing disability risk.

Source: https://cdn.growtha.dev/65bd13293ddfda03cda9a849/67f612553549271fcacc0d01_tmpinxiq3fs.jpeg.

Test Your Knowledge

1. What are key features of polymyositis and dermatomyositis in middle age?
2. What rheumatic diseases are associated with interstitial lung disease in this age group?

4.4. Clinical Presentations in the Elderly

Learning Outcome

1. Appreciate the prevalence of rheumatic diseases in elderly;
2. Describe peculiar clinical features in elderly;
3. Recognize challenges in diagnosis because of comorbidities;
4. Recognize symptoms and their influence on quality of life;
5. Explain treatment considerations and polypharmacy;
6. Discuss the role of caregivers in management;
7. Appreciate the need for a multidisciplinary approach;
8. Learn the psychological impact of chronic disease in the elderly;
9. Highlight future directions in research and care.

Clinical presentations of rheumatic diseases in older patients are generally compounded by the convergence of a number of comorbidities that can mask or mimic the rheumatic presentation. As age increases, cardiovascular disease is more frequent, and hypertension and congestive heart failure are frequent complications that make the clinical picture complicated. Specifically, cardiovascular disease was a cause of significant morbidity and hospitalization among older adults, emphasizing the importance of complete screening for this condition even in patients presenting with non-cardiac complaints (Kisenge, 2011). Additionally, the burden of chronic conditions , such as arthritis and osteoporosis makes diagnosis and treatment more complex, necessitating particular intervention programs to reduce preventable hospitalizations among this high-risk group (Bywood et al., 2016). Therefore, understanding the multifaceted clinical presentations in the elderly is crucial to optimizing care and improving health outcomes in this group of patients.

4.4.1. Prevalence of Rheumatic Diseases in Older Adults

Incidence of rheumatic diseases in older adults is a daunting clinical problem since it reflects the intricate interplay between chronic inflammation and aging. As the age of the world population advances, osteoarthritis, rheumatoid arthritis, and gout are becoming more prevalent conditions, with ill effects on mobility and quality of life. Importantly, younger age groups presenting with similar conditions are not necessarily going to present with the same clinical features, suggesting that age-related diagnostic and therapeutic strategies are required.

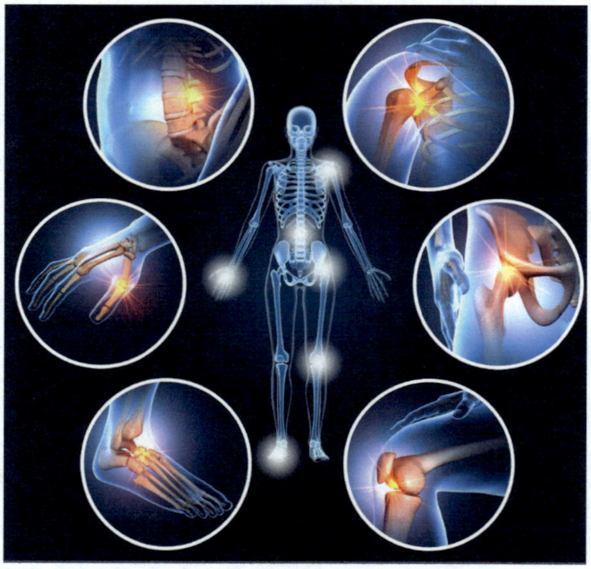

Figure 4.15. Conditions , such as osteoarthritis, rheumatoid arthritis, and gout become increasingly common, with adverse implications for mobility and quality of life.

Source: https://painandspinespecialists.com/wp-content/uploads/AdobeStock_492255186-scaled.jpeg.

Studies have indicated that comorbid conditions like cardiovascular disease and obesity aggravate the consequences of rheumatic disease in the elderly, leading to more disability and less physical function (Kisenge, 2011). Secondly, differences in clinical presentations among the elderly highlight the necessity for a tailored management strategy, particularly among those with multiple comorbid conditions, as has been demonstrated in research on knee osteoarthritis and its phenotypic heterogeneity (Bramble et al., 2019). This emphasizes the necessity of individualized interventions to improve functional outcomes and overall well-being among the elderly (Figure 4.15).

4.4.2. Unique Clinical Features in the Elderly

The presentation of rheumatic disease in the elderly has some specific differentiating features from other age groups. For instance, older patients usually have atypical symptoms, such as decreased pain and inflammation, and these can lead to delayed diagnosis or treatment. The immune changes that occur with aging also make the clinical picture more challenging since inflammation in elderly individuals is not the same. Also, the presence of multiple comorbidities can influence the severity and course of rheumatic diseases in older people, making more in-depth information about treatment algorithms indispensable. This is particularly pertinent because some treatments may be less efficient or pose additional risks in older patients, who generally have a different pharmacological response due to age-related changes in their physiology. These unique characteristics of the clinical presentation need to be addressed in order to optimize care and maximize outcomes for older patients with rheumatic diseases, as per the findings reported by Bolland et al. (2021); Bywood et al. (2016).

4.4.3. Challenges in Diagnosis Due to Comorbidities

Comorbidities make the diagnosis of rheumatic disease very challenging, particularly in demographically diverse populations. RA diagnosis in persons with greater than one comorbid condition has the potential to obscure clinical presentation with ensuing delayed or misdiagnosis. For instance, one of the studies on 500 South African black patients suffering from RA had an incredible 98% prevalence of comorbidity, with three per patient on average, like anemia and high blood pressure, both of which are prevalent among the elderly. This overlap in symptomatology makes it hard to identify the primary condition, while age and disability also impact the variety of such comorbidities, and thus, clinical assessment is challenging (Lala, 1996). The interaction between rheumatic diseases and comorbidities not only affects diagnostic accuracy but also clinical management approach, necessitating a sophisticated evaluation strategy that accounts for these intricacies in order to maximize patient outcomes regardless of age (Figure 4.16).

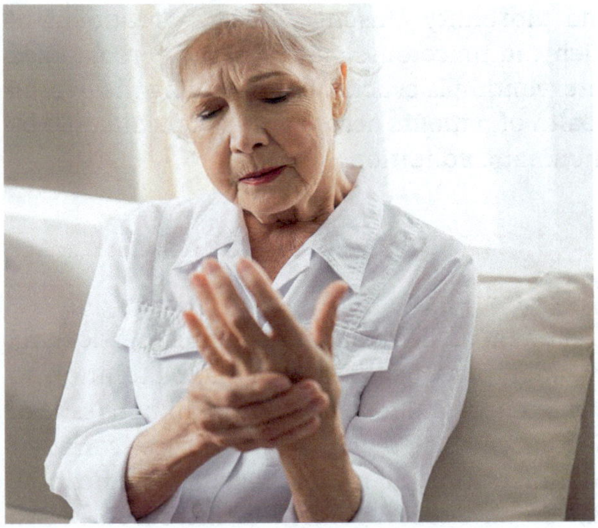

Figure 4.16. Overlapping symptomatology makes it challenging to discern the primary condition, as age and disability further influence the spectrum of these comorbidities, complicating clinical assessments.

Source: https://www.hss.edu/images/socialmedia/woman-ra-ia-hand-pain-1200X628.jpg.

4.4.4. Symptoms and Their Impact on Quality of Life

Rheumatic disease symptoms have a significant influence on the quality of life in patients, affecting both physical and mental well-being. The most frequent presentations are musculoskeletal pain, muscle stiffness, and fatigue that can significantly impair daily function and decrease functional capacity, with social isolation as an aftermath. For instance, rheumatoid arthritis patients will often have comorbid anxiety, which exacerbates the physical symptoms and creates a vicious pain-emotion cycle; in others, this manifests in greater functional disability and increased disease activity (Blaney, 2021). Further, the prevalence of comorbid illnesses, such as cardiovascular diseases among elderly patients, underscores a key need for comprehensive care strategies that aim to minimize risks because the complications not only aggravate the disease condition but also contribute to disability and morbidity (Kisenge, 2011). Treatment of such multifaceted symptoms via personalized intervention is crucial for enhancing the overall health of patients across age groups affected by rheumatic conditions.

4.4.5. Treatment Considerations and Polypharmacy

Treatment of the rheumatic diseases, particularly in older persons, entails vigilant attention to treatment regimens due to the common issue of polypharmacy. Polypharmacy, the concomitant administration of more than one medication, can be an encouragement of increased health hazard, especially in the elderly, who often have multiple comorbid conditions , such as diabetes. Diabetic elderly are found to have a much greater incidence of polypharmacy (41.1% as against 14.8% in the non-diabetic) and this increases the complexity of the treatment regimen for minimizing rheumatic symptoms with fewer adverse effects (Huang et al., 2022). Moreover, the introduction of new therapeutic drugs like belimumab for treating conditions , such as systemic lupus erythematosus signifies the continued advancement in treatments offered; however, balancing such therapies against existing medication use is still crucial (Castro et al., 2017). Thus, doctors ought to adopt a patient-centered model that thoroughly evaluates the safety and benefits of polypharmacy in treating rheumatic disorders across various age groups (Figure 4.17).

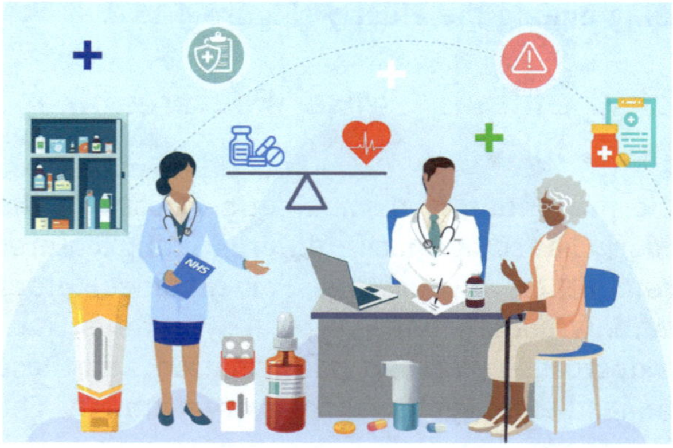

Figure 4.17. Polypharmacy, defined as the concurrent use of multiple medications, can lead to increased health risks, especially among older adults who often manage multiple comorbidities , such as diabetes.

Source: https://coreprescribingsolutions.co.uk/wp-content/uploads/2024/01/MANAGING-POLYPHARMACY-IN-ELDERLY-CARE-scaled.jpg.

4.4.6. Role of Caregivers in Management

Caregivers' roles in the management of patients with rheumatic disease are significant in light of the various clinical presentations across all ages. Caregivers not only aid in daily routine management but also play an essential part in symptom observation and treatment adherence. Involvement by a caregiver is important in identifying early complications that are highly variable in children and aged adults. Kawasaki disease, a disorder prevalent in young people, has a tendency to present typical features , such as persistent fever and conjunctivitis, and thus, some special care measures are essential (Colmegna et al., 2024). In comparison, the older patient may face challenges brought about by comorbid conditions as well as the complexity of polypharmacy, making it critical for caregivers to adjust their approach based on the patient's age and needs (Dodd et al., 2022). It is therefore important to create an environment that enables caregivers to facilitate better outcomes for patients with rheumatic diseases.

4.4.7. Importance of Multidisciplinary Approaches

In the management of the clinical features of rheumatic diseases across all ages, the multifaceted intervention cannot be emphasized enough. The rheumatic diseases occur differently in every age group of patients and thus demand an array of expertise to implement effective intervention management. Multidisciplinary team members consisting of rheumatologists, family practitioners, physical therapists, and mental health professionals offer a comprehensive assessment of what the patient needs. This kind of approach is particularly critical in the prevention of potentially avoidable hospitalizations (PAHs), which are regarded by the Australian Institute of Health and Welfare as avoidable through proper care (Anikeeva et al., 2012). Moreover, the application of focused intervention programs relying on a multidisciplinary model has proven effective in reducing PAHs and emergency department presentations, especially among vulnerable populations , such as Indigenous Australians and individuals who face socioeconomic adversity (Bywood et al., 2016). Therefore, developing a team healthcare culture is essential to optimize the outcomes for patients with rheumatic diseases over the course of their lifetime (Figure 4.18).

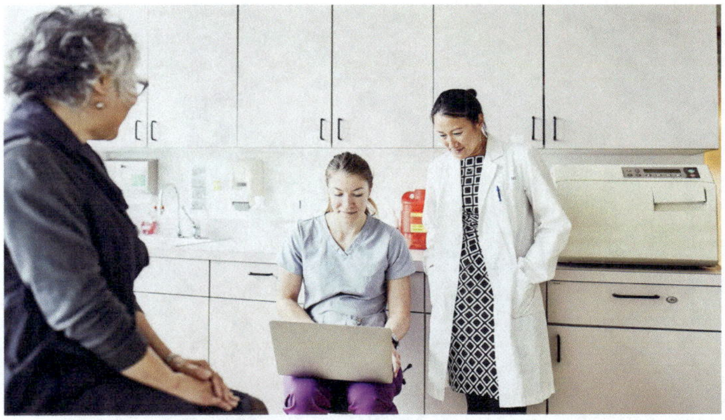

Figure 4.18. Rheumatic conditions often manifest differently depending on the age of the patient, necessitating diverse expertise to tailor effective management strategies.

Source: https://images.everydayhealth.com/images/news/ra-undertreated-in-adults-65-and-over-1440x810.jpg?sfvrsn=7c2f142d_5.

4.4.8. Psychological Effects of Chronic Illness in the Elderly

The psychological effect of chronic disease in the elderly population also raises significant issues that can worsen physical health conditions and impair overall quality of life. Chronic diseases , such as rheumatoid arthritis and osteoarthritis, are prevalent in older adults and frequently lead to comorbid psychiatric disorders , such as depression and anxiety. For instance, research indicates that anxiety is very common among rheumatic patients and has a detrimental impact on functional ability and pain severity, thus creating a cycle of escalating health effects (Blaney, 2021). Similarly, increasing age, body mass index, and comorbidities are variables that have important parts to play in the characterization of levels of physical activity within this population, again testifying to the interconnectedness of mental and physical well-being (Bramble et al., 2019). Formulating effective interventions to optimize mental as much as physical health in the elderly with chronic illness involves comprehending these psychological effects.

4.4.9. Future Directions for Research and Care

Advancing future treatment and research in rheumatic diseases requires a multimodal approach, particularly with the incorporation of age-related clinical presentations. As clinical manifestations and prognosis can widely differ among various ages, studies need to include heterogeneous populations in order to ascertain patterns and responses by age. For instance, understanding the prevalence of neuropsychiatric symptoms in younger systemic lupus erythematosus patients, such as those reported among the Pakistani population, where 84% of the people suffered from these issues, indicates a place of need for interventions (Adil et al., 2024). Besides, the inclusion of management of mental health, including the high percentage of anxiety among rheumatoid arthritis patients and its negative effect on general health, could enhance treatment intervention (Blaney, 2021). By embracing a biopsychosocial approach to care involving psychological support as well as standard biomedical therapies, doctors can optimize patient outcomes and tailor approaches to the unique needs of various age groups with rheumatic diseases (Figure 4.19).

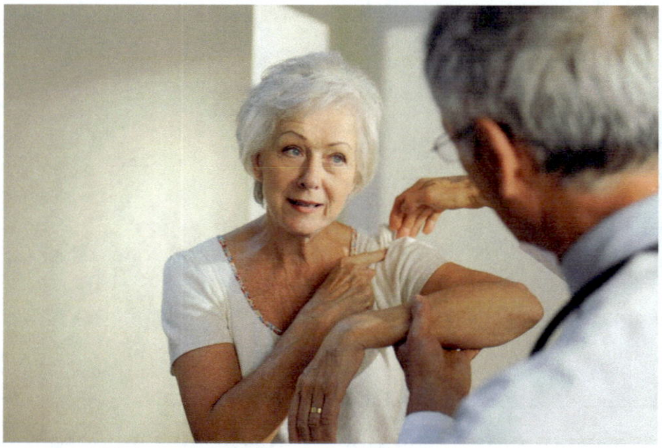

Figure 4.19. Advancing future research and care in rheumatic diseases requires a multifaceted approach, particularly addressing the distinct clinical presentations characterized by age.

Source: https://www.chihealth.com/content/dam/chihealthcom/images/services/shoulderpain.jpg/_jcr_content/renditions/cq5dam.web.1440.959.jpeg.

Test Your Knowledge

1. What rheumatic diseases can be presented atypically in the elderly and mimic infections or malignancies?
2. How is osteoporosis entwined with inflammatory rheumatologic disease in the geriatric age group?

Summary

In summarizing the review of clinical presentation of rheumatologic diseases in various age groups, what appears is that presentation and severity of the diseases are under the dominion of the patient's stage of development. The observations attest to notable age-related differences in symptoms, diagnostic challenges, and sensitivity to therapy. For instance, younger groups have less specific symptoms and must be interpreted very carefully lest the diagnosis be missed, while those from older patients are more intense and multifaceted due to comorbidities. Clinicians need to understand these nuances if they are to respond appropriately. In addition, similar patterns in other illnesses, such as heart complications within various age groups, demonstrate the significance of general, age-based treatment strategies (Gauhar et al., 2025; Zhou et al., 2025). Knowledge of such variations will enable medical doctors to enhance diagnostic accuracy and optimize management among rheumatic disease patients.

Clinical presentation of rheumatoid disease among different age groups, in a study, outlines patterns and resemblances that significantly impact healthcare routines as follows: hypertension, congestive heart failure, and left ventricular hypertrophy are common in older patients, which account for important morbidity and necessitate screening even in non-cardiovascular complaints (Kisenge, 2011). Conversely, in children, the presence of testing tools like pGALSplus reflects the need for accurate diagnosis of severe musculoskeletal issues. It is designed to enhance clinical assessment and decision-making for practitioners, and subsequently, prompt referrals to specialists (Foster et al., 2024). All these findings emphasize the necessity for age-specific interventions in the diagnosis and management of rheumatic disorders, for the improvement of patient health and well-suited health care interventions throughout life.

KEY TERMS FROM THIS CHAPTER

- Rheumatic heart disease
- Evaluation
- Antinuclear antibody (ANA)
- Knowledge
- Treatment
- Fatigue
- Joint deformity
- Osteopenia
- Cardiovascular diseases
- Clinical management
- Acute Rheumatic Fever (ARF)
- Diagnosis
- Juvenile idiopathic arthritis (JIA)
- Disability
- Puberty
- Corticosteroids

Critical Thinking Questions

1. **Which of the following is the most frequent chronic rheumatic disease in children?**
   a. Systemic lupus erythematosus (SLE)
   b. Rheumatoid arthritis
   c. Juvenile idiopathic arthritis (JIA)
   d. Psoriatic arthritis
2. **A 5-year-old child has morning stiffness, joint swelling, and reduced motion lasting more than 6 weeks. The diagnosis most likely is:**
   a. Osteoarthritis
   b. Juvenile idiopathic arthritis
   c. Growing pains
   d. Rheumatic fever
3. **In elderly people, polymyalgia rheumatica most often is characterized by:**
   a. Swollen ankles and knees
   b. Weakness and rash of muscles
   c. Shoulder and hip pain and stiffness, particularly upon arising in the morning
   d. Migratory joint pain and fever
4. **Which rheumatic condition commonly affects adolescent females with photosensitivity, oral ulcers, and positive ANA test?**
   a. Rheumatic fever
   b. Systemic lupus erythematosus
   c. Psoriatic arthritis
   d. Fibromyalgia
5. **Rheumatic fever is most commonly seen in which age group?**
   a. Infants under 1 year
   b. Children aged 5–15 years
   c. Adults aged 30–50 years
   d. Elderly over 65

Short Answer Questions

1. What are the typical manifestations of juvenile idiopathic arthritis (JIA)?
2. How is systemic JIA different from oligoarticular JIA in terms of clinical presentation and prognosis?
3. What are the typical early manifestations of systemic lupus erythematosus (SLE) in young adults?
4. How does ankylosing spondylitis usually present in this age group?
5. How does rheumatoid arthritis usually present in middle-aged patients?
6. What are the differences between seropositive and seronegative RA in clinical presentation?
7. What are the characteristic signs and symptoms of polymyalgia rheumatica (PMR)?
8. How does giant cell arteritis (GCA) usually present in older patients?

Answers to Critical Thinking Questions

1. (c); 2. (b); 3. (c); 4. (b); 5. (b)

References

1. Puzanov, I., Diab, A., Abdallah, K., Bingham, C. O., 3rd, Brogdon, C., Dadu, R., Hamad, L., Kim, S., Lacouture, M. E., LeBoeuf, N. R., Lenihan, D., Onofrei, C., Shannon, V., Sharma, R., Silk, A. W., Skondra, D., Suarez-Almazor, M. E., Wang, Y., Wiley, K., Kaufman, H. L., ... Society for Immunotherapy of Cancer Toxicity Management Working Group (2017). Managing toxicities associated with immune checkpoint inhibitors: consensus recommendations from the Society for Immunotherapy of Cancer (SITC) Toxicity Management Working Group. *Journal for immunotherapy of cancer*, *5*(1), 95. https://doi.org/10.1186/s40425-017-0300-z(accessed on 17th June 2025).
2. Hahn, Y. S., & Kim, J. G. (2010). Pathogenesis and clinical manifestations of juvenile rheumatoid arthritis. *Korean journal of pediatrics*, *53*(11), 921–930. https://doi.org/10.3345/kjp.2010.53.11.921 (accessed on 17th June 2025).
3. Ralli, M., D'Aguanno, V., Di Stadio, A., De Virgilio, A., Croce, A., Longo, L., Greco, A., & de Vincentiis, M. (2018). Audiovestibular Symptoms in Systemic Autoimmune Diseases. *Journal of immunology research*, *2018*, 5798103. https://doi.org/10.1155/2018/5798103 (accessed on 17th June 2025).
4. Adil, M. H., Malik, J., Manzoor, M. S., Maqbool, A., et al. (2024). Varied presentations of patients with systemic lupus erythematosus–What makes Pakistani lupus patients different. https://core.ac.uk/download/616940553.pdf (accessed on 17th June 2025).
5. Ahwireng, N., Bradford, C. M., Ciurtin, C., Gandhi, R., et al. (2021). Stratification of patients with Sjögren's syndrome and patients with systemic lupus erythematosus according to two shared immune cell signatures, with potential therapeutic implications. https://core.ac.uk/download/388714770.pdf (accessed on 17th June 2025).
6. Anikeeva, O., Brown, L., Butler, C., Bywood, P., et al. (2012). Potentially avoidable hospitalizations in Australia: Causes for hospitalizations and primary health care interventions. https://core.ac.uk/download/14947500.pdf (accessed on 17th June 2025).
7. Phillips, R., Williams, D., Bowen, D., Morris, D., Grant, A., Pell, B., Sanders, J., Taylor, A., Choy, E., & Edwards, A. (2018). Reaching a consensus on research priorities for supporting women with autoimmune rheumatic diseases during pre-conception, pregnancy and early parenting: A Nominal Group Technique exercise with lay and professional stakeholders. *Wellcome open research*, *3*, 75. https://doi.org/10.12688/wellcomeopenres.14658.1 (accessed on 17th June 2025).
8. Bakker, M., Boonman, D. C. G., de Vries-vander Zwan, H. M., Hoekman, R., et al. (2004). A system of networks and continuing education for physical therapists in rheumatology: A feasibility study. https://core.ac.uk/download/pdf/3896213.pdf (accessed on 17th June 2025).
9. Balanescu, A., Gwinnutt, J. M., Rodríguez Carrio, J., Wieczorek, M., et al. (2022). 2021 EULAR recommendations regarding lifestyle behaviors and work participation to prevent progression of rheumatic and musculoskeletal diseases. https://core.ac.uk/download/635115938.pdf (accessed on 17th June 2025).
10. Barnett, T. C., Bennett, J., Benothman, R., Bosco, J., et al. (2021). Searching for a technology-driven acute rheumatic fever test: The START study protocol. https://core.ac.uk/download/479568187.pdf (accessed on 17th June 2025).

11. Battini, R., Bonuccelli, A., Consolini, R., Cordelli, D. M., Costagliola, G., D'Elios, S., De Benedetti, F., et al. (2024). Management, treatment, and clinical approach of Sydenham's chorea in children: Italian survey on expert-based experience. https://core.ac.uk/download/638785235.pdf (accessed on 17th June 2025).

12. Blaney, C. (2021). Anxiety in rheumatoid arthritis (RA): Support for a biopsychosocial approach to the management of RA. A Thesis submitted to the Faculty of Graduate Studies of The University of Manitoba In partial fulfillment of the requirements of the degree of DOCTOR OF PHILOSOPHY Department of Psychology University of Manitoba Winnipeg https://core.ac.uk/download/644027821.pdf (accessed on 17th June 2025).

13. Bolland, W., Cherepanov, P., Ciurtin, C., Cornish, T., et al. (2021). Favorable antibody responses to human coronaviruses in children and adolescents with autoimmune rheumatic diseases. https://core.ac.uk/download/477692348.pdf (accessed on 17th June 2025).

14. Bramble, L. A. A. (2019). Physical activity in adults with knee osteoarthritis. https://core.ac.uk/download/210999746.pdf (accessed on 17th June 2025).

15. Bywood, P. T., Erny-Albrecht, K., & Oliver-Baxter, J. (2016). Primary health care-based programmes targeting potentially avoidable hospitalizations in vulnerable groups with chronic disease. https://core.ac.uk/download/43335684.pdf (accessed on 17th June 2025).

16. Casellas Jordá, F., de Toro, J., FusterRuizdeApodaca, M. J., Galindo, A., et al. (2019). Healthcare experience and their relationship with demographic, disease and healthcare-related variables: A cross-sectional survey of patients with chronic diseases using the IEXPAC scale. https://core.ac.uk/download/420060470.pdf (accessed on 17th June 2025).

17. Chiang, B. L., Lee, J. H., Lin, Y. T., Sun, Y., et al. (2015). Juvenile dermatomyositis: A 20-year retrospective analysis of treatment and clinical outcomes. https://core.ac.uk/download/pdf/82409744.pdf (accessed on 17th June 2025).

18. Colmegna, L., Migowa, A., Ngwiri, T., Njeri, E., et al. (2024). Kawasaki disease in Kenya and review of the African literature. https://core.ac.uk/download/613050848.pdf (accessed on 17th June 2025).

19. de Loizaga, S. R., & Gokanapudy Hahn, L. R. (2021). Rheumatic heart disease in the United States: Forgotten but not gone: Results of a 10-year multicenter review. https://core.ac.uk/download/480388854.pdf (accessed on 17th June 2025).

20. Dodd, R., John, R., Kafoa, B., Lung, T., et al. (2022). Promoting evidence-based policies, programs and services for ageing and health in Fiji. https://unsworks.unsw.edu.au/bitstreams/11b611fa-7e97-404d-b303-6eb541a2948a/download (accessed on 17th June 2025).

21. Eglite, J., Gardovska, D., Shantere, R., Sochnevs, A., et al. (2003). HLA class II associations with rheumatic heart disease among clinically homogeneous patients in children in Latvia. https://core.ac.uk/download/pdf/3405302.pdf (accessed on 17th June 2025).

22. Eichenfield, A. H., Rosenberg, A. M., Lee, A. N., Cabral, D. A., Saulsbury, F. T., Cuesta, I., Mauldin, J., et al. (2008). Commentary–Ordering lab tests for suspected rheumatic disease. https://core.ac.uk/download/pdf/8218733.pdf (accessed on 17th June 2025).

23. Foster, H. E., Guglieri, M., Jandial, S., Jones, S. A., Mercer, V., Parr, J. R., & Smith, N. (2024). The development of pGALSplus: Evaluating feasibility and acceptability of an assessment to facilitate the identification and triage of children with musculoskeletal presentations. https://core.ac.uk/download/615278835.pdf (accessed on 17th June 2025).

24. Fritzler, J. (2018). Incidence, clinical manifestations and risk factors of acute rheumatic fever: A systematic review and meta-analysis of the global perspective. https://core.ac.uk/download/220123811.pdf (accessed on 17th June 2025).
25. Gauhar, T. M., Mahmud, T., Khanum, R., Khan, S. U., Ahmed, W., & Jutt, N. (2025). Breast lump patterns across different age groups among female patients presenting to surgical outpatient department of a tertiary care hospital in District Malir Karachi. *Pakistan Journal of Health Sciences*. https://www.semanticscholar.org/paper/f24ba5020d6461d5130eb7c2079d701dc6ce828b (accessed on 17th June 2025).
26. Giancane, G. (2019). Pharmacovigilance in juvenile idiopathic arthritis patients (Pharmachild) treated with biologic agents and/or methotrexate. A Pediatric Rheumatology International Trials Organization (PRINTO)/Pediatric Rheumatology European Society (PRES) registry. https://core.ac.uk/download/201719507.pdf (accessed on 17th June 2025).
27. Murphy, D. L., Timpano, K. R., Wheaton, M. G., Greenberg, B. D., & Miguel, E. C. (2010). Obsessive-compulsive disorder and its related disorders: a reappraisal of obsessive-compulsive spectrum concepts. *Dialogues in clinical neuroscience, 12*(2), 131–148. https://doi.org/10.31887/DCNS.2010.12.2/dmurphy (accessed on 17th June 2025).
28. Guerreiro Castro, S., & Isenberg, D. (2017). Belimumab in systemic lupus erythematosus (SLE): Evidence-to-date and clinical usefulness. https://core.ac.uk/download/83113624.pdf (accessed on 17th June 2025).
29. Hanly, J. G., Skedgel, C., & Thompson, K. (2015). The use of administrative health care databases to identify patients with rheumatoid arthritis. https://core.ac.uk/download/41991036.pdf (accessed on 17th June 2025).
30. Huang, Y. T. (2022). Polypharmacy in older adults–prevalence, risk factors, and associations with mortality–and the role of diabetes. https://core.ac.uk/download/519717468.pdf (accessed on 17th June 2025).
31. Kisenge, P. R. (2011). Pattern of cardiovascular diseases among elderly patients admitted in medical wards at Muhimbili National Hospital Dar es Salaam, Tanzania. Kisenge, Peter R (Muhimbili University of Health and Allied Sciences, 2011). https://core.ac.uk/download/pdf/16666639.pdf (accessed on 17th June 2025).
32. Lala, V. G. (1996). Comorbidities in Black South Africans with rheumatoid arthritis. https://core.ac.uk/download/pdf/188770619.pdf (accessed on 17th June 2025).
33. Livermore, P. (2021). Understanding the lived experience and psychosocial needs of children and young people with juvenile dermatomyositis: A mixed methods study. https://core.ac.uk/download/390094302.pdf (accessed on 17th June 2025).
34. Mok, T. M. Y. (2014). Immunosuppressants in systemic lupus erythematosus–Treatment options and potential toxicity. https://core.ac.uk/download/38055590.pdf (accessed on 17th June 2025).
35. Thomson Mangnall, L. J. (2017). Outcomes of adolescents and younger adults who have mechanical valve replacement surgery for rheumatic heart disease in a low-middle-income country. https://core.ac.uk/download/212692600.pdf (accessed on 17th June 2025).
36. Zhou, Z., Qiu, M., Zhang, R., Li, Y., Tian, M., Tu, J., Han, L., et al. (2025). Clinical features of non-compaction cardiomyopathy across age groups: A retrospective study of 415 patients. *Open Heart, 12*. https://www.semanticscholar.org/paper/b273386e07bd6bcb854968649d1685977ede5039 (accessed on 17th June 2025).

CLINICAL EVALUATION OF THE RHEUMATOLOGIC PATIENT

5

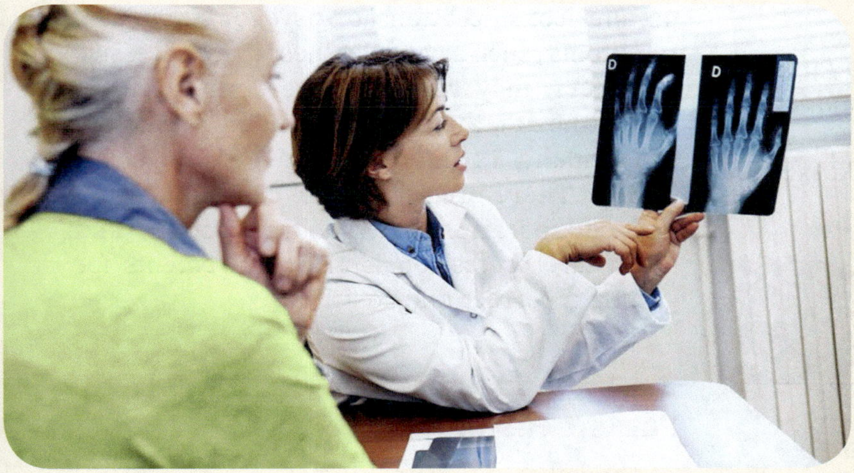

LEARNING OBJECTIVES

After studying this chapter, you will be able to:

1. Identify patient history and symptoms;
2. Understand physical examination techniques;
3. Define laboratory and imaging tests;
4. Define differential diagnosis and treatment.

Introduction

Clinical evaluation of rheumatologic patients is a multimodal process that involves clinical assessment as well as advanced imaging techniques to make the right diagnosis and monitor therapy. Upstream developments in magnetic resonance imaging (MRI) and musculoskeletal ultrasonography (US) have revolutionized the ability to quantify cartilage thickness and disease activity, facilitating greater assessment of treatment response (Barbulescu et al., 2019). Furthermore, multicenter registries and biobanks for individual rare diseases , such as juvenile idiopathic inflammatory myopathies, point toward the benefit of cooperative study in promoting knowledge and outcome. Such studies provide valuable information that may be utilized to guide treatment regimens and pathophysiology of diseases (Bohan et al., 2011). As rheumatologic diseases often present with multifaceted symptoms affecting multiple systems, it is a must to provide a detailed evaluation in order to devise effective management strategies that are tailored to individual patient needs (Figure 5.1).

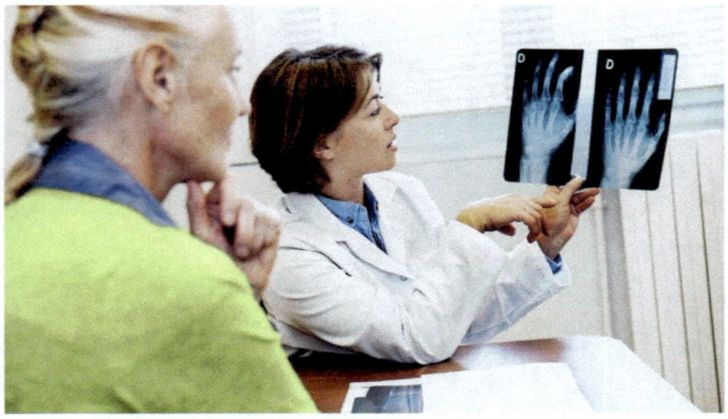

Figure 5.1. Clinical evaluation of rheumatologic patients.

Source: https://i0.wp.com/post.medicalnewstoday.com/wp-content/uploads/sites/3/2021/11/rheumatologist_diagnose_GettyImages697568781_Header-1-1024x575.jpg?w=1155&h=1528.

5.1. Patient History and Symptoms

Learning Outcome

1. Understand the importance of comprehensive patient history;
2. Identify presenting symptoms in rheumatologic patients;
3. Highlight duration and nature of symptoms;
4. Describe the family history of rheumatologic diseases;
5. Take note of the impact of symptoms on daily living;
6. Take note of previous treatments and response thereto;
7. Discuss accompaniment of systemic symptoms;
8. Review of medications and drug allergies;
9. Identify environmental and social determinants.

Perception of patient history and symptoms is important in clinical evaluation of rheumatologic patients due to the fact that it serves as the foundation for accurate diagnosis and treatment. A complete history must cover not just the patients' current symptoms, for example, joint pain or tiredness, but their history, including past conditions or previous rheumatologic diagnoses. It is this method that enables physicians to differentiate between similar presentations of dissimilar disorders. For instance, in the evaluation of Sjögren's syndrome symptoms in patients treated with immune checkpoint inhibitors, most importantly, one must perform a proper examination and the respective diagnostic tests, such as salivary and lacrimal gland function (Karagodina et al., 2023). Furthermore, parallel considerations of psychopathological symptoms , such as hopelessness and depressive disorders, may reveal greater intricacies in patient health, thereby emphasizing predictors of suicidality in this group (Riera-Serra et al., 2023). Therefore, effective communication and collaboration between the patient and healthcare professionals are requirements for getting a correct diagnosis.

5.1.1. Importance of Comprehensive Patient History

A thorough patient history is of critical significance during the clinical evaluation of rheumatologic patients because it enables professionals to tailor their examinations and develop appropriate management plans. A complete history not only involves the patients' current symptoms but also addresses their past clinical experience, family background, and psychosocial factors potentially influencing their condition. For instance, an appreciation of the severity of patients' pain and fatigue will enable in a position to distinguish fibromyalgia from other rheumatologic diseases, backed by evidence that there is overwhelmingly impaired quality of life among children with fibromyalgia compared to children with other diseases (Burwinkle et al., 2007). Further, the incorporation of patient-reported outcome measures (PROMs) into the evaluation process, as a case in point in one study of psoriatic arthritis, also underscores the worth of subjective information in assessing impact on disease and formulating treatment plans that optimize overall patient well-being (Argano et al., 2024). As such, a thorough patient history is the foundation of effective rheumatologic practice (Figure 5.2).

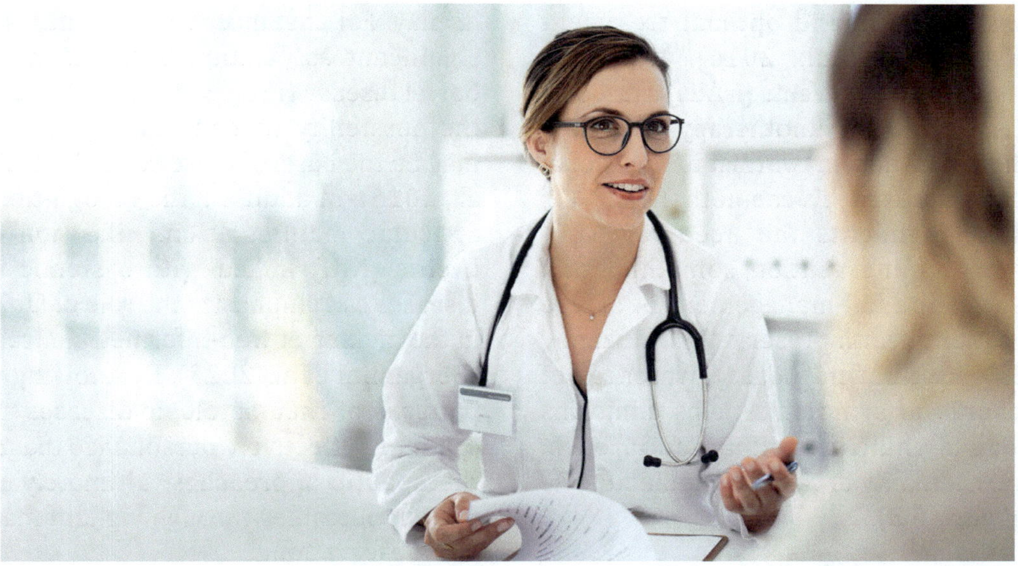

Figure 5.2. Capturing a detailed history not only includes the patient's current symptoms but also delves into their past medical history, family background, and psychosocial factors that may influence their condition.

Source: https://s7d9.scene7.com/is/image/labcorp/GettyImages-1207212199-1201x658-ab13ae9%20(2).

5.1.2. Common Symptoms in Rheumatologic Patients

The clinical examination of the rheumatologic patients usually starts with a complete assessment of common symptoms, which could reveal underlying musculoskeletal diseases. Patients typically present with joint pain and stiffness, which are classic features of inflammatory processes. Additionally, malaise and fatigue may accompany joint symptoms and reflect systemic disease, thus affecting patients' quality of life. Swelling and tenderness in affected joints are also valuable diagnostic clues, making clinicians consider particular rheumatologic diseases. Finally, the time pattern of symptoms, i.e., how they begin and change over time, may be highly helpful in differential diagnosis. The addition of diagnostic decision support software (DDSS) has also been promising to enhance non-specialist accuracy, reducing error by 28%–15% with support (Athreya et al., 2016). Also, consensus guidelines emphasize the evaluation of symptoms, including reaction to therapies like Spa therapy for musculoskeletal pathology, in ideally managing these complex diseases (Paoloni et al., 2017).

5.1.3. Duration and Pattern of Symptoms

The symptom pattern and duration in rheumatologic patients are particularly significant in diagnosis and treatment. The symptoms tend to come and go in cycles, with flares of pain followed by periods of remission, making it a complicated clinical scenario. For instance, chronic conditions , such as spondyloarthritis (SpA) have a heterogeneous pattern of symptoms, both peripheral and axial, that demand careful and detailed assessment to avoid misdiagnosis and optimal treatment planning (Ascolani et al., 2016). Moreover, immune-related adverse events (irAEs) caused by therapies, especially immunotherapy, are of late onset and long duration, in contrast to traditional adverse effects caused by chemotherapy. This characteristic highlights the need for early identification and intervention, something that is essential for optimal management of severe irAEs and patient health preservation (Puzanov et al., 2017). Last but not least, awareness of the time course of symptoms helps clinicians individualize a multidisciplinary approach, maximizing the quality of care for rheumatologic patients (Figure 5.3).

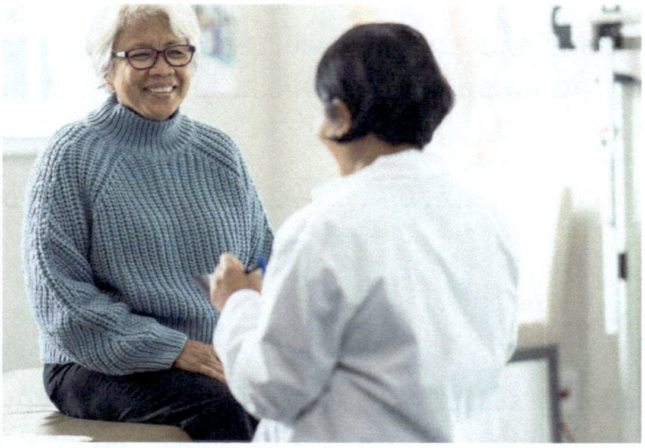

Figure 5.3. Symptoms often manifest in phases, with periods of exacerbation followed by remission, complicating the clinical picture.

Source: https://www.hss.edu/images/socialmedia/doctor-visit_1200x630.jpg.

5.1.4. Family History of Rheumatologic Diseases

Systematic questioning of a patient's family history is crucial in clinical evaluation of patients with rheumatology because it may reveal an inherited basis for most autoimmune and inflammatory conditions. When there are multiple cases of rheumatologic diseases among family members, the likelihood of relatives having the same conditions is quite significant, indicating potential genetic and environmental factors at play. For instance, evidence has indicated a significant association between inflammatory bowel disease (IBD) and spondyloarthritis, with the possibility that the same pathophysiology may be the basis of these conditions (Ascolani et al., 2016). In addition, the recognition of extra-articular manifestations like non-infectious uveitis (NIU) linked with systemic rheumatic diseases can emphasize the role of family history in the making of well-informed clinical decisions (Bergamini et al., 2023). By knowing the family patterns of rheumatologic diseases, physicians can more effectively personalize diagnostic and therapeutic approaches, ultimately improving patient outcomes through vigilant management and observation.

5.1.5. Impact of Symptoms on Daily Life

Symptoms of rheumatologic diseases can directly affect the daily lives of patients, not just their physical condition, but also their mental state and quality of life. Most patients present disabling symptoms , such as pain, tiredness, and sleep disorders that can hinder them from performing daily activities and social interaction. In primary Sjögren's syndrome, for instance, sleep disorder has been correlated with impaired quality of life, highlighting the importance of sleep disorder in disease management (Antonazzo et al., 2016). Moreover, the incidence of immune-related adverse events in diseases that are being treated with immunotherapies poses a delicate dimension of symptom management since they can lead to severe and, in some cases, life-threatening health conditions, and prompt identification and timely response are required (Puzanov et al., 2017). Therefore, it is necessary to understand the multi-dimensional impact of such symptoms during the clinical evaluation of rheumatologic patients so that treatment protocols may become more comprehensive in nature and responsive (Figure 5.4).

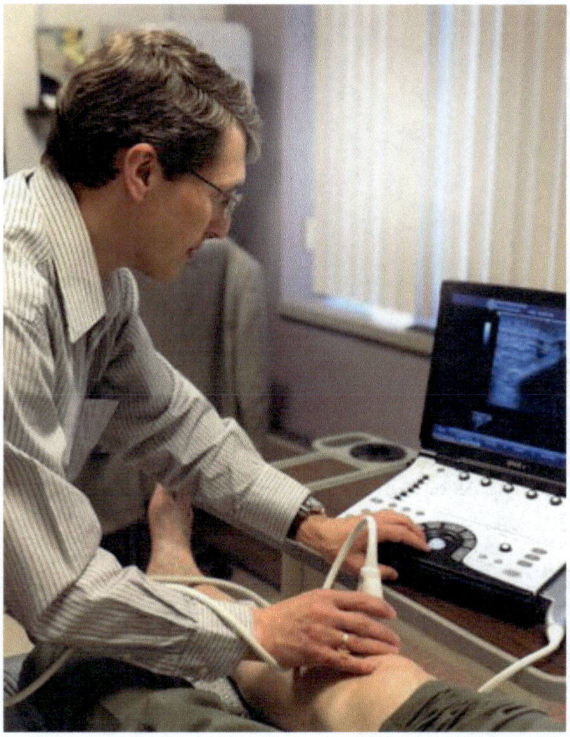

Figure 5.4. Many patients experience debilitating symptoms , such as pain, fatigue, and sleep disturbances, which can hinder their ability to perform routine activities and maintain social relationships.

Source: https://www.healio.com/~/media/images/news/print/healio-rheumatology/2019/07_july/kissin_eugene.jpg.

5.1.6. Previous Treatments and Responses

Past responses and therapy are crucial when evaluating rheumatologic patients in guiding effective clinical measures. Patients have been traditionally treated with disease-modifying antirheumatic drugs (DMARDs) and nonsteroidal anti-inflammatory drugs (NSAIDs) with variable success. More recently, the use of biologics has transformed paradigms for treatment, particularly in cases of acute inflammation or failure of conventional therapy. For instance, anti-IL-1 and anti-IL-6 therapies were found to be successful in avoiding cytokine storms in infections-complicated conditions , such as COVID-19, where an highly calibrated immune response is imperative (Ansari et al., 2020). In addition, new technologies , such as SpA therapy have also found consensus from experts regarding being effective for the treatment of musculoskeletal disorders and for speeding up patient recovery (Paoloni et al., 2017). Therefore, previous treatment histories not only influence clinical management but also highlight the dynamic character of therapy in rheumatology.

5.1.7. Associated Systemic Symptoms

Assessment of rheumatologic patients in the clinic frequently reveals related systemic symptoms that can complicate diagnosis and treatment. The symptoms, such as fatigue, fever, and sleep disturbances, are indicative of basic inflammatory processes. For instance, in primary Sjögren's syndrome, the patients have poor quality of sleep, and this is reflected by a significantly higher PSQI score compared to matched controls, thus depicting the prevalence of daily disturbances and subjective poor quality of sleep in the cohort (Antonazzo et al., 2016).

Not only do they lower the quality of life, but also symptoms may mimic or present in the form of other systemic diseases, and hence the clinical presentation becomes more complicated. Moreover, systemic symptoms can be expressed as immune-related adverse events in patients on therapy like immune checkpoint inhibitors, emphasizing the necessity of vigilant monitoring and multimodal approaches in managing these concomitant symptoms (Puzanov et al., 2017). These systemic symptoms are knowledge that is crucial for complete patient care in rheumatologic practice (Figure 5.5).

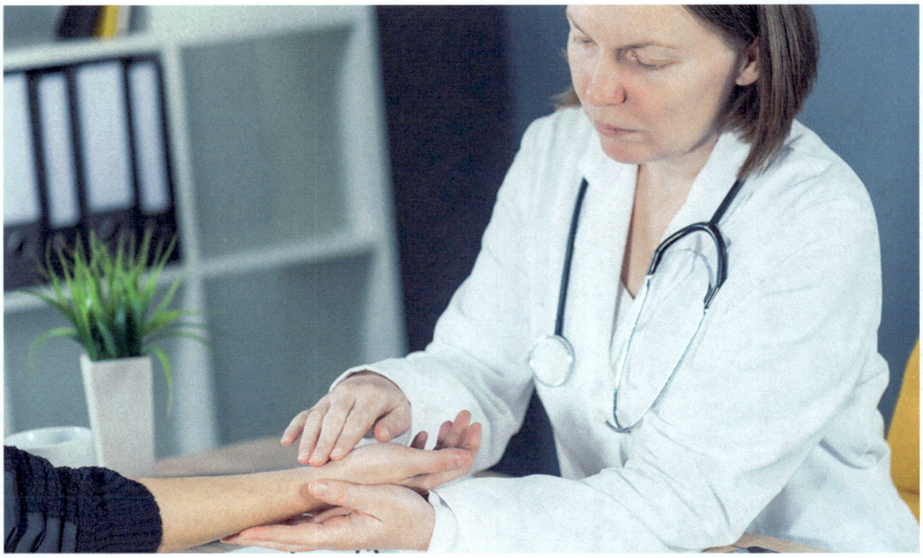

Figure 5.5. The clinical evaluation of rheumatologic patients frequently reveals associated systemic symptoms that can complicate diagnosis and management.

Source: https://www.iinn.com/wp-content/uploads/2024/05/2.jpg.

5.1.8. Review of Medications and Allergies

Comprehensive medication review and allergy evaluation are a critical component of the rheumatologic patient's clinical assessment, directly affecting treatment safety profiles and outcome efficacy. Some of the rheumatologic conditions require the use of immunosuppressives, biologics, and corticosteroids that may interact with a patient's ongoing drugs or exacerbate underlying allergies. For instance, in-depth assessment can detect potential allergic reactions to drugs often given, which in any other case would cause drug-side effects (Ferenz et al., 2021). In addition, knowledge of the patient's drug history is essential in the detection of response and resistance patterns of treatment, thus facilitating the tailoring of more efficient therapeutic regimens (Businger et al., 2014). Thus, clinicians would do well to prioritize a systematic method of drug and allergy reviews in a bid to enhance patient outcomes as well as minimize complications. This practice not only enhances evidence-based clinical decision-making but also encourages patient involvement in care management.

5.1.9. Social and Environmental Factors

Environmental and social factors are a critical component of the clinical evaluation of rheumatologic patients, particularly as they pertain to gaining an understanding of their level of physical activity and overall health. Evidence has indicated that young people and children with juvenile idiopathic arthritis (JIA) are likely not to meet the World Health Organization's guidelines for physical activity, and significant differences have been found depending on gender and disease category (Berendes et al., 2024). This demonstrates that clinicians should consider the social environment in which such patients are living since family support, peer interaction, and socioeconomic status are strong predictors of taking part in physical activity. In addition, dietary habits have emerged as yet another social determinant of health outcomes; emerging evidence suggests a potential relationship between acne vulgaris, an illness potentially disrupting the compliance of rheumatologic patients to therapy and mental health, and food intake, in particular, dairy (Patton, 2016). Thus, effective evaluation of these social determinants can help develop interventions that are maximally patient-centered (Figure 5.6).

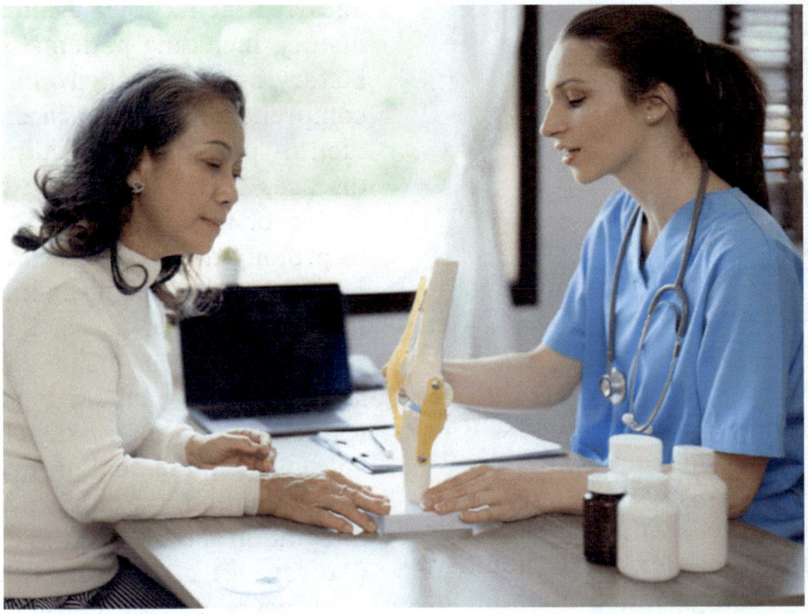

Figure 5.6. Social and environmental factors play a pivotal role in the clinical evaluation of rheumatologic patients, particularly in understanding their physical activity levels and overall health.

Source: https://orthopedicnj.com/attachments/News/169/gallery/what-is-a-rheumatologist_thumb-detail.png.

Test Your Knowledge

1. Why is morning stiffness significant, and how is morning stiffness duration utilized in diagnosis?
2. What family history is critical in risk determination for rheumatic or autoimmune disease?

5.2. Physical Examination Techniques

Learning Outcome

1. Know general patient assessment;
2. Focus on joint examination techniques;
3. Define range of motion evaluation;
4. Perform evaluation of swelling and tenderness;
5. Learn skin examination for rashes and lesions;
6. Highlight neurological examination;
7. Define musculoskeletal examination;
8. Recognize vital signs and systemic evaluation;
9. Highlight documentation of observations.

Physical examination is the most important in the clinical evaluation of rheumatologic patients in an effort to reach correct diagnoses and facilitate treatment. This evaluation includes a comprehensive testing for joint mobility, tenderness, and swelling, and evaluation of extra-articular manifestations in accordance with various autoimmune disorders.

For instance, co-occurrence of SpA and IBD emphasizes the need for a specific multidisciplinary approach, because arthralgia in these patients can also significantly benefit from rheumatological consultation and timely treatment, including reduction of diagnostic delay due to such comorbidities (Ascolani et al., 2016). Additionally, diseases like fibromyalgia require specific methods of examination in order to differentiate them from other rheumatologic disorders, employing sophisticated diagnostic aids like ATR-FTIR spectroscopy for non-invasive testing (Carvalho et al., 2020). Thus, applying appropriate physical examination techniques is crucial to ensure improved patient outcomes in rheumatologic practice.

5.2.1. General Assessment of the Patient

Global assessment of the patient is critical in clinical evaluation of rheumatologic disorders because it sets the stage for effective diagnosis and treatment. Total evaluation involves total history, including patients' symptoms, medical history, and socio-environmental features. This comprehensive approach enables clinicians to identify possible risk factors for rheumatologic diseases, such as congestive heart disease or the taking of medications that have been proven to prolong the QTc interval, specifically among patients who are being administered methadone for pain (Brown et al., 2017). Furthermore, the application of diagnostic decision support software has been found to produce a significant reduction in diagnostic errors among non-specialists in the field of rheumatologic disease determination, the implication of which is the integration of technology in clinical examinations (Athreya et al., 2016). With determinations made acutely, medical professionals can enhance their accuracy rate in diagnosis and ultimately improve patient outcomes in the practice of rheumatology (Figure 5.7).

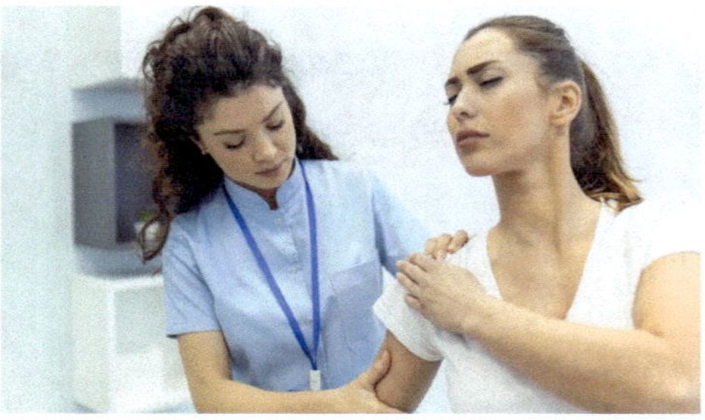

Figure 5.7. A thorough assessment includes a comprehensive history that encompasses the patient's symptoms, medical history, and socio-environmental factors.

5.2.2. Joint Examination Techniques

Appropriate joint examination techniques are crucial components in clinical rheumatologic patient assessment, providing insight regarding the nature and extent of musculoskeletal disease. A thorough physical examination, in addition to advanced imaging modalities , such as musculoskeletal ultrasonography (US) and magnetic resonance imaging (MRI), enables a better evaluation of cartilage integrity and joint involvement. These modalities have revolutionized the assessment of diseases like osteoarthritis, where clinicians can quantify cartilage thickness and evaluate treatment efficacy over time; e.g., US has shown dramatic differences in cartilage thickness following therapy for knee osteoarthritis, which reflects changes not discerned by traditional evaluation (Barbulescu et al., 2019). Besides, in approaching such complex conditions as Enteropathic-related Spondyloarthritis, a multidisciplinary approach combining joint assessments with gastroenterological examinations has proven to enhance diagnostic accuracy and reduce treatment delay, finally offering better patient outcomes (Ascolani et al., 2016).

5.2.3. Assessment of Range of Motion

Comprehensive ROM evaluation is critical for the assessment of rheumatologic patients' functional status as it is directly correlated with their quality of life and being able to perform activities on a daily basis. Clinical evaluation frequently employs the utilization of multiple measures for the evaluation of ROM, one of which is the Signals of Functional Impairment (SOFI) measure, which is routinely employed. However, studies indicate that SOFI may have a reduced responsivity to change detection over time, particularly after surgery for conditions like inflammatory rheumatic disorders (Carswell et al., 2009). It is essential to be aware of the limitations of ROM measurement, especially against the background of an estimated shortfall in rheumatologists, which can exacerbate waiting lists for patients requiring specialist treatment (Layton, 2015). Thus, using multiple measures to provide a full assessment enhances the validity of ROM measurements and, by extension, facilitates enhanced clinical decision-making leading to enhanced patient outcomes (Figure 5.8).

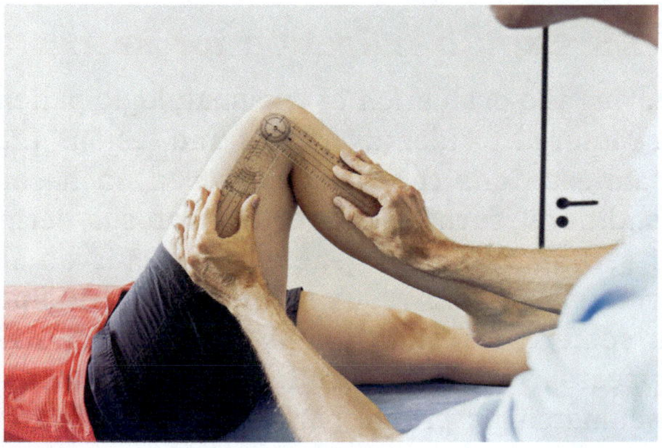

Figure 5.8. Clinical evaluations frequently utilize various instruments to measure ROM, among which the Signals of Functional Impairment (SOFI) tool is commonly employed.

Source: https://www.verywellhealth.com/thmb/owWUJ7QN8t64luEI7m-N7LxE7GQ=/1500x0/filters:no_upscale():max_bytes(150000):strip_icc()/IMG_1113-5890d45b5f9b5874ee6c7ce3.JPG.

5.2.4. Evaluation of Swelling and Tenderness

Swelling and tenderness assessment are significant components of the rheumatologic disease patient's clinical evaluation. Systematic assessment of these symptoms is important because they could be evidence of an underlying disease activity or complication, particularly in conditions , such as rheumatoid arthritis. A thorough musculoskeletal examination that prioritizes the most commonly affected joints, like the wrists and metacarpophalangeal joints, is essential in determining the extent of inflammation and joint involvement. The clinicians need to be vigilant for presentations of immune-related adverse events when patients are on therapies , such as immune checkpoint inhibitors, which can cause joint and soft tissue symptoms in addition to the therapeutic effect (Puzanov et al., 2017). By integrating these evaluations, health care providers can make informative management decisions and modify treatment interventions directed at both swelling and tenderness, ultimately resulting in better patient outcomes.

5.2.5. Skin Examination for Rashes and Lesions

During the evaluation of rheumatologic patients in the clinical setting, a careful skin examination is required to identify rashes and lesions that may indicate hidden systemic diseases. The skin manifestations can be very varied, in harmony with the heterogeneity of the rheumatologic conditions , such as lupus erythematosus, dermatomyositis, or vasculitis. Interestingly, the diagnosis of secondary illness generally depends on skin manifestations, which emphasizes that medical professionals are required to possess an amazing eye for detail while conducting examinations. In some cases, skin lesions may be indicative of viral infection, such as cytomegalovirus, that appears in the form of retinitis in immunocompromised patients and, in addition, complicates the rheumatologic profile (Ardekani et al., 2016). Thus, when incorporating skin assessments with history and laboratory findings, it gives a more comprehensive picture of the patient's health to enable on-time interventions and care plans considering both cutaneous and systemic conditions (Berg et al., 2016) (Figure 5.9).

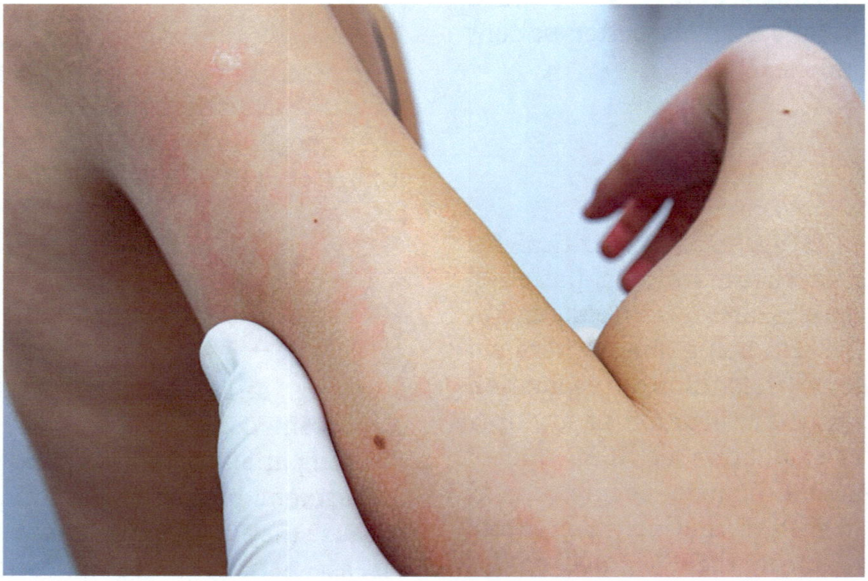

Figure 5.9. In the clinical evaluation of rheumatologic patients, a meticulous skin examination is crucial for identifying rashes and lesions that may indicate underlying systemic conditions.

Source: https://drmaggieyu.com/wp-content/uploads/2023/10/autoimmune-skin-conditions-diagnosis-treatment.jpg.

5.2.6. Neurological Assessment

Neurological examination is necessary in the clinical examination of rheumatologic patients because most autoimmune diseases have serious neurological implications. Cognitive impairment symptoms, peripheral neuropathy, and encephalopathy can be indicative of an underlying systemic disease that needs to be immediately identified and treated. For instance, infusion of monoclonal antibodies like rituximab in the management of rheumatologic disorders is problematic with respect to transfer to breast milk and infant exposure, as indicated by studies reporting trace concentrations in mature breast milk (Anderson et al., 2020). In addition, cancer therapy may cause neurologic adverse events, such as immune-related adverse events, of which neurologic toxicity is one (Brém et al., 2020). Therefore, it not only enhances diagnostic accuracy but also assists in directing the treatment strategy and monitoring for potential complications, ultimately improving the patient's outcome with rheumatologic diseases.

5.2.7. Musculoskeletal Examination

An adequate musculoskeletal examination must be conducted to adequately assess rheumatologic diseases because it provides critical information about the patients' extra-articular and articular findings. The musculoskeletal examination starts with a detailed patient history, such as symptom onset and duration, severity, and functional impairment. The physician then conducts a systematic physical examination, evaluating joint tenderness and swelling, range of motion, and deformities because these symptoms may indicate specific rheumatologic diseases. The significance of this process is also underscored by the prevalence of musculoskeletal symptoms within the population; diseases , such as rheumatoid arthritis, osteoarthritis, and psoriatic arthritis can profoundly influence patients' quality of life. Proper and timely diagnosis hinges on this meticulous examination, so therapeutic management may be targeted accordingly. Appreciation of the diversity of possible musculoskeletal presentations will help clinicians create whole-person management plans that address the unique needs of each patient (Puzanov et al., 2017) (Figure 5.10).

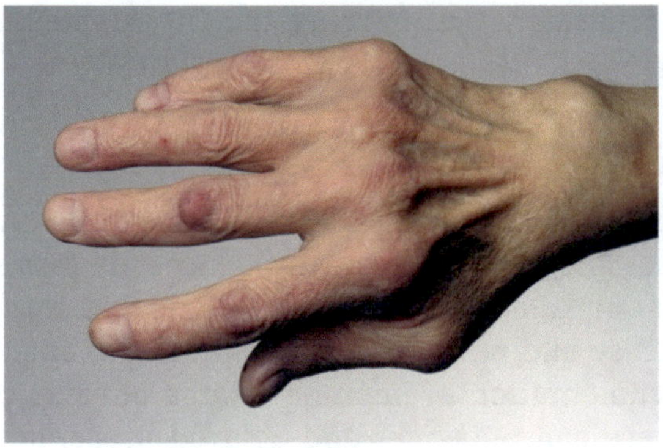

Figure 5.10. An effective musculoskeletal examination is essential for accurately assessing rheumatologic conditions, as it provides critical insights into the patient's articular and extra-articular manifestations.

Source: https://www.rheumatologyadvisor.com/wp-content/uploads/sites/18/2019/01/scisourcess5896resize01_900202.jpg.

5.2.8. Vital Signs and Systemic Evaluation

Vital sign measurement is a critical component of systemic examination in rheumatologic patients, as it indicates the patient's overall well-being and can implicate underlying complications of their illness. An increase in temperature, change in heart rate, or abnormal blood pressure can signal inflammation or infection, which are by no means rare findings in autoimmune patients. Second, a thorough assessment includes meticulous musculoskeletal examination, as emphasized in recent rheumatology textbooks, which supports the identification of localized joint involvement and functional impairment.

Third, monitoring of vital signs typically precedes indicators of disease activity and response to therapy, supporting clinicians in their adjustment of therapeutic intervention accordingly. For instance, in a study of the effectiveness of treatment, significant improvement in inflammatory markers was observed concurrently with enhanced control of vital signs, reinforcing the interdependency of systemic evaluation and clinical outcome in rheumatic diseases (Ayala et al., 2017).

5.2.9. Documentation of Findings

Proper documentation of findings forms an integral part of the rheumatologic patient's clinical assessment, as it directly influences diagnosis, management, and patient outcome. Accurate records not only address the patient's clinical history and presenting symptoms but also the progress of the disease and response to therapy. In patients treated with immunotherapy, for example, meticulous documentation of immune-related adverse events (irAEs) is essential because of their potentially severe consequences and delayed presentation, as underlined by the Society for Immunotherapy of Cancer (Puzanov et al., 2017). In addition, comparative analysis between SLE patients and other systemic rheumatic patients emphasizes the importance of careful documentation of organ dysfunctions and resolution, and in the process, can play an important role in clinical decision-making and management intervention (Azevedo et al., 2011). Ultimately, accurate documentation is a fundamental cornerstone in delivering high-quality, patient-centered care in rheumatology (Figure 5.11).

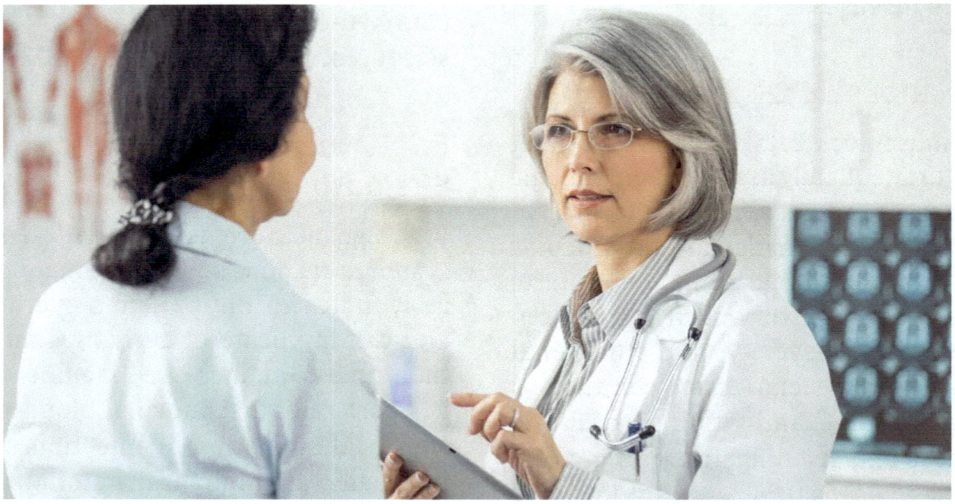

Figure 5.11. Effective documentation of findings is a crucial aspect of the clinical evaluation of rheumatologic patients, as it directly influences diagnosis, treatment decisions, and patient outcomes.

Source: https://cdn.pfizer.com/pfizercom/styles/convert_to_webp/s3/is-it-rheumatoid-arthritis-ask-a-rheumatologist_0.jpg.webp?VersionId=fxBMcY3zow06SIvtqAzWNN7YGmZEMC1f&itok=cMx4D7aH.

Test Your Knowledge

1. What are the physical exam findings of synovitis?
2. What cutaneous findings are important in rheumatic conditions (e.g., malar rash, Gottron's papules, livedo reticularis)?

5.3. Laboratory and Imaging Studies

Learning Outcome

1. Understand the role of laboratory tests in diagnosis;
2. Highlight the prevalence of standard blood tests in rheumatologic assessment;
3. Identify the importance of imaging tests;
4. Understand types of imaging used in rheumatology;
5. Describe the interpretation of laboratory results;
6. Discuss biomarkers in diseases of rheumatology;
7. Highlight genetic testing issues;
8. Identify imaging and laboratory study limitations;
9. Describe the incorporation of test results into clinical evaluation.

Laboratory and imaging tests are significant in both diagnosis and treatment follow-up in the clinical assessment of rheumatologic patients. Imaging techniques , such as Ultrasound Tissue Characterization (UTC) have proven to be effective diagnostic instruments in the assessment of tendon structures in conditions , such as psoriatic arthritis, whose patients exhibit evident pain and functional impairment, in addition to evident walking speed and tendon strength deficiencies (Busso et al., 2025). Diagnostic imaging modalities , such as PET-CT are also significant in diagnosing isolated aortitis, which may be independent of systemic vasculitis. This approach enhances understanding of the presentation and course of conditions, thus directing therapeutic planning (Jain et al., 2024). Last but not least, combined laboratory assessment with new imaging technologies allows a rich insight into rheumatologic disorders, leading to ideal patient management and improving clinical outcomes.

5.3.1. Role of Laboratory Tests in Diagnosis

Laboratory tests in clinical evaluation of rheumatologic patients are a cornerstone of accurate diagnosis and management. These tests provide valuable biomarkers that differentiate various rheumatologic conditions, such as rheumatoid arthritis, systemic lupus erythematosus, and remitting seronegative symmetric synovitis with pitting edema (RS3PE) (Filippou et al., 2021). The complexity of rheumatic disease typically necessitates a multidisciplinary strategy, where laboratory examination, for example, autoantibody profiles and inflammatory markers, complements clinical assessment and imaging investigations. Particularly for RS3PE, laboratory tests play a significant role in establishing a diagnosis based on the occurrence of specific clinical symptoms and seronegativity for autoimmunity (Filippou et al., 2021). Additionally, as clinical practice progresses, the incidence of immune-related adverse events of treatments , such as immunotherapy highlights the need for ongoing laboratory assessment to effectively monitor and manage possible side effects (Figure 5.12).

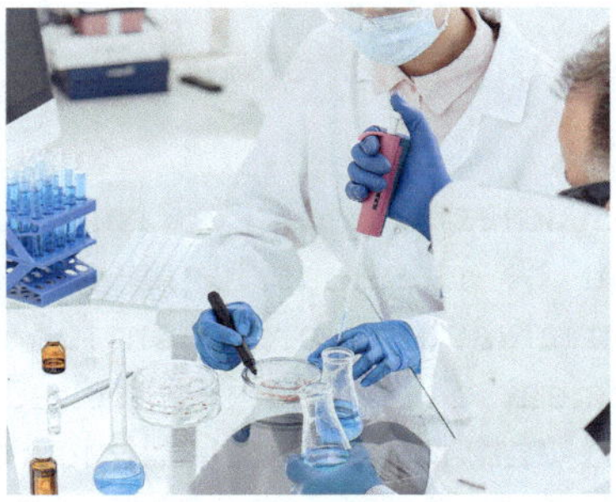

Figure 5.12. In the clinical evaluation of rheumatologic patients, laboratory tests serve as a cornerstone for accurate diagnosis and management.

Source: https://ascendimagingcenter.com/wp-content/uploads/2024/09/lab-technicians-carefully-performing-laboratory-tests-with-safety-precautions-in-the-lab.jpg.

5.3.2. Common Blood Tests for Rheumatologic Evaluation

Comprehensive rheumatologic assessment usually involves a routine panel of typical blood tests that provide useful information on a patient's autoimmune condition and inflammatory process. These tests typically include assessment for rheumatoid factor (RF), anti-citrullinated protein antibodies (ACPAs), and anti-nuclear antibodies (ANAs) that are utilized in the diagnosis of specific rheumatic diseases , such as rheumatoid arthritis and systemic lupus erythematosus. Moreover, inflammatory parameters like erythrocyte sedimentation rate (ESR) and C-reactive protein (CRP) are included in assessing disease activity and treatment response. The patient case study of an 83-year-old male, experiencing anemia and hyper-sedimentation, highlights the usefulness of these tests in the diagnostic differentiation between diseases like RS3PE and other rheumatic diseases (Emamifar et al., 2016). Early identification by these blood tests not only has diagnostic applications but also directs targeted therapeutic planning (Puzanov et al., 2017).

5.3.3. Importance of Imaging Studies

Imaging studies play a key role in clinical evaluation of rheumatologic patients and provide invaluable information for diagnosis and treatment. Such imaging technologies as ultrasound and MRI enable clinicians to see inflammation in joints and soft tissues, thus enabling an early diagnosis of such diseases as rheumatoid arthritis and systemic lupus erythematosus. The integration of imaging findings with clinical data significantly enhances differential diagnosis accuracy, thereby reducing misdiagnosis chances. In fact, studies have shown that decision support systems coupled with traditional imaging enhance the chances of identifying rheumatologic disorders to a significant level, representing a significant reduction of errors of diagnosis among generalists and specialists (Athreya et al., 2016). Moreover, continuous technological growth in the field of imaging enables better monitoring of disease onset and therapy efficacy, thereby allowing timely interventions for better patient outcomes (Puzanov et al., 2017) (Figure 5.13).

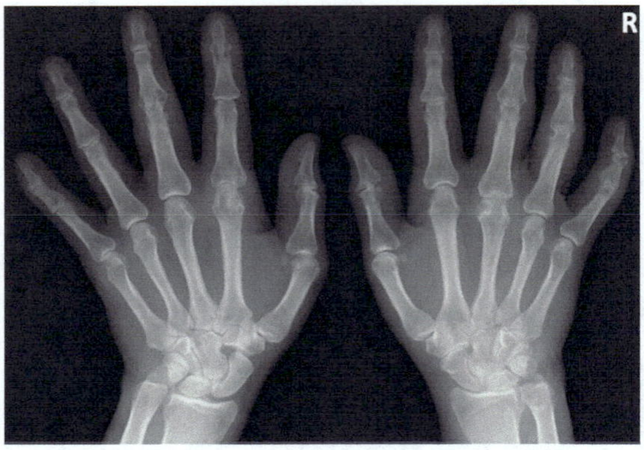

Figure 5.13. Imaging studies play a pivotal role in the clinical evaluation of rheumatologic patients, providing essential insights that aid in diagnosis and management.

Source: https://www.radiologic.theclinics.com/cms/10.1016/j.rcl.2024.03.005/asset/5ab77a28-451e-4830-babd-d05b8c4bcb11/main.assets/gr10_lrg.jpg.

5.3.4. Types of Imaging used in Rheumatology

Rheumatological imaging modalities play a key role in the accurate evaluation of musculoskeletal disorders, diagnosis, as well as treatment monitoring. Although widely utilized, traditional radiography is generally suboptimal in soft tissues as well as in the assessment of early joint abnormality; newer modalities , such as MRI and musculoskeletal US, have gained prominence. MRI offers high-resolution imaging of synovial tissue and cartilage and has the capacity to detect inflammatory alterations in the early stages, which are significant in diseases like rheumatoid arthritis. Conversely, the US has the capability of dynamic assessment and has been found to be effective in the measurement of cartilage thickness, as confirmed in a study demonstrating that it can assess treatment outcomes in knee osteoarthritis (Barbulescu et al., 2019). Moreover, US has an important role in detecting inflammatory lesions among juvenile idiopathic arthritis patients, outlining its applications in varied clinical scenarios (Manca et al., 2009). In conclusion, these imaging methods enhance the rheumatologic patient's clinical evaluation by enabling comprehensive information regarding the joint status of health.

5.3.5. Interpretation of Laboratory Results

Interpretation of the lab results is a critical aspect of rheumatologic patient clinical examination, providing useful information about the inflammatory condition and potential underlying disease. Elevated inflammatory markers, for example, are significant in the diagnosis of diseases , such as adult-onset Stills disease (AOSD), where elevated systemic scores have been correlated with poor outcomes and higher mortality (Berardicurti et al., 2016). Further, in diseases like RS3PE, careful examination of symptoms coupled with laboratory parameters can result in recognition of associations with other underlying disorders. For example, malignancies (Emamifar et al., 2016). Cautious laboratory investigations, for instance, complete blood counts (CBC) and inflammatory markers, thereby identify relevant clinical features, ultimately guiding both diagnosis and treatment protocols. By incorporating these laboratory results within the framework of the overall clinical presentation, rheumatologists can formulate directed management plans, maximizing patient outcome and prognosis (Figure 5.14).

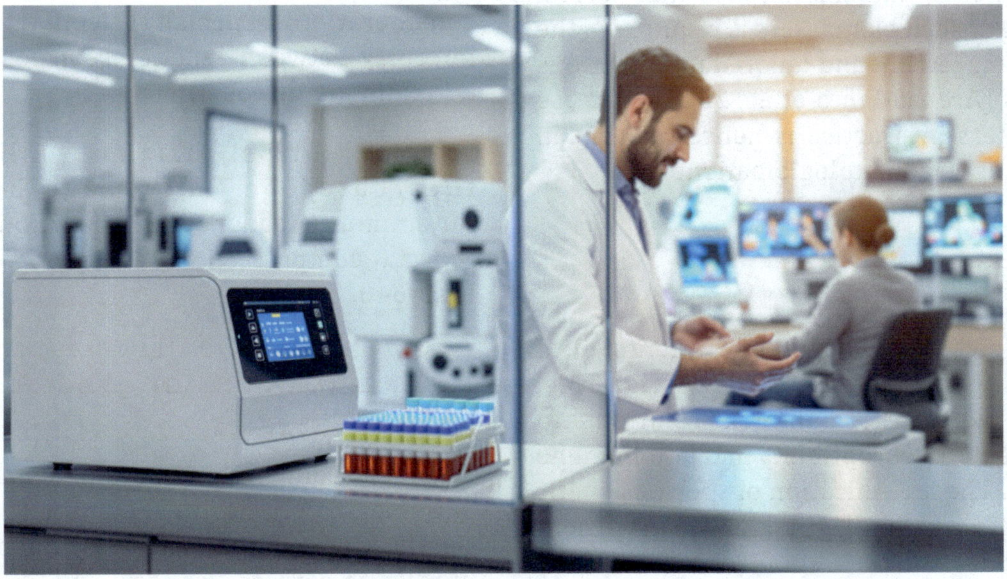

Figure 5.14. The interpretation of laboratory results is a critical element in the clinical evaluation of rheumatologic patients.

Source: https://media.licdn.com/dms/image/v2/D5612AQEidBaoKXxF3Q/article-cover_image-shrink_720_1280/B56ZZ3XH2lGUAI-/0/1745759280627?e=2147483647&v=beta&t=5lIt_XfeSlVG6kUhbdd8Btu0YPFPFbYQn_FUI-2aGA4.

5.3.6. Biomarkers in Rheumatologic Diseases

Identification and use of biomarkers in rheumatologic diseases hold great promise for maximizing the clinical evaluation of patients. These biomarkers can provide useful insights into disease diagnosis, prognosis, and treatment response, ultimately guiding personalized treatment regimens. By enabling early, sensitive, and specific diagnosis, biomarkers assist in the timely intervention with disease-modifying antirheumatic drugs (bDMARDs), which have revolutionized the management of inflammatory rheumatic diseases. However, treatment failure with bDMARDs remains an issue with 30%–40% of patients exhibiting suboptimal response or unacceptable side effects, highlighting the need for predictive biomarkers to maximize treatment success (Glintborg et al., 2018). Also, high biomarkers of systemic inflammation have been linked to untoward events even in treated patients, and this implies that careful monitoring of such biomarkers is required in the optimal management and tailored interventions of patients (Arenas-Pinto et al., 2015). The use of biomarkers in practice is hence relevant in transforming rheumatologic patient care.

5.3.7. Genetic Testing Considerations

In the clinical evaluation of patients with rheumatology, genetics plays a vital role, especially with the complex relationship between genetic susceptibility and autoimmune conditions. The identification of specific genetic markers can aid in the diagnosis and management of conditions , such as spondyloarthritis and inflammatory bowel disease, which have a tendency to occur in association and share similar genetic causes (Ascolani et al., 2016). Clarification of these interactions can have a strong influence on outcomes in patients by enabling intentional therapeutic interventions. Moreover, with the technological advancement of genetic testing, clinicians can use the results to forecast disease development and tailor individualized treatment plans. However, beyond the clinical and economic implications of genetic testing, there are also ethical issues related to informed consent and potential psychosocial repercussions that need to be addressed in order for patients to have a complete understanding of the implications of their results (Brém et al., 2020). Ultimately, judicious integration of genetic testing into rheumatologic assessment can streamline clinical practice and improve the overall quality of care (Figure 5.15).

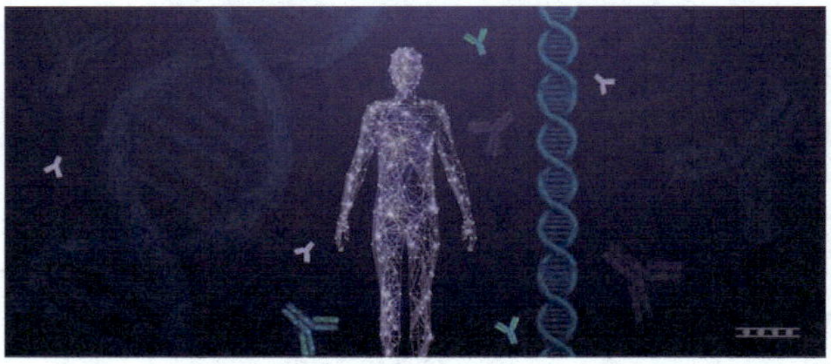

Figure 5.15. Genetic testing emerges as a vital consideration, especially given the complex interplay between genetic predispositions and autoimmune diseases.

Source: https://img.mlo-online.com/files/base/ebm/mlo/image/2022/03/AutoimmuneHeader.6233762c0736d.png?auto=format,compress&fit=max&q=45&w=640&width=640.

5.3.8. Limitations of Laboratory and Imaging Studies

Although useful in clinical evaluation, laboratory and imaging studies in rheumatology do have significant limitations, and these can prove to be hurdles to correct diagnosis and management. Laboratory tests, such as serological markers, may yield false positives or false negatives depending on various reasons , such as the overlapping presentation of diseases and comorbid conditions. In addition, imaging studies, though very useful for the visualization of joint damage and inflammation, do not correlate with clinical symptom severity in most cases, leading to potential misinterpretation of a patient's status. For example, pulmonary histoplasmosis research emphasizes that early imaging will conceal background pathologies, resulting in misdiagnosis and improper treatment strategies, hence the need for careful assessment beyond such modalities (Britto, 2018). Further, the absence of standard protocols in result interpretation of imaging results can give rise to heterogeneity in clinical decision-making. Hence, a multichannel strategy with integration of clinical judgement with imaging and laboratory data is important to effective rheumatologic patient management (Puzanov et al., 2017).

5.3.9. Integration of Test Results into Clinical Evaluation

Integration of test results into clinical evaluation remains very important for effective diagnosis and management of rheumatologic diseases. After a thorough review of laboratory and imaging data, clinicians are in a position to better understand disease progression and the efficacy of therapy. This convergence is particularly crucial in cases of equivocal clinical presentations and the necessity to make decisions on the basis of objective measures. A case in point is the application of technology-assisted rehabilitative tools, which have shown promising results in tracking functional improvement over time and proving that integrated assessments result in better patient outcomes (Amirabdollahian et al., 2016). Further, understanding the environment of clinical research within rheumatology clarifies the importance of continued investigation into processes of disease and therapy. As new knowledge reveals the necessity of new research, integrating test results with existing clinical research becomes imperative in maximizing therapeutic strategies and improving patient care (Desjardins et al., 2009) (Figure 5.16).

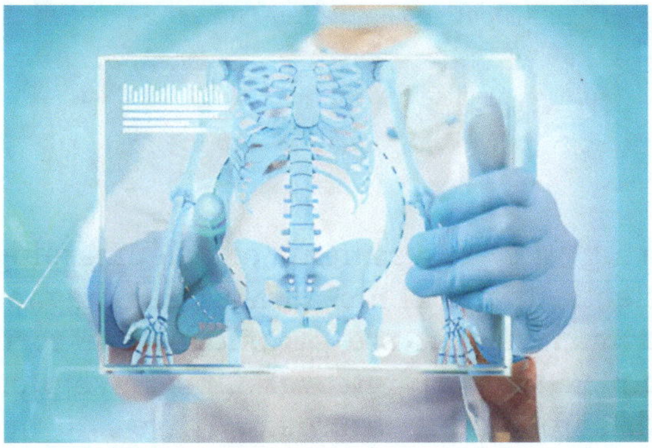

Figure 5.16. The integration of test results into clinical evaluation is paramount for accurately diagnosing and managing rheumatologic conditions.

Source: https://conquest.health/wp-content/uploads/2024/06/Role-of-PETCT-in-diagnosing-and-monitoring-disease-activity-in-rheumatoid-arthritis-A-review.webp.

Test Your Knowledge

1. What are the characteristic imaging findings of osteoarthritis versus rheumatoid arthritis?
2. How useful is MRI in the prompt identification of erosions of joints or inflammation of soft tissues?

5.4. Differential Diagnosis and Management

Learning Outcome

1. Understand the importance of differential diagnosis;
2. Discuss common conditions to exclude;
3. Understand the criteria for some of the rheumatologic diseases;
4. Learn rheumatologic condition treatment;
5. Discuss the physical therapy and rehabilitation role;
6. Highlight patient education and self-management;
7. Monitoring disease course;
8. Learn follow-up evaluation importance.

During the assessment of rheumatologic patients in the clinic, differential diagnosis and management are paramount due to the complex interplay of overlapping symptoms with autoimmune disorders. There is a need for an organized approach because diverse presentations owe their beginnings to subclinical inflammatory, infectious, or neoplastic disease. For instance, the recent understanding of cancer immunotherapy-related immune-related adverse events (irAEs) makes it specifically important to be aware of these disorders. As reported, severe irAEs, although less common, have serious implications for patient outcomes and require immediate intervention to avoid severe life-threatening complications (Puzanov et al., 2017). Secondly, the association between primary immunodeficiencies and related autoimmune phenomena requires a personalized management approach, weighing immune support against suppression (Cooper et al., 2016). Through a multidisciplinary approach, clinicians can increase accuracy in diagnosis and treatment effectiveness, ultimately contributing to enhanced patient care and quality of life.

5.4.1. Importance of Differential Diagnosis

The role of differential diagnosis in the clinical evaluation of rheumatology patients cannot be overstated since it plays a critical role in isolating most diseases that may share similar characteristics. Accurate diagnosis is not only crucial to facilitate effective treatment but to prevent possibly fatal reactions to mismanagement of rheumatologic illness. For instance, immune-related adverse effects (irAEs) of treatments like immune checkpoint inhibitors often need a meticulous assessment to differentiate these side effects from actual disease manifestations, particularly in autoimmune diseases (Schneider et al., 2021). Proper and prompt therapy of irAEs, like in the skin, gut, or musculoskeletal systems, relies on an early understanding of the involved immunologic mechanisms (Puzanov et al., 2017). Thus, differential diagnosis systematically assists healthcare workers in devising individualized treatment plans while ensuring comprehensive patient care (Figure 5.17).

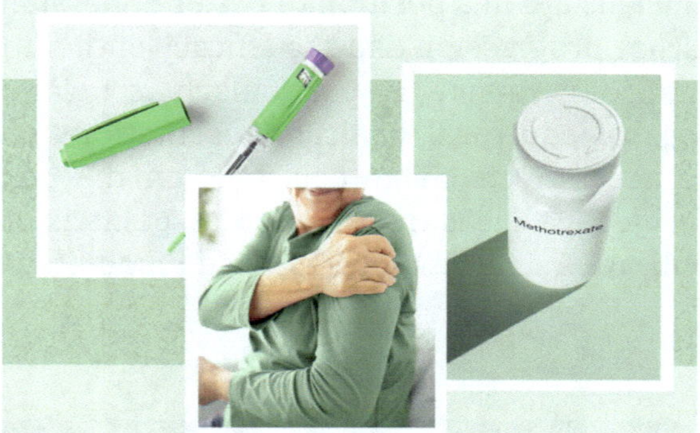

Figure 5.17. Accurate diagnosis is essential for optimizing treatment, and for preventing potentially severe complications arising from mismanagement of rheumatologic disorders.

Source: https://images.everydayhealth.com/images/arthritis/rheumatic-diseases/treatment-guide-for-polymyalgia-rheumatica-1440x810.jpg?sfvrsn=72011d0d_3.

5.4.2. Common Conditions to Differentiate

In clinical evaluation of rheumatologic patients, differentiation among common conditions is important for accurate diagnosis and successful treatment. For instance, the convergence of SpA and IBD captures the complexities that clinicians face in establishing joint pain. Studies have shown that nearly half of the IBD patients who experience joint pain also show features of Enteropathic-related Spondyloarthritis (ESpA), a condition needing full management with rheumatologists and gastroenterologists (Ascolani et al., 2016). Additionally, the management of immune-mediated inflammatory diseases (IMID) with chronic anti-TNF therapy has been shown to affect T cell function, complicating differential diagnosis further due to shared immunological mechanisms (Mastroianni et al., 2018). Therefore, detection of the characteristics of such interconnected conditions highlights the requirement for a multidisciplinary management approach to clinical evaluations for improved patient outcomes.

5.4.3. Criteria for Specific Rheumatologic Diseases

The clinical evaluation of rheumatologic patients necessitates a thorough understanding of the criteria specific to various diseases, which aids in diagnosis and management. For instance, with Adult-onset Still's disease (AOSD), identification of central clinical features—, such as frequent fevers, arthritis, and systemic inflammation—is especially critical due to the threat of dangerous complications like macrophage activation syndrome that can be harmful to patient outcome (Berardicurti et al., 2016). Also, with patients who are on methadone for pain relief, there has to be identification of factors for QTc prolongation, particularly where rheumatologic disease has been present, as it will contribute to their complex regimen (Brown et al., 2017). The use of some criteria for various rheumatologic disorders not only makes diagnosis easier but also maximizes therapeutic approaches, ultimately leading to improved patient care and outcomes in an extremely heterogeneous patient group (Figure 5.18).

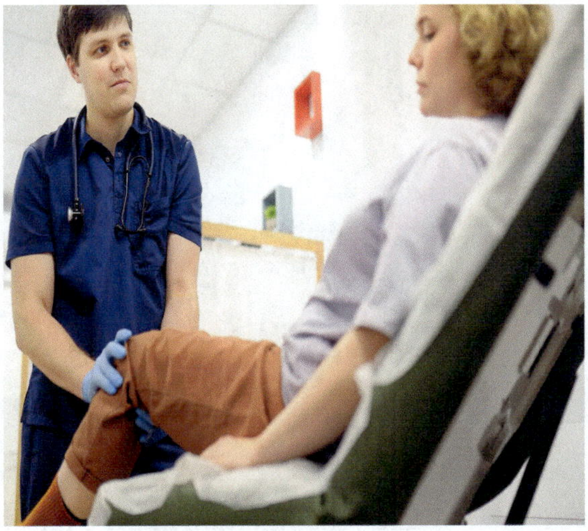

Figure 5.18. The clinical evaluation of rheumatologic patients necessitates a thorough understanding of the criteria specific to various diseases, which aids in diagnosis and management.

Source: https://www.inspirahealthnetwork.org/sites/default/files/2025-04/getty5.jpg.

5.4.4. Treatment Options for Rheumatologic Conditions

The therapeutic pattern of rheumatologic diseases has significantly shifted with the introduction of newer medications, particularly biologics and targeted agents. Among those, Janus kinase (JAK) inhibitors , such as tofacitinib have been under the limelight as they can also manage conditions like rheumatoid arthritis and have had exemplary efficacy in symptom relief and in the disease course (Alikhan et al., 2020). Nevertheless, the apparently contradictory development of diseases , such as vitiligo during therapy serves to underscore the value of careful patient monitoring and further investigation of the underlying mechanisms. Concurrent with these advances, application of radiopharmaceuticals for imaging has been instrumental in assessing the effectiveness of treatment and monitoring disease activity, increasing the precision of clinical evaluations (Auletta et al., 2016). As more therapies are on the horizon, it is increasingly crucial for clinicians to balance the benefit of treatment against potential side effects and retain a well-rounded practice in rheumatology patient care.

5.4.5. Role of Physical Therapy and Rehabilitation

Physical therapy and rehabilitation play a pivotal role in the clinical evaluation of rheumatologic patients to optimize functional capacity and improve quality of life. By utilizing tailored exercises and therapy interventions, physical therapists assist patients in managing symptoms as well as regaining movement, which can be particularly beneficial for sufferers of disease conditions , such as rheumatoid arthritis or lupus. Studies have indicated that rehabilitation modalities facilitated through technology, such as in the case of telerehabilitation, can facilitate patients to conduct self-management therapy at home, thereby increasing the dosage of practice and compliance with rehabilitation regimens they experience (Amirabdollahian et al., 2016).

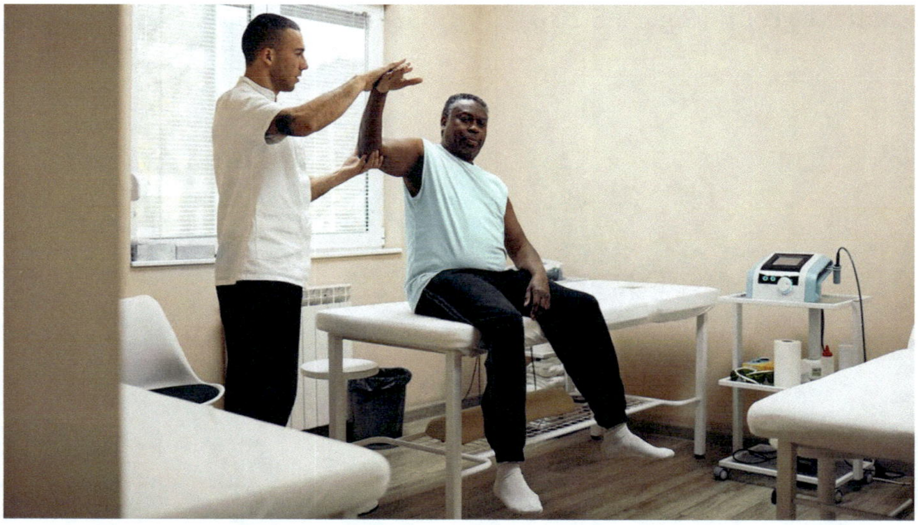

Figure 5.19. The role of physical therapy and rehabilitation in the clinical evaluation of rheumatologic patients is critical for enhancing functional capacity and improving quality of life.

Source: https://i0.wp.com/post.healthline.com/wp-content/uploads/2022/09/mature-male-physical-therapy-1296-728-header.jpg?w=1155&h=1528.

Furthermore, familiarity with the various models of service delivery for the treatment of rheumatoid arthritis is significant, as this allows for the implementation of effective rehabilitation interventions based on patients' specific needs (Finn et al., 2009). Finally, the strategies not only aid in physical healing but also provide emotional stability, hence facilitating a more holistic process of recovery in rheumatologic patients (Figure 5.19).

5.4.6. Patient Education and Self-management

Effective patient education and self-management are integral parts in the clinical evaluation of rheumatologic patients, particularly in the treatment of chronic disease , such as rheumatoid arthritis and other autoimmune disorders. As there is a growing need for the service of rheumatology due to an aging population and possible shortage of rheumatologists, it has never been more crucial for patients to be more involved in their own care (Layton, 2015). Preparing patients thoroughly not only enhances their level of understanding about their condition, but also promotes the taking of medication and adopting lifestyle modification. The latest research focuses on self-management strategies, which can minimize symptoms and improve the quality of life. On top of that, early identification of adverse events and implementation of correct self-care interventions can significantly influence treatment results (Puzanov et al., 2017). Putting patient education first and facilitating self-management has the possibility to improve the efficiency of care as well as optimize patient experiences in the increasingly tightened rheumatology environment.

5.4.7. Monitoring Disease Progression

Disease surveillance in rheumatologic patients is crucial to fully optimize treatment regimens and maximize patient outcomes. Effective management is contingent on an adequate knowledge of evolving clinical manifestations of the diseases. For instance, musculoskeletal ultrasound (MSUS) has emerged as a key element in such situations, with a capability to evaluate intra-articular and periarticular structures in real time, thereby allowing it to make accurate judgments regarding disease activity and joint involvement (Iagnocco et al., 2016). Further, as the use of immune checkpoint inhibitors in the treatment of specific conditions is becoming more widespread, surveillance for irAEs of delayed onset and long duration must be conducted. Early recognition of such toxicities is significant for early management and best treatment and thus endorses the multi-dimensional nature of disease assessment and its management and complications (Puzanov et al., 2017). With these monitoring mechanisms, rheumatological patient care can be significantly enhanced (Figure 5.20).

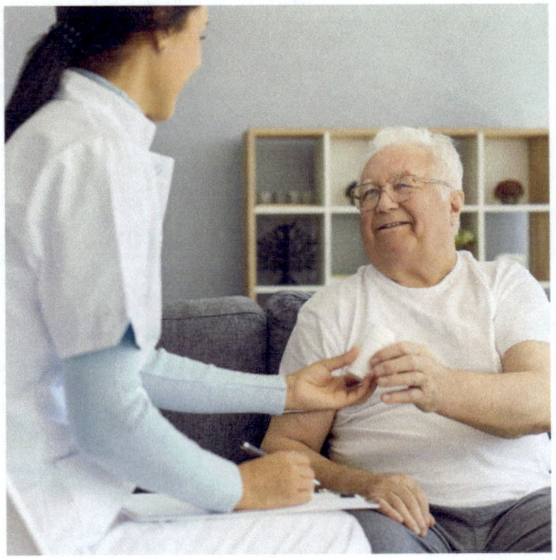

Figure 5.20. Monitoring disease progression in rheumatologic patients is crucial for optimizing treatment regimens and improving patient outcomes.

Source: https://islandrheumatology.com/wp-content/uploads/2024/11/Untitled-design-13.jpg.

5.4.8. Importance of Follow-up Evaluations

Follow-up evaluations are valuable in clinical care of rheumatologic patients since they provide the opportunity to follow up on disease progression, monitor response to treatment, and adjust therapeutic approach as needed. The evaluations are particularly valuable in such conditions as rheumatoid arthritis, in which early intervention can potentially alter the long-term course profoundly. The primary goal in follow-ups is preserving clinical remission and preventing irreversible joint destruction, an issue that has evolved with improvements in diagnosis and treatment modalities in the recent years (Diaconu et al., 2018). Moreover, regular evaluations allow clinicians to gain important information that can optimize knowledge of disease behavior and therapeutic responses and therefore contribute to evidence-based rheumatological interventions (Desjardins et al., 2009). Thus, a systematized follow-up procedure not only stimulates patient care in a single patient but also enhances the overall field of investigative rheumatology by influencing ongoing research and therapeutic advances.

Test Your Knowledge

1. When is urgent referral to rheumatology indicated?
2. How do you assess disease activity and treatment response in rheumatologic diseases?

Summary

Rheumatologic patient clinical evaluation is a complex process that mandates an understanding of the interaction between various risk factors and treatment protocols. Studies reveal that co-morbid states , such as congestive heart failure and rheumatologic disorders, considerably enhance the risk of QTc interval prolongation in patients being treated with methadone, emphasizing rigorous monitoring in pain management interventions (Brown et al., 2017). Also, the use of tumor necrosis factor antagonists, as a therapeutic for the management of inflammatory conditions, is linked with an increased risk of tuberculosis reactivation, particularly when compounded by the use of drugs like methotrexate or azathioprine (Armuzzi et al., 2014). Practitioners must hence use a careful evaluation and personalized treatment approach that not only manages the rheumatologic disease but also comorbidities, maximally protecting the patient and therapeutic outcome.

While clinically evaluating rheumatologic patients, several significant aspects come to light that enhance the understanding and management of such complex conditions. Firstly, the implementation of point-of-care testing (POCT) has begun transforming diagnostic workflows, making them efficient and accessible in patient care while simultaneously putting more onus on its regulation and training in order to prevent misinterpretation of the findings (Banfi et al., 2024). Besides, the utilization of adjunct therapies , such as injectable platelet-rich fibrin (i-PRF) with conventional treatment has been documented to provide positive results in the management of common comorbidities found among rheumatologic patients, particularly those with long-term disorders like diabetes (Shunmuga et al., 2023). This implies the necessity of customized treatment modalities that consider both rheumatologic as well as related health issues. Collectively, these advances highlight the importance of a multi-disciplinary approach to offer global care and therefore optimize patient outcomes in diverse clinical practice.

KEY TERMS FROM THIS CHAPTER

- Clinical assessment
- Magnetic resonance imaging (MRI)
- Juvenile idiopathic inflammatory myopathies
- Symptoms
- Patient-reported outcome measures (PROMs)
- Misdiagnosis
- Inflammatory bowel disease (IBD)
- Therapy
- Musculoskeletal ultrasonography (US)
- Pathophysiology
- Clinical evaluation
- Diagnostic decision support software
- Immune-related adverse events (irAEs)
- Spondyloarthritis

Critical Thinking Questions

1. Of the following symptoms, which is most characteristic of inflammatory arthritis?

a. Pain that increases with movement and decreases with rest

b. Morning stiffness for >1 hour

c. Lack of swelling of the affected joints

d. Acute onset of joint pain without systemic symptoms

2. Which of the following laboratory tests is most specific for the diagnosis of systemic lupus erythematosus (SLE)?

a. Rheumatoid factor (RF)

b. Antinuclear antibody (ANA)

c. Anti-dsDNA antibody

d. C-reactive protein (CRP)

3. Which of the following is included in the routine physical examination in a patient with suspected inflammatory arthritis?

a. Auscultation of bowel sounds

b. Joint palpation for swelling and tenderness

c. Fundoscopic eye examination

d. Neurological reflex testing in isolation

4. In a suspected case of rheumatoid arthritis, the initial joints most frequently affected are:

a. Hips and knees

b. Spine and shoulders

c. Wrists and small hand joints

d. Ankles and feet in isolation

5. Which joint pattern of involvement is most typical of osteoarthritis?

a. Symmetric MCP and PIP joint involvement

b. Symmetric DIP joints and first CMC joint involvement

c. Asymmetric oligoarthritis of the large joints

d. Migratory arthritis with systemic manifestations

Short Answer Questions

1. What are the main questions to ask when assessing joint pain (location, onset, duration, symmetry)?
2. How can inflammatory and non-inflammatory joint pain be distinguished on history taking?
3. What are the key components of a simple musculoskeletal examination?
4. How can joint swelling be distinguished from bony enlargement or deformity?

5. Why is antinuclear antibody (ANA) testing useful in autoimmune disease?
6. In what ways are rheumatoid factor (RF) and anti-CCP antibodies used in the diagnosis of RA?
7. How do you differentiate between rheumatoid arthritis and osteoarthritis on the basis of clinical and laboratory features?
8. What are the key clinical findings that point towards a connective tissue disease versus a mechanical joint disorder?

Answers to Critical Thinking Questions

1. (b); 2. (c); 3. (b); 4. (c); 5. (b)

References

1. Puzanov, I., Diab, A., Abdallah, K., Bingham, C. O., 3rd, Brogdon, C., Dadu, R., Hamad, L., Kim, S., Lacouture, M. E., LeBoeuf, N. R., Lenihan, D., Onofrei, C., Shannon, V., Sharma, R., Silk, A. W., Skondra, D., Suarez-Almazor, M. E., Wang, Y., Wiley, K., Kaufman, H. L., ... Society for Immunotherapy of Cancer Toxicity Management Working Group (2017). Managing toxicities associated with immune checkpoint inhibitors: consensus recommendations from the Society for Immunotherapy of Cancer (SITC) Toxicity Management Working Group. *Journal for immunotherapy of cancer*, *5*(1), 95. https://doi.org/10.1186/s40425-017-0300-z(accessed on 17th June 2025).
2. Alikhan, M., Jogi, R., Nguyen, J. K., Patel, A., et al. (2020). A case of new-onset vitiligo in a patient on tofacitinib and brief review of paradoxical presentations with other novel targeted therapies. https://core.ac.uk/download/322493870.pdf (accessed on 17th June 2025).
3. Amirabdollahian, F., Buurke, J. H., Infarinato, F., Nijenhuis, S. M., et al. (2016). Feasibility of a second iteration wrist and hand supported training system for self-administered training at home in chronic stroke. https://core.ac.uk/download/287582589.pdf (accessed on 17th June 2025).
4. Anderson, A., Bevan, C., Bove, R., Hale, T., et al. (2020). Minimal breast milk transfer of rituximab, a monoclonal antibody used in neurological conditions. https://core.ac.uk/download/323075107.pdf (accessed on 17th June 2025).
5. Ansari, A. A., Ceribelli, A., De Santis, M., Gershwin, M. E., et al. (2020). Recommendations for coronavirus infection in rheumatic diseases treated with biologic therapy. https://core.ac.uk/download/323069262.pdf (accessed on 17th June 2025).
6. Antonazzo, B., Curcio, G., Fusconi, M., Minniti, A., et al. (2016). Sleep quality in patients with primary Sjögren's syndrome. https://core.ac.uk/download/54537328.pdf (accessed on 17th June 2025).
7. Ardekani, M. S., Fazel, F., Hakamifard, A., Shirani, M., et al. (2016). Cytomegalovirus retinitis in an immunocompetent pregnant woman. https://core.ac.uk/download/478304087.pdf (accessed on 17th June 2025).
8. Arenas-Pinto, A., Gilson, R., Maini, M., McKendry, C., et al. (2015). Systemic inflammation and residual viraemia in HIV-positive adults on protease inhibitor monotherapy: A cross-sectional study. https://core.ac.uk/download/29414641.pdf (accessed on 17th June 2025).
9. Argano, C., Cangemi, I., Corrao, S., Giardina, E. G., et al. (2024). Critical importance of patient-reported outcomes for a comprehensive assessment of psoriatic arthritis patients. https://core.ac.uk/download/614225412.pdf (accessed on 17th June 2025).
10. Armuzzi, A., Bruzzese, V., Gatta, L., Hassan, C., et al. (2014). Higher risk of tuberculosis reactivation when anti-TNF is combined with immunosuppressive agents: A systematic review of randomized controlled trials. https://core.ac.uk/download/153366740.pdf (accessed on 17th June 2025).
11. Ascolani, M., Biancone, L., Calabrese, E., Chimenti, S., et al. (2016). Impact of a multidisciplinary approach in enteropathy spondylarthritis patients. https://core.ac.uk/download/pdf/53869326.pdf (accessed on 17th June 2025).
12. Athreya, B., Newgard, C. D., Correll, C. K., Deal, C. L., Zurakowski, D., Vittinghoff, E., Ang, E.

Y. N., et al. (2016). Evidence-based decision support for pediatric rheumatology reduces diagnostic errors. https://core.ac.uk/download/83049477.pdf (accessed on 17th June 2025).

13. Auletta, S., Carideo, L., Galli, F., Lauri, C., et al. (2016). Immunoscintigraphic for therapy decision making and follow-up of biological therapies. https://core.ac.uk/download/153364883.pdf (accessed on 17th June 2025).

14. Ayala, F., Balato, A., Balato, N., Caso, F., et al. (2017). Minimal disease activity in patients with psoriatic arthritis treated with Ustekinumab: Results from a 24-week real-world study. https://core.ac.uk/download/pdf/84248778.pdf (accessed on 17th June 2025).

15. Azevedo, L. C. P., Battaini, L. C., Giannini, F. P., Moraes, M. B., et al. (2011). Outcomes and organ dysfunctions of critically ill patients with systemic lupus erythematosus and other systemic rheumatic diseases. https://core.ac.uk/download/pdf/37456269.pdf (accessed on 17th June 2025).

16. Banfi, G., Božič, B., Cihan, M., Pašalić, D., Pennestrì, F., & Plebani, M. (2024). Point-of-care testing, near-patient testing and patient self-testing: Warning points. *Clinical Chemistry and Laboratory Medicine (CCLM), 62*, 2388–2392. https://www.semanticscholar.org/paper/421cd2edd4563af301bb8ad69cbe1bfe6fb20874 (accessed on 17th June 2025).

17. Barbulescu, A. L., Chisalau, B. A., Ciurea, P. L., Criveanu, M., et al. (2019). The effect of glucosamine, chondroitin and *Harpagophytum procumbens* on femoral hyaline cartilage thickness in patients with knee osteoarthritis: An MRI versus ultrasonography study. https://core.ac.uk/download/216811083.pdf (accessed on 17th June 2025).

18. Benfaremo, D., Bolognini, L., Ciccia, F., Ciferri, M., et al. (2017). Adalimumab efficacy in enteropathy spondylarthritis: A 12-mo observational multidisciplinary study. https://core.ac.uk/download/127501902.pdf (accessed on 17th June 2025).

19. Berardicurti, O., Carubbi, F., Ciccia, F., Cipriani, P., Di Benedetto, P., Giacomelli, R., Guggino, G., et al. (2016). Adult-onset Still's disease: Evaluation of prognostic tools and validation of the systemic score by analysis of 100 cases from three centers. https://core.ac.uk/download/287858923.pdf (accessed on 17th June 2025).

20. Berendes, R., Dressler, F., Haas, J. P., Hansmann, S., et al. (2024). Level and correlates of physical activity among children and adolescents with juvenile idiopathic arthritis compared to controls: Results from a German nationwide prospective observational cohort study. https://core.ac.uk/download/619988117.pdf (accessed on 17th June 2025).

21. Berg, A., Brotman, D. J., Chan, M. P., Houchens, R., et al. (2016). Painful losses. http://deepblue.lib.umich.edu/bitstream/2027.42/134073/7/jhm2610_am.pdf (accessed on 17th June 2025).

22. Bergamini, A., Cantarini, L., Caso, F., Chimenti, M. S., Conigliaro, P., Costa, L., D'Antonio, A., et al. (2023). Rheumatologist's perspective on non-infectious uveitis: Patterns from tertiary referral rheumatologic clinics in Italy. https://core.ac.uk/download/618720077.pdf (accessed on 17th June 2025).

23. Bohan, B., Brown, G., Chinoy, H., Christen-Zaech, S., Pilkington, C. A., et al. (2011). A national registry for juvenile dermatomyositis and other pediatric idiopathic inflammatory myopathies: 10 years' experience; the Juvenile Dermatomyositis National (UK and Ireland) Cohort Biomarker Study and Repository for Idiopathic Inflammatory Myopathies. https://core.ac.uk/download/10413.pdf (accessed on 17th June 2025).

24. Brém, E., Koyfman, A., & Long, B. J. (2020). Oncologic emergencies: Immune-based cancer therapies and complications. https://core.ac.uk/download/305124082.pdf (accessed on 17th June 2025).

25. Britto, J. (2018). Pulmonary histoplasmosis in a patient with cough, dyspnea, pulmonary nodule and rheumatologic manifestations: Case report and review. https://core.ac.uk/download/217211020.pdf (accessed on 17th June 2025).

26. Brown, J., Hutchinson, D., Juba, K., Khadem, A., et al. (2017). Methadone and corrected QT prolongation in pain and palliative care patients: A case–control study. https://core.ac.uk/download/81665714.pdf (accessed on 17th June 2025).

27. Burwinkle, T. M., Limbers, C. A., Szer, I. S., Varni, J. W., et al. (2007). The PedsQL™ as a patient-reported outcome in children and adolescents with fibromyalgia: An analysis of OMERACT domains. https://core.ac.uk/download/pdf/7546464.pdf (accessed on 17th June 2025).

28. Businger, A. C., Dempsey, P. P., Linder, J. A., Whaley, C. M., et al. (2014). Visit complexity, diagnostic uncertainty, and antibiotic prescribing for acute cough in primary care: A retrospective study. https://core.ac.uk/download/28946602.pdf (accessed on 17th June 2025).

29. Busso, C., Parisi, S., Andrighetti, M., Ditto, M. C., Massazza, G., Fusaro, E., & Minetto, M. (2025). Ultrasound tissue characterization and function of Achilles tendon in psoriatic arthritis patients: A cross-sectional study. *European Journal of Physical and Rehabilitation Medicine, 61*, 109–118. https://www.semanticscholar.org/paper/36e1b2d031823828ec2a6145a2e49272be2071ba (accessed on 17th June 2025).

30. Carswell, A., Sturesson, A. L., Dellhag, B., Backamn, C., Ekdahl, C., Dixon, D., Beaton, D. E., et al. (2009). Measures and time point relevant for post-surgical follow-up in patients with inflammatory arthritis: A pilot study. https://core.ac.uk/download/pdf/8294002.pdf (accessed on 17th June 2025).

31. Carvalho, J. L., Cavalcante, A. F., dos Santos Alves, M. V., Freitas, D. S., et al. (2020). Spectrochemical analysis in blood plasma combined with subsequent chemometrics for fibromyalgia detection. https://core.ac.uk/download/327061388.pdf (accessed on 17th June 2025).

32. Cooper, M. A., Farmer, J. R., Foldvari, Z., Torgerson, T. R., et al. (2016). Mechanism-based strategies for the management of autoimmunity and immune dysregulation in primary immunodeficiencies. https://core.ac.uk/download/129070181.pdf (accessed on 17th June 2025).

33. Desjardins, C., Ehrenberg, R. G., & St. Clair, E. W. (2009). The scope and scale of clinical research accomplished by rheumatologists early in their careers. https://core.ac.uk/download/5131729.pdf (accessed on 17th June 2025).

34. Diaconu, C. C., Hainarosie, R., Iancu, M. A., Iftimie, N., et al. (2018). The importance of early arthritis in patients with rheumatoid arthritis. https://core.ac.uk/download/216809651.pdf (accessed on 17th June 2025).

35. Emamifar, A., Gildberg-Mortensen, R., Hess, S., Jensen Hansen, I. M., et al. (2016). Association of remitting seronegative symmetrical synovitis with pitting edema, polymyalgia rheumatica, and adenocarcinoma of the prostate. https://core.ac.uk/download/pdf/50713364.pdf (accessed on 17th June 2025).

36. Ferenz, S., Glicksman, C., Haws, M., Kadin, M. E., et al. (2021). Impact of capsulectomy type on post-explantation systemic symptom improvement: Findings from the ASERF systemic symptoms in Women-Biospecimen Analysis Study: Part 1. https://core.ac.uk/download/552340697.pdf (accessed on 17th June 2025).

37. Filippou, G., Romano, M., Sarzi-Puttini, P., Sirotti, S., et al. (2021). RS3PE and the role of ultrasound: A case report and brief review of the literature. https://core.ac.uk/download/478967652.pdf (accessed on 17th June 2025).

38. Finn, H., King, J., Lauzon, C., Li, M., et al. (2009). Development of a framework for reporting health service models for managing rheumatoid arthritis. https://core.ac.uk/download/pdf/8361996.pdf (accessed on 17th June 2025).

39. Glintborg, B., Hetland, M. L., Hogdall, E. V., Johansen, J. S., et al. (2018). Identification of new biomarkers to promote personalized treatment of patients with inflammatory rheumatic disease: Protocol for an open cohort study. https://core.ac.uk/download/269306619.pdf (accessed on 17th June 2025).

40. Naredo, E., & Iagnocco, A. (2016). One year in review: ultrasound in arthritis. *Clinical and experimental rheumatology*, *34*(1), 1–10.(accessed on 17th June 2025).

41. Jain, S., Muñoz-Urbano, M., Khormi, A., Sangle, S., & D'Cruz, D. (2024). P181 Clinical assessment of radiologically defined clinically isolated aortitis in a single center study. *Rheumatology*. https://www.semanticscholar.org/paper/0da0bcaac3789fd41ff934196d85e6e477c159ce (accessed on 17th June 2025).

42. Karagodina, Y. B., Ruban, M., Savchina, V. V., Bolotina, L., Fedenko, A., & Kornietskaya, A. (2023). Rare immune-related adverse events: A clinical case of Sjögren's syndrome on the background of immunotherapy in a patient with lung adenocarcinoma. *Effective Pharmacotherapy*. https://www.semanticscholar.org/paper/3162f65c3f8ae8b3ef8ea885dee71e5a01ef6315 (accessed on 17th June 2025).

43. Layton, K. R. (2015). Evaluation of a rheumatology patient prioritization triage system. https://core.ac.uk/download/232575604.pdf (accessed on 17th June 2025).

44. Manca, A., Mavidrou, A., Premkumar, A., Karmazyn, B., Wallace, C. A., Sherry, D. D., Turner, D. E., et al. (2009). Protocol for the Foot in Juvenile Idiopathic Arthritis trial (FiJIA): A randomized controlled trial of an integrated foot care programmed for foot problems in JIA. https://core.ac.uk/download/1396388.pdf (accessed on 17th June 2025).

45. Mastroianni, C. M., Mengoni, F., Sauzullo, I., Scrivo, R., et al. (2018). Changes in T cell effector functions over an 8-year period with TNF antagonists in patients with chronic inflammatory rheumatic diseases. https://core.ac.uk/download/158328089.pdf (accessed on 17th June 2025).

46. Paoloni, M., Bernetti, A., Brignoli, O., Coclite, G. M., et al. (2017). Appropriateness and efficacy of spa therapy for musculoskeletal disorders: A Delphi method consensus initiative among experts in Italy. https://core.ac.uk/download/84928671.pdf (accessed on 17th June 2025).

47. Patton, E. E. (2016). Nutritional factors associated with acne vulgaris. https://open.bu.edu/bitstream/2144/19444/1/Patton_bu_0017N_12304.pdf (accessed on 17th June 2025).

48. Riera-Serra, P., Navarra-Ventura, G., Castro, A., Gili, M., Salazar-Cedillo, A., Ricci-Cabello, I., Roldán-Espínola, L., et al. (2023). Clinical predictors of suicidal ideation, suicide attempts

and suicide death in depressive disorder: A systematic review and meta-analysis. *European Archives of Psychiatry and Clinical Neuroscience, 274*, 1543–1563. https://www.semanticscholar.org/paper/0f811670aebabd0ede07d7fc068822e6cb151e55 (accessed on 17th June 2025).

49. Schneider, B. J., Naidoo, J., Santomasso, B., Lacchetti, C., Adkins, S., Anadkat, M. J., Atkins, M. B., et al. (2021). Management of immune-related adverse events in patients treated with immune checkpoint inhibitor therapy: ASCO guideline update. *Journal of Clinical Oncology, 39*, 4073–4126. https://doi.org/10.1200/jco.21.01440 (accessed on 17th June 2025).

50. Shunmuga, P. D., Tadepalli, A., Parthasarathy, H., Ponnaiyan, D., Cholan, P. K., & Ramachandran, L. (2023). Clinical evaluation of the combined efficacy of injectable platelet-rich fibrin along with scaling and root planning in the non-surgical periodontal therapy of stage III and grade C periodontitis patients having type 2 diabetes mellitus: A randomized controlled trial. *Clinical Advances in Periodontics*. https://www.semanticscholar.org/paper/fa426aafa1fe9de141869650587056ccccf9b1c0 (accessed on 17th June 2025).

GENE-ENVIRONMENT INTERACTION IN RHEUMATOLOGY

6

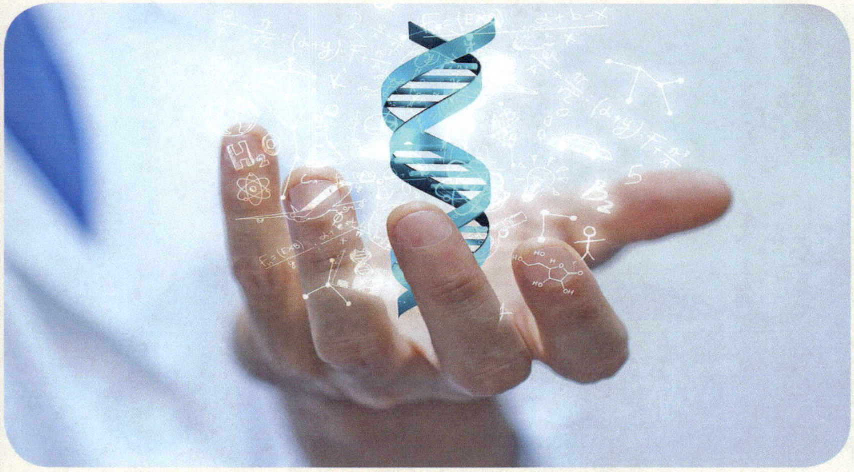

LEARNING OBJECTIVES

After studying this chapter, you will be able to:

1. Identify rheumatological genetic factors;
2. Discuss environmental influence on rheumatic diseases;
3. Highlight gene-environment interactions.

Introduction

Gene-environment interaction is a unifying theme in human understanding of rheumatological disease, which has a widespread influence on patient morbidity. Rheumatological conditions , such as rheumatoid arthritis (RA) and systemic sclerosis (SSc), are strongly variable in prevalence and severity across populations, which suggests an interaction between genetic predisposition and environmental exposures. For instance, research has recognized that some genetic locations, specifically the HLA-DRB1 alleles, confer varying susceptibilities to RA across varying ethnic populations, indicating that genetic susceptibility could confer disparate risks in such groups as those studied in Malaysia (Too, 2012). Moreover, longitudinal observations , such as the Genetics versus Environment in Scleroderma Outcomes Study (GENISOS), have identified modifiable psychosocial and clinical predictors of severity of fatigue in initial SSc and emphasize the need to consider both environmental factors and genetic predisposition when addressing progression of disease (Assassi et al., 2011). As a whole, this two-pronged focus provides an exhaustive framework for researching and treating such complex illnesses.

6.1. Genetic Factors in Rheumatology

Learning Outcome

1. Give an overview of genetic predisposition;
2. Understand the role of some genes in rheumatic conditions;
3. Highlight family history and heritability studies;
4. Identify genetic markers and the role they play;
5. Clarify epigenetics and gene control;
6. Describe genetic testing and its implications;
7. Understand the interaction of many genes in disease expression;
8. Discuss advances in genetic research technology;
9. Outline future research directions.

The intricate interaction among genetic factors and rheumatological disease pathogenesis highlights the importance of understanding inherited susceptibility in rheumatological diseases. Inherited susceptibility is observed in diseases , such as autoimmune hepatitis, where particular autoantibodies and immune mechanisms highlight the importance of genetics in identifying autoantigens and triggering chronic inflammation within the liver (Muratori et al., 2023). Similarly, diseases like fibromyalgia exhibit a strong hereditary component, evidenced by overlapping patterns of symptoms with co-morbid disorders and the disproportionate prevalence of such comorbidities as depression, which carries genetic risk factors as well (Yépez et al., 2022). Such evidence suggests that exploring the genetic causes of rheumatological diseases can enhance current diagnostics and treatment protocols. Lastly, detection of genetic predispositions aids not only in the detection of vulnerable populations but also in paving the way for personalized medicine strategies where treatment protocols can be adjusted to the patient's own unique genetic makeup, thereby improving patient outcomes (Figure 6.1).

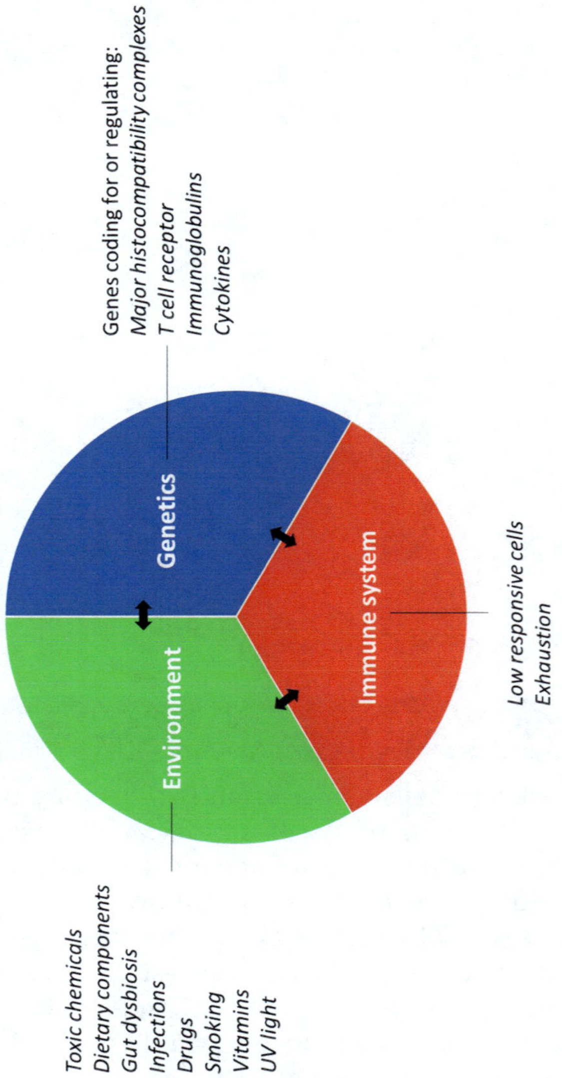

Figure 6.1. The intricate interplay between genetic factors and the pathogenesis of rheumatological conditions underscores the importance of understanding inherited predispositions in these diseases.

Source: https://www.mdpi.com/ijms/ijms-24-13609/article_deploy/html/images/ijms-24-13609-g001.png.

6.1.1. Overview of Genetic Predisposition

Genetic susceptibility to rheumatological diseases, particularly rheumatoid arthritis (RA), plays a crucial role in determining an individual's susceptibility to the disease. Various studies have found some genetic markers , such as the HLA-DRB1 shared epitope alleles, to have a critical role in increasing the susceptibility to ACPA-positive RA, particularly in diverse populations , such as in Asia, where certain genetic differences , such as DRB1*0405, are prevalent (Too, 2012). Besides, data prove that polymorphisms in the peptidylarginine deiminase type IV (PADI4) gene are implicated in RA susceptibility among Asian populations, thereby underscoring the gene's contribution to populations (Too, 2012). Such a genetic composition illustrates the complexity of RA since genetic susceptibility is not unilateral but combines with environmental stimuli, such as smoking, to further confuse disease onset. Explanation of these interactions is most important for the development of targeted prevention and treatment strategies in rheumatology.

6.1.2. Role of Specific Genes in Rheumatic Diseases

During the discovery of the genetic basis of rheumatic diseases, researchers found some particular genes that are involved in susceptibility and disease progression. For instance, certain alleles of the HLA-DRB1 gene have been associated with an increased risk of developing RA, particularly in Asian populations, whereby such genes as DRB1*0405 confer a higher susceptibility to ACPA-positive RA. This is a representation of population genetic heterogeneity in that the presence of distinct risk alleles will generate variation in disease phenotypes and outcome, for example, in studies that highlighted the gene-environment interaction, most particularly with tobacco use augmenting risk among those who were seropositive. Besides, gene polymorphisms , such as PADI4 have been strongly linked to RA susceptibility among Asians but not Europeans, illustrating the importance of research in heterogeneous populations in uncovering the complex genetic architecture of rheumatic conditions (Too, 2012; Reynisdottir, 2015). This discovery opens the door to personalized therapeutic treatments of such conditions (Figure 6.2).

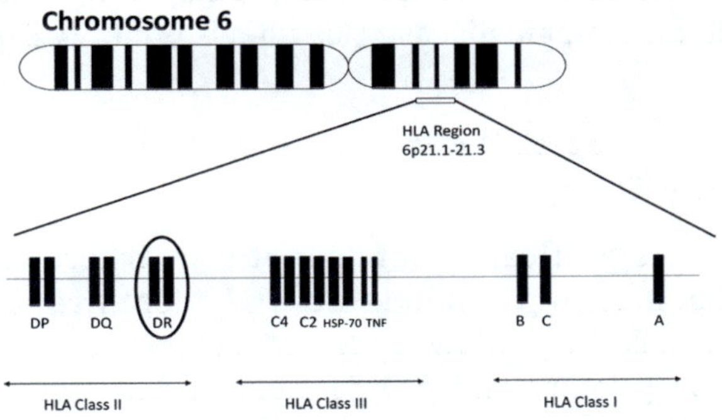

Figure 6.2. While understanding the genetic basis of rheumatic diseases, researchers have pinpointed specific genes that significantly influence susceptibility and disease progression.

Source: https://pub.mdpi-res.com/cells/cells-09-01127/article_deploy/html/images/cells-09-01127-g001.png?1590677826.

6.1.3. Family History and Heritability Studies

Family history and heritability need to be valued when researching rheumatologic disease because they significantly influence disease predisposition. A number of studies reveal an important heritable component for conditions , such as rheumatoid arthritis, whereby some genetic variants can increase risk even before symptom onset. For instance, recent research quoted connections between gut microbiota profiles and known rheumatoid arthritis risk alleles, which suggests that genetic and environmental components work together to affect disease risk in genetically predisposed individuals (Wells et al., 2020). Also, a study of local health inequalities determines the manner in which environmental factors can enhance genetic vulnerabilities. People living in rural areas are likely to have lower access to healthcare services and higher-risk behaviors and hence more cases of chronic conditions, like the joint-related conditions. This information highlights the need for a dual consideration of environmental and genetic factors while making the assessment of familial predispositions of rheumatologic disease (Matthews et al., 2017).

6.1.4. Genetic Markers and their Significance

The significance of genetic markers in rheumatology extends beyond identification because they allow us to differentiate disease susceptibility and progression. Recent studies have indicated that specific genetic variations, particularly in the MHC locus, are significant in diseases , such as rheumatoid arthritis and systemic juvenile idiopathic arthritis (sJIA).

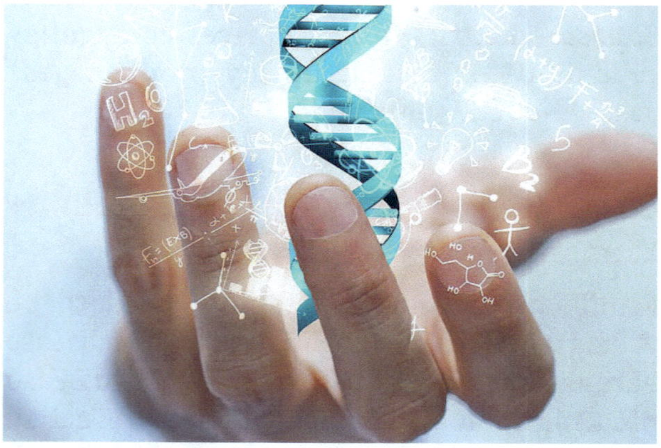

Figure 6.3. The significance of genetic markers in rheumatology extends beyond mere identification, as they contribute to our understanding of disease susceptibility and progression.

Source: https://consumer.healthday.com/media-library/eyJ0eXAiOiJKV1QiLCJhbGciOiJIUzI1NiJ9.LnJibC5tcy8yOTM3ODE1Ny9vcmlnaW4uanBnIiwiZXhwaXJlc19hdCI6MTcxMjUxODg3MH0.nlDqINDDZ2woSn7CxB7bosagvknvl1EgGNl3rO_p2nI/image.jpg?width=1245&height=700&coordinates=0%2C270%2C0%2C270.

For example, a genome-wide association study determined that the SNP rs151043342 is highly correlated with sJIA risk, pointing to the contribution of adaptive immune systems to disease etiology (Ombrello et al., 2015). Similarly, evidence has been presented that there are certain gut microbiota, such as *Prevotella* spp., which correlate with rheumatoid arthritis genetic predispositions, pointing to the intricate interplay of genetic and environmental factors (Wells et al., 2020). Thus, elucidating these genetic markers not only demystifies our understanding of rheumatological disease but also creates avenues for targeted therapy and personalized medicine, finally for the benefit of the patient (Figure 6.3).

6.1.5. Epigenetics and Gene Expression

The interplay between epigenetics and gene expression is increasingly being recognized as an important factor in the research of the pathogenesis of autoimmune diseases in rheumatology. Epigenetic modifications , such as DNA methylation and histone modification, can potentially have a significant impact on gene expression without altering the underlying genetic code. The process can lead to aberrant immune responses and tissue inflammation that mirrors diseases like rheumatoid arthritis. For instance, activation and infiltration of monocytes and macrophages have epigenetic regulation that appears crucial in the establishment of these diseases. Not only are such cells involved in immune response, but also tissue repair and hence are a good target for therapy through their epigenetic makeup (Ma et al., 2019). Moreover, longitudinal studies , such as those carried out in the TwinsUK cohort are beneficial in understanding the multifaceted interaction between environmental exposures and epigenetic adjustment, casting more light on the complex dynamics involved in genetic susceptibility to autoimmune diseases (Verdi et al., 2019).

6.1.6. Genetic Testing and Its Implications

Implications of genetic testing in rheumatology are extensive, particularly if they extend to diseases , such as autoimmune diseases in the context of RA. As more evidence is discovered supporting the heritability of RA, the potential for genetic tests to offer insight into diagnoses and treatment regimens becomes more apparent.

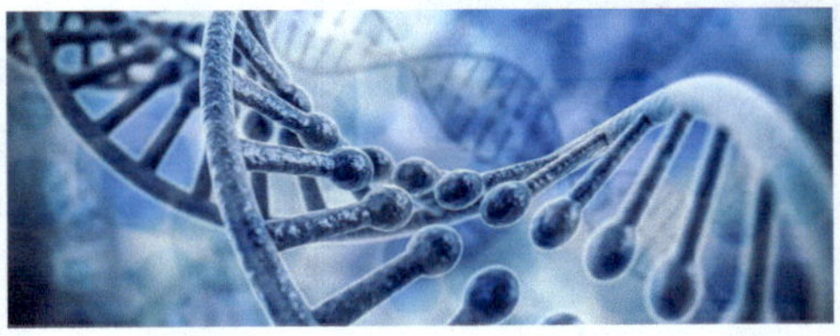

Figure 6.4. The implications of genetic testing in the context of rheumatology are profound.

Source: https://medizinonline.com/wp-content/uploads/2017/09/dna_genetik_2.jpg.

For instance, genetic alterations, i.e., in HLA-DRB1 alleles, have been identified as significant associations with RA susceptibility across populations globally, thus suggesting that disease-directed testing will be valuable for furthering personalized medicine programs. Further, studies indicate that gene factors may have an interaction with environmental stimuli, e.g., cigarette smoking, and modulate the risk of disease, illustrating the complexity of RA's etiology (Lahore et al., 2021). Also, data from animal models underscore the functional significance of some gene polymorphisms in the disease process and open up new possibilities for therapeutic intervention (Lahore et al., 2021). Thus, genetic testing not only facilitates risk estimation but can also improve our knowledge about the intricate interactions between genes and environmental factors in rheumatology (Figure 6.4).

6.1.7. Interaction of Multiple Genes in Disease Manifestation

The pathogenesis of autoimmune diseases , such as RA, emphasizes the role of interactions between genes in disease expression. Multiple studies have demonstrated that gene-gene interactions contribute significantly to RA susceptibility, an indication of the role of particular genetic variants in disease pathogenesis. A case is SELS gene variant interaction with cytokine gene polymorphisms like IL1β, which has generated strong epistatic effects to modify disease risk and demonstrate how such genetic variants act in inflammatory pathways (Binks et al., 2009). Moreover, research within diverse populations, including Malaysian cohorts, has shown that particular HLA-DRB1 alleles impart RA susceptibility on an ethnic heterogeneity basis, suggesting that the genetic makeup is not equal (Too, 2012). Such discoveries encourage subtle analysis of the interaction among different genes since they all interact to create the heterogeneous character of RA, ultimately directing therapy to targeted approaches.

6.1.8. Advances in Genetic Research Technologies

The profession of rheumatology is being transformed with the evolution of genetic research technologies, leading to a new era of disease diagnosis and treatment of conditions like RA. With the germinative rates of genotyping and sophisticated analytical techniques, multiple genetic risk factors have been discovered for RA, thereby enhancing diagnostic and predictive capabilities. As noted, "Enhanced knowledge of the underlying pathogenesis of the disease promises better diagnostic and predictive tools based on this knowledge". In addition, these advances allow for the examination of gene-environment interactions, emphasizing the complexity of this autoimmune disorder. However, even with such technological advancements, there are obstacles, particularly in the translation of genetic findings to clinical practice. An inter-disciplinary approach that merges genetic data with clinical assessment will definitely play an important part in optimizing individualized treatment regimens for patients (Smolen et al., 2016) (Figure 6.5).

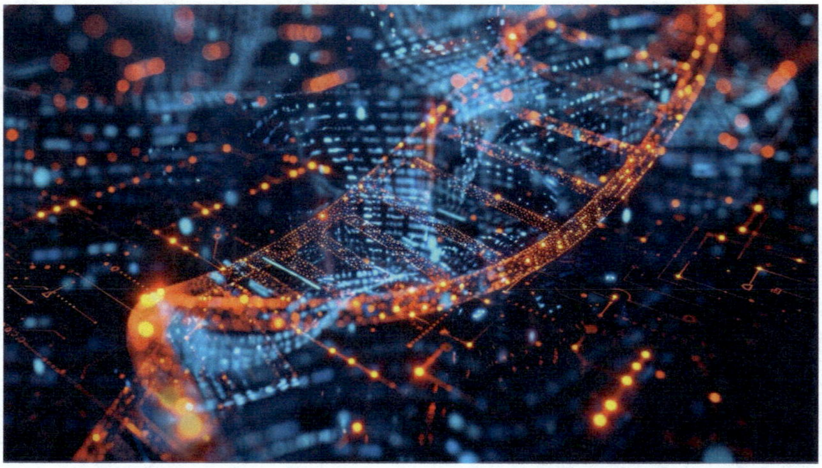

Figure 6.5. Rapid developments in genotyping, coupled with sophisticated analytical techniques, have led to the discovery of numerous genetic risk factors associated with RA, thereby enhancing diagnostic and prognostic capabilities.

Source: https://www.whatisbiotechnology.org/assets/images/science/pages/3dgenomics.jpg.

6.1.9. Future Directions in Genetic Studies

As further breakthroughs are made with genetic research, research directions in the future hold great potential for rheumatology research, particularly as far as the gene-environment interaction is concerned. Studies are moving more towards integrating genomic data with environmental factors, potentially redefining our concept of rheumatic diseases. New tools , such as genome-wide association studies (GWAS) and graph neural networks, allow researchers to decipher the code of complex interactions between environmental stimuli and genetic susceptibility, as seen in cancer research methodologies , such as those presented by Mendel et al. (2025). These tools would enable one to visualize how different genetic variants influence disease susceptibility in various environments. Further, epigenetic profiling and utilization of multi-omics technology may uncover novel therapeutic and personalized medicine targets and thus simplify existing treatment strategies to rheumatic ailments. Thus, the convergence of all these intricate scientific techniques will be crucial in enhancing our understanding of genetics in rheumatology and personalizing future treatments.

Test Your Knowledge

1. What is the role of family history in risk stratification for rheumatologic diseases?
2. What is the role of genetic testing in the diagnosis or treatment of rheumatologic diseases?

6.2. Environmental Influences on Rheumatic Diseases

Learning Outcome

1. Understand the definition of environmental factors;
2. Focus on the role of lifestyle choices;
3. Know the impact of pollutants and toxins;
4. Describe climate and geographical conditions;
5. Explain infections and their relationship to rheumatic diseases;
6. Discuss stress and psychosocial factors;
7. Focus on occupational hazards and risks;
8. Identify environmental precipitants in disease development.

The interplay between environmental agents and the pathogenesis of rheumatic illnesses has been under intense scrutiny in recent years. Specific environmental triggers, such as exposure to toxins, smoking, and microbial infection, have been implicated in initiating and perpetuating diseases like rheumatoid arthritis and lupus. Lifestyle factors, too, determined by the immediate environment, diet, activity levels, and stress, are also found to modulate disease activity and outcome. For instance, individuals residing in rural areas are likely to be more susceptible to certain rheumatic diseases via a deficiency of access to health care and health-promoting services that might hinder early diagnosis and intervention (Matthews et al., 2017). Moreover, the COVID-19 pandemic has emphasized the importance of maintaining health care access, as interruption would compound symptoms for patients with established rheumatic illness (Bashshur et al., 2020). Thus, it is paramount to know such environmental influences for rational management and prevention in rheumatology.

6.2.1. Definition of Environmental Factors

Environmental factors are defined as a range of non-genetic influences that can potentially exert a significant effect on health consequences and disease susceptibility, particularly in rheumatology. Examples of these are physical exposures like pollutants and infectious agents, as well as lifestyle determinants like diet and exercise. Up-to-date studies highlight the necessity of knowing how external factors affect genetic predisposition in conditions like giant cell arteritis and uterine fibroids. In giant cell arteritis, for instance, the external factors might be predisposing factors that, in association with genetic predisposition, contribute to the pathogenesis of the disease (González-Gay et al., 2025). Similarly, the prevalence of uterine fibroids has been linked with alterations in microbiota, by which they may influence tumorigenesis via epigenetic alterations, establishing an extremely strong interaction between the environment and genetic mechanisms (Senbadejo et al., 2024). Understanding such interactions is crucial to further enhance treatment and prevention of rheumatological conditions (Figure 6.6).

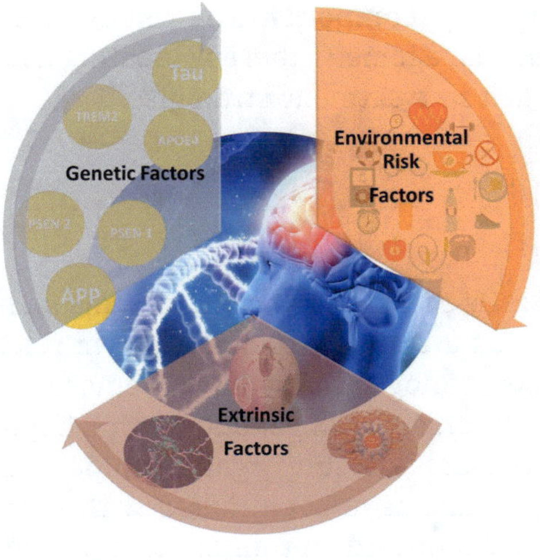

Figure 6.6. Environmental factors encompass a range of non-genetic influences that can significantly affect health outcomes and disease susceptibility, particularly in the field of rheumatology.

Source: https://www.frontiersin.org/files/Articles/1303111/fneur-14-1303111-HTML/image_m/fneur-14-1303111-g004.jpg.

6.2.2. Role of Lifestyle Choices (Diet, Exercise)

The interplay between lifestyle choices, particularly diet and exercise, and rheumatological conditions is increasingly being recognized as a significant factor in prevention and management. A balanced diet of anti-inflammatory foods, such as omega-3 fatty acids, vegetables, and fruits, can relieve symptoms and improve overall health in patients who present with diseases like RA. Evidence suggests that regular physical activity not only benefits physical function but also reduces the prevalence of comorbidities common among rheumatic diseases, including cardiovascular disease and chronic pain syndromes like fibromyalgia (Hamilton et al., 2013). Secondly, the multifaceted aspect of RA, with demonstration of systemic inflammation across multiple joints, further lays down the need for overall lifestyle modifications (Cole, 2016). With mounting evidence for the contribution of diet and physical activity, lifestyle interventions become key components in rheumatological disease management, thereby creating a holistic approach in treatment strategies.

6.2.3. Impact of Pollutants and Toxins

The effects of toxins and contaminants on health have been a big issue, particularly in reference to rheumatological disease, as environmental factors intersect with genetic factors. Exposures to particulates, volatile organic compounds, and heavy metals have been linked with increased inflammation and autoimmunity, which may exacerbate diseases , such as lupus and rheumatoid arthritis. Advanced chemical sensing instruments have been most beneficial in monitoring these environmental contaminants, providing vital data on the quantity and types of toxins present (Ojomo, 2025). Furthermore, rhizosphere bacteria bioremediation offers effective alternatives to reverse the effect of toxins on the environment since the microbes can effectively degrade poisonous materials and enhance soil fertility (Balkrishna et al., 2024). Learning about toxic exposure and genetic susceptibility is important for developing effective prevention measures in rheumatology, given the imperative to address environmental health (Figure 6.7).

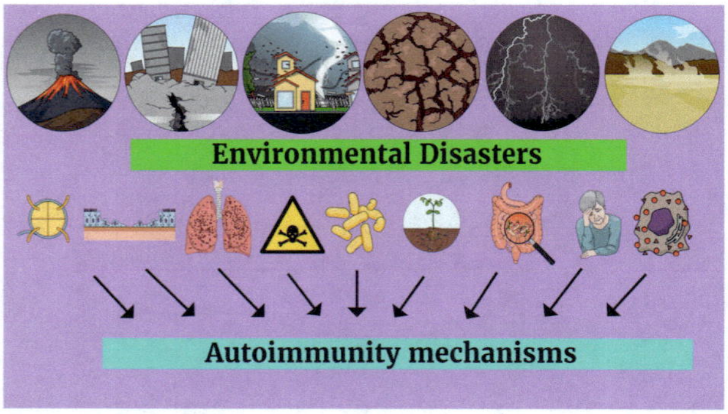

Figure 6.7. Exposure to heavy metals, volatile organic compounds, and particulate matter has been linked to increased inflammation and autoimmunity, potentially exacerbating conditions , such as rheumatoid arthritis and lupus.

Source: https://pub.mdpi-res.com/healthcare/healthcare-12-01767/article_deploy/html/images/healthcare-12-01767-ag.png?1725436186.

6.2.4. Climate and Geographical Influences

Geographic and climatic determinants have been implicated in playing a significant role in the development and expression of rheumatologic disease, which further suggests the intricate interplay between genetic susceptibility and environmental stresses. For instance, investigations have revealed that Sjögrens syndrome patients from countries that are under challenging climate-related threats exhibit varying clinical manifestations, e.g., age of diagnosis and symptom severity, thereby suggesting that environmental damage is able to modulate disease progression. Similarly, geographic heterogeneity has been linked with phenotypic variation in systemic sclerosis, where Southern Italian patients had more severe disease compared to Northern European patients. This difference may be due to interaction between genetic susceptibility and local environmental factors, including climate and access to healthcare (Giuggioli et al., 2022). Identification of these dynamics is vital to the design of specific therapeutic strategies and maximization of patient outcomes based on geographical and climatic conditions in rheumatology.

6.2.5. Infections and Their Relationship to Rheumatic Diseases

This interaction of infections and rheumatic diseases is increasingly recognized in rheumatology research, including environmental factors in the disease process and its development. Infections may act as triggers for autoimmune responses, particularly in genetically susceptible individuals, to lead to autoimmune diseases , such as RA. It has been shown that some pathogens have the potential to induce an inflammatory process that ultimately progresses to autoimmunity because some autoantibodies, such as anti-citrullinated protein antibodies (ACPAs), may arise from immune responses generated by infections of the lungs before the onset of clinical signs of joint symptoms (Reynisdottir, 2015). In addition, the chronic nature of rheumatoid diseases enhances the susceptibility to infection, thus ultimately making treatment outcomes complicated (Chaplain et al., 2019). Consequently, it is important to understand the interactive complexity of environmental factors , such as infections with genetic susceptibilities, towards an attempt at developing targeted therapy strategies that not only manage symptoms but also halt disease progression in susceptible populations (Figure 6.8).

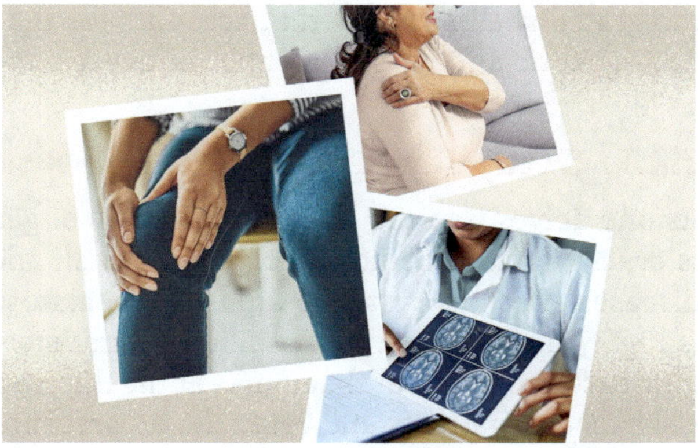

Figure 6.8. Infections may serve as triggers for autoimmune responses, particularly in genetically predisposed individuals, leading to conditions , such as rheumatoid arthritis (RA).

Source: https://images.everydayhealth.com/images/autoimmune-diseases/autoimmune-disorders-of-the-joints-and-nerves-1440x810.jpg?sfvrsn=a523a5ee_5.

6.2.6. Stress and Psychosocial Factors

An understanding of the interaction between stress, psychosocial issues, and rheumatological diseases is important to design comprehensive treatment plans. Stress, and particularly chronic stress, has a strong influence on physical well-being, and it may exacerbate conditions , such as osteoarthritis and complicate their therapy even further. The evidence indicates that stress of psychological origin influences not only the individual's pain experience but also influences inflammatory responses within the body, and thus accelerates diseases like knee osteoarthritis (KOA) (Geng et al., 2023). The psychosocial context also plays a significant role in influencing a patient's response to illness, e.g., coping and adherence to treatment regimens (Óskarsdóttir et al., 2023). For instance, effective stress management can be beneficial in reducing pain and improving the quality of life for patients with chronic rheumatic disorders. Intervention for psychosocial aspects is, therefore, part of an integrated rheumatology that accounts for the fact that the prognosis of the disease is affected by both genetic and environmental influences, including stress.

6.2.7. Occupational Hazards and Risks

As one delves into the complex interplay of genetics and the environment within rheumatology, it is crucial to analyze how occupational risk and hazard play a role in the etiology of autoimmune diseases , such as systemic lupus erythematosus (SLE). Current research underlines that SLE risk is highly increased within families with a known history of the condition, suggesting a genetically influenced component that meets at the intersection with environmental factors. Specifically, relative risks among patients and relatives, as presented in the research findings of 43.9% heritability for SLE, point towards environmental, including occupational, exposures playing the predominant role. Also, studies of occupational workers with exposure to ergonomic problems, such as workers in the textile industry, point to very high rates of MSDs contributing to lost productivity and increased health risk. In this case, understanding the intricacy of occupational exposure becomes crucial in risk reduction regarding autoimmune diseases (Doherty et al., 2015; Starovoytova, 2017) (Figure 6.9).

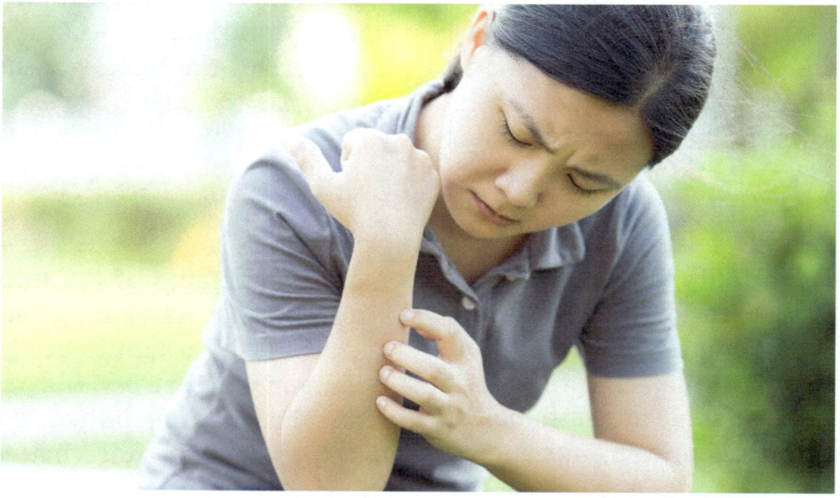

Figure 6.9. Occupational hazards and risks contribute to the prevalence of autoimmune diseases.

Source: https://womenshealth.gov/sites/default/files/heading-images/Autoimmunediseases.jpg.

6.2.8. Environmental Triggers in Disease Onset

Recognition of the place of the environmental trigger in disease causation is important in rheumatology, a specialty where complex interaction between genetic predisposition and environment plays a major role in determining the trajectory of disease. Autoimmune hepatitis is a good example of how environmental influence can precipitate immune responses leading to inflammatory disease. In this case, there is a pathological immune response against liver autoantigens, with persistent inflammation, if untreated, evolving into severe complications , such as cirrhosis (Muratori et al., 2023). Furthermore, research has explained that gene–environment interactions play a central role in most disease pathologies and outlined how exposures like pollution or pathogens can cause disease in genetically susceptible individuals (Virolainen et al., 2022). This overlap between environmental and genetic factors reaffirms the complexity of rheumatological diseases and highlights the importance of combined research to improve diagnostic and therapeutic processes.

Test Your Knowledge

1. What role does stress play in autoimmune rheumatic condition exacerbations?
2. How may dietary patterns (e.g., high salt, Western diet) affect inflammation in autoimmune disease?

6.3. Gene-Environment Interactions

Learning Outcome

1. Learn definition of gene-environment interactions;
2. Provide examples of interactions in specific diseases;
3. Understand mechanism of interaction;
4. Highlight research methods for studying interactions;
5. Discuss implications for personalized medicine;
6. Identify challenges in research on gene-environment interactions;
7. Explain public health implications;
8. Know directions for future research in this area.

The relationship between environmental elements and genetic predispositions is significant in the identification of etiology in a variety of rheumatological diseases, such as in Juvenile Idiopathic Arthritis (JIA) and Meniere's disease. It is demonstrated that some genetic markers, particularly those for immune response genes, can exert strong effects on susceptibility to such illnesses, with environmental stimuli like infection and lifestyle being involved in aggravating their occurrence. For instance, studies have discovered that certain HLA alleles predispose to JIA, showing how genetic variation can set a person up for autoimmunity in the face of challenge from the environment (Saleh, 2024). Similarly, in Meniere's disease, multiple gene variants have been involved in the immune system as well as the systemic process, pointing to a complex system of gene-environment interaction that gives rise to the disease expression (Arweiler-Harbeck et al., 2020). Thus, the characterization of these interactions is imperative to the development of targeted interventions and improved patient outcomes in rheumatology.

6.3.1. Definition of Gene-environment Interactions

Gene-environment interactions emphasize the dynamic nature of disease causation, particularly in conditions , such as RA. Gene-environment interactions explain how genetic predisposition is tempered by environmental factors and results in disease severity and progression. Research has indicated the presence of certain gene variants, i.e., the HLA-DRB1 shared epitope alleles, that are linked with increased risk of ACPA-positive RA, particularly when combined with lifestyle factors , such as smoking (Too, 2012). Gene polymorphisms that relate to autoimmune responses have varied impacts on various populations, a factor which highlights the significance of both genetic and environmental background (Croen et al., 2006). This intricate interaction necessitates that the prevention and treatment interventions incorporate not only the genetic markers but also environmental determinants most likely to trigger or exacerbate rheumatological conditions. Gene-environment interactions are thus essential to advancing personalized medicine for rheumatology (Figure 6.10).

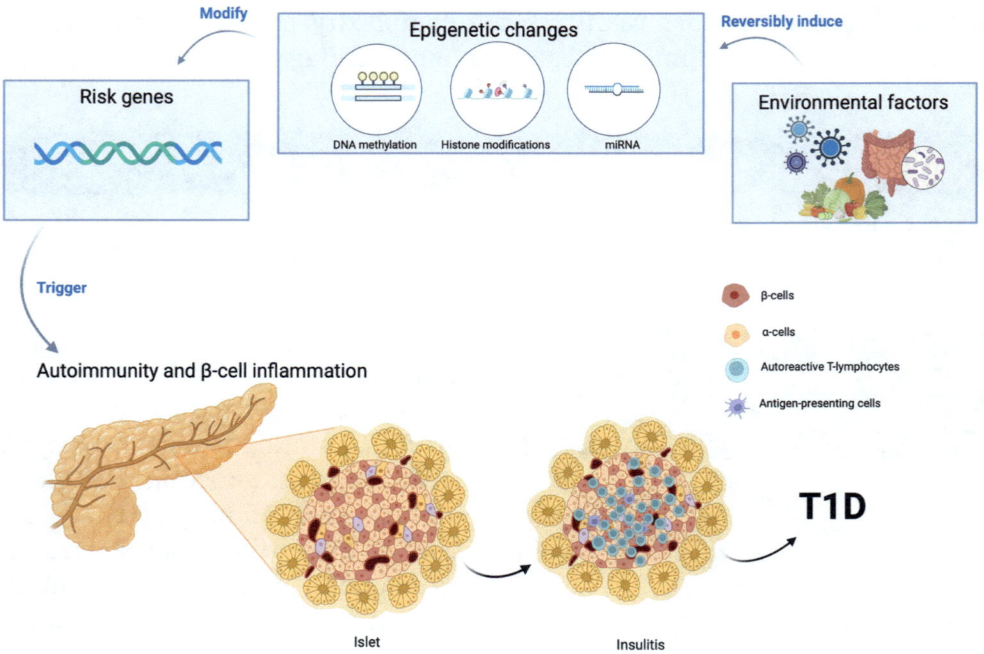

Figure 6.10. The concept of gene-environment interactions underscores the complexity of disease etiology, particularly in conditions , such as rheumatoid arthritis (RA).

Source: https://www.frontiersin.org/files/Articles/1335435/fendo-15-1335435-HTML/image_m/fendo-15-1335435-g001.jpg.

6.3.2. Examples of Interactions in Specific Diseases

The complex interplay between the genetic and environmental factors is the clue to the pathogenesis of rheumatic disorders, such as observed in conditions like atopic dermatitis (AD). The skin disorder is a prime example of how inbuilt genetic susceptibility can interact with microbial populations to enhance inflammation. Research indicates AD patients have a profoundly altered dermal microbiota from healthy controls, with various bacterial genera like Staphylococcus and Cutibacterium having significant differences in relation to disease severity (Bay et al., 2025). Lastly, states of mental health, usually comorbid with rheumatic diseases, demonstrate the involvement of nuclear receptors in gene-environment interactions and neuropsychiatric burden modulation relating to them (Donskov et al., 2021). These observations make it important to comprehend such intricate interactions because they will result in personalized treatments addressing both genetic vulnerabilities and environmental triggers, ultimately enhancing patient management in rheumatology.

6.3.3. Mechanisms of Interaction

Comprehension of the interaction mechanisms between genes and environment is central to deconstructing the intricacy of rheumatological diseases, particularly RA. Substantial evidence of large genetic susceptibility to RA exists, with heritability of approximately 60% indicating significant contributions by specific genes and gene-environment interactions. For instance, a number of single nucleotide polymorphisms (SNPs) in the NADPH-oxidase (NOX) complex have been identified with significant association in male patients with RA. These genetic differences have the potential to affect the production of reactive oxygen species, the severity and course of disease, and therefore demonstrate how genetic pathways may intermingle with environmental stimulants, such as infection or smoking, to trigger RA pathology. Treatment strategies now also show awareness of these interactions, as clinicians aim at both genetic susceptibility and environmental factors for disease activity, showing the need for a multidimensional therapeutic strategy in rheumatology for improving patient outcomes (Alfredsson et al., 2007; Smolen et al., 2016) (Figure 6.11).

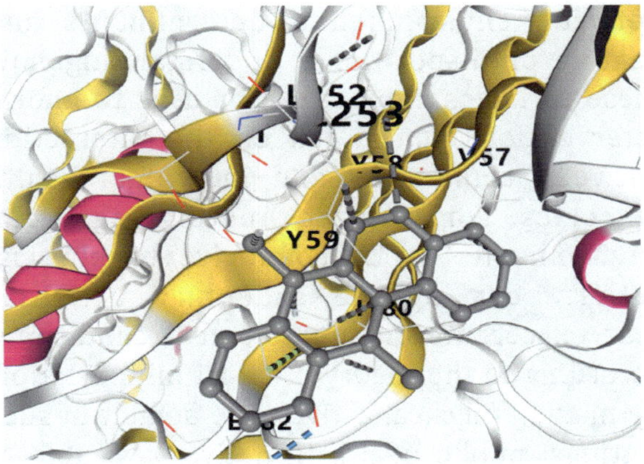

Figure 6.11. Understanding the mechanisms of interaction between genetic factors and environmental influences is crucial in elucidating the complexities of rheumatological diseases, particularly rheumatoid arthritis (RA).

Source: https://media.springernature.com/lw685/springer-static/image/art%3A10.1038%2Fs41598-025-94053-7/MediaObjects/41598_2025_94053_Fig27_HTML.png.

6.3.4. Research Methodologies for Studying Interactions

Research into interactions between environmental pressures and genetics in rheumatology demands good and multidimensional research methodologies. These strategies use a combination of genetic screening and environmental quantification to reverse-engineer gene-by-environment (G×E) interactions, which underpin disease susceptibility and progression. For instance, genomic data correlation with phenotypic data has been extremely valuable in identifying some traits that will react differently under various environments, as in the review of breeding schemes in cattle (Neto et al., 2024). Furthermore, polygenic risk scores (PRS) and multilocus genetic profile scores (MGPS) are the frontline instruments for the key purpose of identifying how genetic susceptibility interacts with environmental stressors to influence outcomes like depression, which is characteristic of the nuances of rheumatic diseases (Grillo, 2024). These integrated approaches highlight that genetic and environmental factors need to be given proper merit consideration if the nuances of rheumatological diseases are to be fully grasped."

6.3.5. Implications for Personalized Medicine

Involving genetics and the environment in personalised medicine carries significant implications for rheumatology, most obviously in the tailoring of therapy to the individual patient. Genetic diversity, especially at a population level, offers new avenues of investigation of disease mechanisms and drug response. For example, newer studies have shown that genetic differences can influence the susceptibility of an individual to autoimmune disorders like rheumatoid arthritis and thus the safety and efficacy of the treatment. Furthermore, as discussed, the African populations are the most genetically heterogeneous on earth and provide new avenues to enhance pharmacogenomics and personalize the therapies. Notwithstanding, challenges still exist in the form of underrepresentation in clinical trials and insufficient relevant genomic references that will enhance personalized healthcare delivery (Bhowmik et al., 2025). Removing these barriers through intensive genomic studies and comprehensive research approaches is crucial to optimizing personalized medical practices in rheumatology as well as delivering balanced outcomes to diverse populations (Bhowmik et al., 2025) (Figure 6.12).

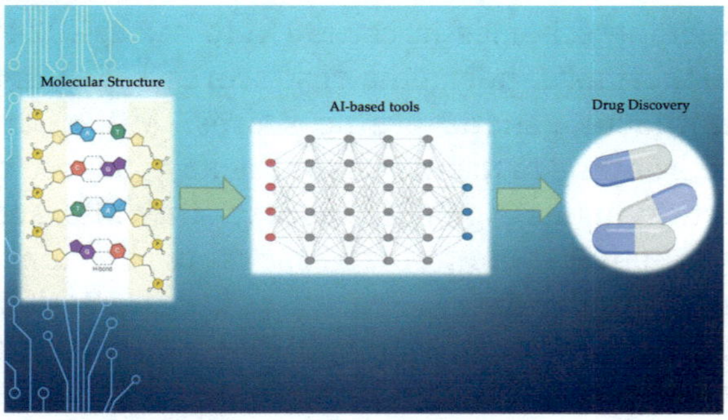

Figure 6.12. Genetic diversity, especially within populations, offers new avenues for understanding disease mechanisms and treatment responses.

Source: https://chemistry-europe.onlinelibrary.wiley.com/cms/asset/f18499e3-91a2-4fbd-a624-5febe8863632/cbic202300816-toc-0001-m.jpg.

6.3.6. Challenges in Studying Gene-environment Interactions

It is a challenging endeavor to study gene-environment interactions, particularly in complex diseases , such as RA. The intricate interaction between genetic susceptibility and many environmental factors can complicate it to become a challenging task to identify specific risk loci and their functional significance. For instance, even though certain alleles like HLA-DRB1 are established genetic risk alleles for ACPA-positive RA in Asian populations, their impact might not be generalizable to heterogeneous ethnic groups, as indicated by findings of varying associations in Malaysian cohorts (Too, 2012). Furthermore, environmental factors , such as smoking have been shown to enhance genetic susceptibility, but the multifactorial nature of RA limits the scope to draw categorical conclusions without extensive and heterogeneous population studies. Consequently, understanding such interactions necessitates robust methodologies that well account for both genetic heterogeneity and environmental heterogeneity, thus making translational studies in rheumatology more demanding (Djouad et al., 2022).

6.3.7. Public Health Implications

Public health problems in rheumatology are explained in critical terms by interactions between environmental determinants and genetic predispositions. Understanding how these variables interact can be used to inform interventions that work on the interaction between community and individual health outcomes. For instance, redesigning urban environments to be conducive to physical activity can oppose sedentary activities that exacerbate rheumatological conditions, according to the theory of effort minimization. By making physical activity the default in such settings, public health initiatives are able to enhance community engagement and overall health (Cheval et al., 2025).

Furthermore, environmental exposure to toxicants and childhood trauma also significantly contribute to the determinants of personal health trajectories, particularly in genetically vulnerable individuals. These environmental toxins can be targeted by public health policy to prevent their negative impact and create a healthier population, and it is thus crucial to include true interventions in the context of rheumatology (Iannaccone et al., 2024). Hence, it becomes crucial to merge genetics with the environment to aid public health efforts (Figure 6.13).

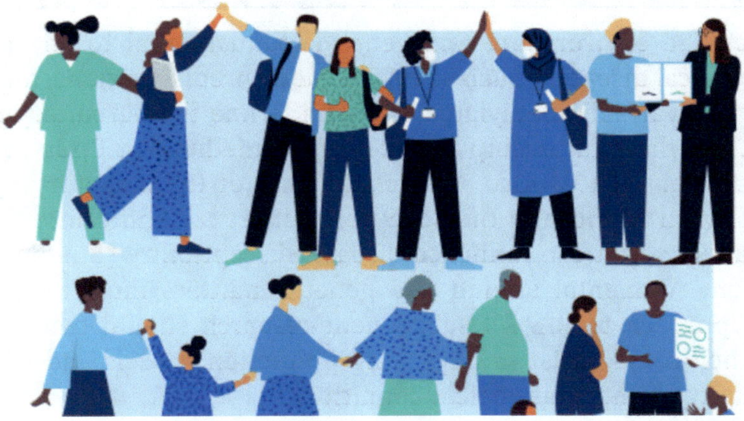

Figure 6.13. Public health initiatives can enhance community engagement and overall well-being.

Source: https://global.comminit.com/sites/default/files/cengagewho4.png.

6.3.8. Future Research Directions in this Area

As the dynamic interplay of genetics and environmental factors in rheumatology gets elucidated, eventual research agendas shall be geared towards the development of precision therapies and bespoke medicine. This can be achieved by the discovery of precision biomarkers that determine response to therapy, particularly in diseases characterized by chronic inflammation, such as connective tissue disease-associated interstitial lung disease (CTD-ILD) and other skin disorders. Resolving these challenges will augment diagnosis and therapeutic approaches, allowing for specific treatment regimens that respect the individualized genetic backgrounds and environmental exposures of the patients. Understanding the mechanism of the chronic inflammation characteristic of these disorders will also shed light on their pathogenesis and may open avenues for novel therapeutic modalities. In conclusion, a multidisciplinary approach of genetic, environmental, and immunological perspectives will be extremely crucial in refining our insight and control of rheumatic disease in the years to come, as seen in the complexities presented by Shao et al. (2021); Ujiie et al. (2022).

Test Your Knowledge

1. How does epigenetic regulation modulate environmental effects on gene expression in autoimmunity?
2. What is the role of the gut microbiome as an environmental mediator in genetically predisposed individuals?

Summary

The interaction between the environment and genes is fundamental to an appreciation of the complexity of rheumatological diseases , such as RA7. Genetic predispositions, for example, through differential biomarkers like variably methylated CpGs, underline the hereditary risk of RA. This is notably illustrated through the relationship between hypermethylated CpGs in peripheral blood with disease (Barcellos et al., 2017). Also, the relationship of inflammatory cytokine pathways with genetic variations , such as those in the SELS gene, offers a significant degree of complexity due to gene-gene interactions that can influence disease susceptibility (Binks et al., 2009). These findings suggest both environmental stimuli and genetic markers must be intervened with to provide an integrated approach to RA. All subsequent research should tend to elucidate , such associations further, which could assist in improving prediction models and treatment protocols for the multidimensionality of rheumatological conditions.

Research on genetic and environmental determinants of RA has shed important light on its multi-factorial pathogenesis. In particular, it has been found that particular HLA-DRB1 alleles, e.g., DRB1*0405, significantly increase the risk for ACPA-positive RA in Asian populations. Conversely, the DRB1*1202 allele provides protective effects against the disease among Malays and Chinese, indicating varying genetic susceptibility among various races (Too, 2012). Further, gene-environment interactions have been reported to include smoking as a significant environmental factor that increases risk among carriers of specific HLA-DRB1 alleles (Too, 2012). In addition, recent reports have pointed to the importance of PADI4 and DCIR gene polymorphisms in susceptibility to RA, particularly ACPA-negative disease, so detection of the heterogeneity of populations in research on the genetic structure of RA must be dealt with more adequately.

KEY TERMS FROM THIS CHAPTER

- Morbidity
- Genetic predisposition
- Depression
- Personalized medicine
- Genetic heterogeneity
- Alleles
- Gut microbiota
- Systemic sclerosis (SSc)
- Genetic locations
- Vulnerable populations
- Genetic makeup
- Gut microbiota
- Systemic juvenile idiopathic arthritis (sJIA)
- Targeted therapy

Critical Thinking Questions

1. **Which HLA allele is most associated with rheumatoid arthritis?**
   a. HLA-B27
   b. HLA-DR4
   c. HLA-A3
   d. HLA-DQ2
2. **Presence of HLA-B27 is most often linked with which group of rheumatic diseases?**
   a. Systemic lupus erythematosus
   b. Osteoarthritis
   c. Spondyloarthropathies
   d. Polymyalgia rheumatica
3. **Which environmental factor has been most closely related to the development and severity of rheumatoid arthritis?**
   a. High-fiber diet
   b. Smoking
   c. Cold weather
   d. Low salt intake
4. **Which of the following is the best description of the interaction between genes and environment in rheumatic diseases?**
   a. Environment determines disease entirely independent of genes
   b. Genes always cause disease independent of environment
   c. Environmental triggers operate on genetically susceptible individuals
   d. Autoimmunity results from lifestyle factors alone
5. **What is the infection that has been suspected to cause reactive arthritis?**
   a. *Streptococcus pneumoniae*
   b. *Chlamydia trachomatis*
   c. Epstein-Barr virus
   d. Varicella zoster virus

Short Answer Questions

1. What is the role of HLA genes (e.g., HLA-DR4, HLA-B27) in autoimmune rheumatic diseases?
2. How does HLA-B27 presence increase ankylosing spondylitis and other spondyloarthropathies?
3. What is the association between smoking and the development of seropositive rheumatoid arthritis?
4. How does exposure to the sun (UV) influence disease activity in systemic lupus erythematosus?
5. How does smoking in HLA-DR4 individuals increase susceptibility to rheumatoid arthritis?
6. What is evidence supporting gene-environment synergy in the pathogenesis of autoimmune diseases?

Answers to Critical Thinking Questions

1. (b); 2. (c); 3. (b); 4. (c); 5. (b)

References

1. Abacar, K., Akasbi, M., Armagan, B., et al. (2023). *Influence of Exposure to Climate-Related Hazards in The Phenotypic Expression of Primary Sjögren's Syndrome*. https://core.ac.uk/download/612187213.pdf (accessed on 17th June 2025).
2. Smolen, J. S., Aletaha, D., & McInnes, I. B. (2016). Rheumatoid arthritis. *Lancet (London, England), 388*(10055), 2023–2038. https://doi.org/10.1016/S0140-6736(16)30173-8 (accessed on 17th June 2025).
3. Alfredsson, L., Burkhardt, H., Holmdahl, R., Klareskog, L., et al. (2007). A case-control study of rheumatoid arthritis identifies an associated single nucleotide polymorphism in the NCF4 gene, supporting a role for the NADPH-oxidase complex in autoimmunity. https://core.ac.uk/download/14505784.pdf (accessed on 17th June 2025).
4. Apparailly, F., Baumans, V., Desaintes, C., Di Santo, J., et al. (2011). *Animal Models for Arthritis: Innovative Tools for Prevention and Treatment*. https://core.ac.uk/download/11279774.pdf (accessed on 17th June 2025).
5. Arweiler-Harbeck, M., Begovich, A., Brama, I., Cabrera, A., Campbell, L., de Lima, M., Doi, K., et al. (2020). Rare variants of putative candidate genes associated with sporadic Meniere's disease in East Asian population. https://core.ac.uk/download/289095089.pdf (accessed on 17th June 2025).
6. Assassi, S., Fischbach, M., GENISOS Study Group, Gonzalez, E. B., et al. (2011). Predictors of fatigue severity in early systemic sclerosis: A prospective longitudinal study of the GENISOS cohort. https://core.ac.uk/download/323073807.pdf (accessed on 17th June 2025).
7. Balkrishna, A., Kaushik, P., Mohini, Arya, V., & Ghosh, S. (2024). Harnessing the power of rhizosphere bacteria for pollution remediation: Strategies, mechanisms, and environmental impact: A review. *Ceylon Journal of Science*. https://www.semanticscholar.org/paper/9e928cce48d06a647a6f7750edf22860db66ee88 (accessed on 17th June 2025).
8. Barcellos, L. F., Chernitskiy, V., Criswell, L. A., Graf, J., et al. (2018). Hypomethylation of CYP2E1 and DUSP22 promoters associated with disease activity and erosive disease among rheumatoid arthritis patients. https://core.ac.uk/download/323073278.pdf (accessed on 17th June 2025).
9. Barcellos, L. F., Cole, M., Criswell, L. A., Firestein, G. S., et al. (2017). Rheumatoid arthritis naive T cells share hypermethylation sites with synoviocytes. https://core.ac.uk/download/323062246.pdf (accessed on 17th June 2025).
10. Bashshur, R. L., Doarn, C. R., Frenk, J., Kvedar, J. C., & Woolliscroft, J. O. (2020). Telemedicine and the COVID-19 pandemic, lessons for the future. *Telemedicine Journal and e-Health, 26*, 571–573. https://doi.org/10.1089/tmj.2020.29040.rb (accessed on 17th June 2025).
11. Bay, L., Barnes, C. J., Fritz, B., Ravnborg, N., Ruge, I., Halling-Sønderby, A. S., Søeborg, S. R., et al. (2025). Unique dermal bacterial signature differentiates atopic dermatitis skin from healthy. *mSphere*. https://www.semanticscholar.org/paper/16c6fe87477e02b698e3e351dfb73ad978a691d7 (accessed on 17th June 2025).
12. Bhowmik, S., Hajra, A., & Bandyopadhyay, D. (2025). Genetic insights in infectious diseases: Insights from a case report and implications for personalized medicine. *World Journal of*

Clinical Cases, 13. https://www.semanticscholar.org/paper/15c73b41f2da1c7aa7178220ece f2040de92a126 (accessed on 17th June 2025).

13. Binks, M. H., Dickson, M. C., Marinou, L., Montgomery, J., et al. (2009). Evidence of epistasis between interleukin-1 and selenoprotein-S with susceptibility to rheumatoid arthritis. https://core.ac.uk/download/49859.pdf (accessed on 17th June 2025).
14. Chaplain, M. A. J., Eftimie, R., & Macfarlane, F. R. (2019). Quantitative predictive modelling approaches to understanding rheumatoid arthritis: A brief review. https://core.ac.uk/download/286356117.pdf (accessed on 17th June 2025).
15. Cheval, B., Maltagliati, S., & Owen, N. (2025). Effort minimization and the built environment: Public health implications. *Journal of Physical Activity & Health.* https://www.semanticscholar.org/paper/31068b41138ca9813625a9e543000bf103ed1fbc (accessed on 17th June 2025).
16. Cole, A. (2016). Comorbidity: A neglected aspect of the burden of RA. https://core.ac.uk/download/71427759.pdf (accessed on 17th June 2025).
17. Croen, L. A., Hansen, R., Hertz-Picciotto, I., Jones, C., et al. (2006). The CHARGE study: An epidemiologic investigation of genetic and environmental factors contributing to autism. https://core.ac.uk/download/323070787.pdf (accessed on 17th June 2025).
18. Djouad, F., Ladel, C., Lang, A., Larkin, J., et al. (2022). Animal models of osteoarthritis part 1–Preclinical small animal models: Challenges and opportunities for drug development. https://core.ac.uk/download/628858819.pdf (accessed on 17th June 2025).
19. Doherty, M., Grainge, M. J., Kuo, C. F., Luo, S., et al. (2015). Familial aggregation of systemic lupus erythematosus and coaggregation of autoimmune diseases in affected families. https://core.ac.uk/download/96620422.pdf (accessed on 17th June 2025).
20. Donskov, J., Starnawska, A., Pallesen, J., Grove, J., Børglum, A., & Qvist, P. (2021). Large-scale genomic data-mining implicates dysregulated nuclear receptor-mediated signaling in mental illness. *Journal of Translational Genetics and Genomics.* https://www.semanticscholar.org/paper/c1158dd98d3a1eb51ae2b5e0c684964e2da21f60 (accessed on 17th June 2025).
21. Fernandez Lahore, G. (2021). Identifying genetic determinants of T cell-dependent autoimmunity using forward genetics. https://core.ac.uk/download/459196066.pdf (accessed on 17th June 2025).
22. Geng, R., Li, J., Yu, C., Zhang, C., Chen, F., Chen, J., Ni, H., et al. (2023). Knee osteoarthritis: Current status and research progress in treatment (Review). *Experimental and Therapeutic Medicine, 26.* https://doi.org/10.3892/etm.2023.12180 (accessed on 17th June 2025).
23. Giuggioli, D., & Bajocchi, G. (2022). Geographical heterogeneity of clinical and serological phenotypes of systemic sclerosis observed at tertiary referral centers: The experience of the Italian SIR-SPRING registry and review of the world literature. https://core.ac.uk/download/543268266.pdf (accessed on 17th June 2025).
24. González-Gay, M. A., Heras-Recuero, E., García-Fernández, A., Blázquez-Sánchez, T., Torres-Roselló, A., Caraballo-Salazar, C., Rengifo-García, F., et al. (2025). Revisiting the epidemiology of giant cell arteritis. *Clinical and Experimental Rheumatology, 43*(4), 742–748. https://www.semanticscholar.org/paper/a4bbb26846fac639852d53668cbd3d5b4620a10b (accessed on 17th June 2025).
25. Grillo, A. R. (2024). Polygene by environment interactions predicting depressive outcomes.

American Journal of Medical Genetics Part B: Neuropsychiatric Genetics, 198. https://www.semanticscholar.org/paper/60796df4399b32c15ca756490388fa6c2614c0b0 (accessed on 17th June 2025).

26. Hamilton, A. D. (2013). *Fibromyalgia Syndrome: A Patho Neurological Basis of Disease.* https://core.ac.uk/download/58824886.pdf (accessed on 17th June 2025).
27. Iannaccone, P. M., Ryznar, R., & Van Winkle, L. J. (2024). Genetics, epigenetics, and the environment: Are precision medicine, provider compassion, and social justice effective public health measures to mitigate disease risk and severity? *International Journal of Environmental Research and Public Health, 21.* https://www.semanticscholar.org/paper/18d88ba79e0d44bce048b2adac8dcb4f9d15ac0f (accessed on 17th June 2025).
28. Ma, W., Gao, F., Gu, K., & Chen, D. (2019). The role of monocytes and macrophages in autoimmune diseases: A comprehensive review. *Frontiers in Immunology, 10.* https://doi.org/10.3389/fimmu.2019.01140 (accessed on 17th June 2025).
29. Matthews, K. A., Croft, J. B., Liu, Y., Lu, H., Kanny, D., Wheaton, A. G., Cunningham, T. J., et al. (2017). Health-related behaviors by urban-rural county classification — United States, 2013. *MMWR Surveillance Summaries, 66*, 1–8. McInnes, I. B., & Schett, G. (2017). Pathogenetic insights from the treatment of rheumatoid arthritis. *Lancet (London, England), 389*(10086), 2328–2337. https://doi.org/10.1016/S0140-6736(17)31472-1(accessed on 17th June 2025).
30. Mendel, O., Sinclair, M. S., Jagodnik, K. M., Krenz, T., Pissinis, J., Stathias, V., Bartal, A., et al. (2025). Abstract 1052: Integrating geographical and socioeconomic data with genomic information for enhanced prediction of cancer risk using large language models and knowledge graphs. *Cancer Research.* https://www.semanticscholar.org/paper/13013f916f15cd7e59f0e793e96793194067a7c2 (accessed on 17th June 2025).
31. Muratori, L., Lohse, A. W., & Lenzi, M. (2023). Diagnosis and management of autoimmune hepatitis. *BMJ.* https://doi.org/10.1136/bmj-2022-070201 (accessed on 17th June 2025).
32. Ojomo, T. (2025). Advanced chemical sensing technologies for environmental monitoring: Developing high-sensitivity sensors for real-time detection of pollutants, toxins, and greenhouse gases to combat climate change. *International Journal of Scientific Research and Management (IJSRM).* https://www.semanticscholar.org/paper/1deca13a359919d4555463ab00393864cc8510b6 (accessed on 17th June 2025).
33. Ombrello, M. J., Remmers, E. F., Tachmazidou, I., Grom, A. A., Foell, D., Haas, J. P., Martini, A., et al. (2015). *HLA-DRB1*11* and variants of the MHC class II locus are strong risk factors for systemic juvenile idiopathic arthritis. *Proceedings of the National Academy of Sciences, 112*, 15970–15975. https://doi.org/10.1073/pnas.1520779112 (accessed on 17th June 2025).
34. Óskarsdóttir, S., Boot, E., Crowley, T. B., Loo, J. C. Y., Arganbright, J. M., Armando, M., Baylis, A. L., et al. (2023). Updated clinical practice recommendations for managing children with 22q11.2 deletion syndrome. *Genetics in Medicine, 25*, 100338–100338. https://doi.org/10.1016/j.gim.2022.11.006 (accessed on 17th June 2025).
35. Reynisdottir, G. B. (2015). *Molecular and Epidemiological Investigations of Lung Involvement in Very Early Rheumatoid Arthritis.* https://core.ac.uk/download/70343796.pdf (accessed on 17th June 2025).
36. Saleh, R. (2024). *Understanding Juvenile Idiopathic Arthritis: A Multidimensional Approach.* https://core.ac.uk/download/599460676.pdf (accessed on 17th June 2025).

37. Senbadejo, T., Abiola, I., & Paemka, L. (2024). Probing genetics and environmental factors underlying uterine fibroid tumorigenesis in Ghana, West Africa. *Research Ideas and Outcomes*. https://www.semanticscholar.org/paper/7a5962788bfd8138405e2ec56946cfbc83f160f2 (accessed on 17th June 2025).

38. Shao, T., Shi, X., Yang, S., Zhang, C., Li, X., Shu, J., Alqalyoobi, S., et al. (2021). Interstitial lung disease in connective tissue disease: A common lesion with heterogeneous mechanisms and treatment considerations. *Frontiers in Immunology, 12*. https://doi.org/10.3389/fimmu.2021.684699 (accessed on 17th June 2025).

39. Sibomana, O. (2024). Genetic diversity landscape in African population: A review of implications for personalized and precision medicine. *Pharmacogenomics and Personalized Medicine, 17*, 487–496. https://www.semanticscholar.org/paper/97083d002b8c89cc625d3793f92a4701a70c218c (accessed on 17th June 2025).

40. Silva Neto, J. B., Mota, L. M. F., Londoño-Gil, M., Schmidt, P. I., Rodrigues, G. R. D., Ligori, V. A., Arikawa, L. M., et al. (2024). Genotype-by-environment interactions in beef and dairy cattle populations: A review of methodologies and perspectives on research and applications. *Animal Genetics*. https://www.semanticscholar.org/paper/62ab7baf2c197c4d829dc023415123e566d510bb (accessed on 17th June 2025).

41. Smirnova, N. V., Timofeenko, I. A., & Krutovsky, K. (2025). Red-leafed lettuces: Genetic variation or epigenetic photomorphogenesis? *Plants, 14*. https://www.semanticscholar.org/paper/878cbb57e4c51917d8686274f267ec236fc1d59a (accessed on 17th June 2025).

42. Starovoytova, D. (2017). *Hazards and Risks at Rotary Screen Printing (Part 1/6): Survey on Musculoskeletal Disorders*. https://core.ac.uk/download/234685650.pdf (accessed on 17th June 2025).

43. Talele, C., Gohil, D., Kumari, M., Shah, N., & Sadhu, P. (2024). Comprehensive review of rheumatoid arthritis: Insights, challenges, and prospects. https://core.ac.uk/download/603897628.pdf (accessed on 17th June 2025).

44. Too, Chun Lai (2012). Genetic predispositions to rheumatoid arthritis in Malaysian population. Karolinska Institutet. Thesis. https://hdl.handle.net/10616/41300(accessed on 17th June 2025).

45. Ujiie, H., Rosmarin, D., Schön, M. P., Ständer, S., Boch, K., Metz, M., Maurer, M., et al. (2022). Unmet medical needs in chronic, non-communicable inflammatory skin diseases. *Frontiers in Medicine, 9*. https://doi.org/10.3389/fmed.2022.875492 (accessed on 17th June 2025).

46. Verdi, S., Abbasian, G., Bowyer, R. C. E., Lachance, G., Yarand, D., Christofidou, P., Mangino, M., et al. (2019). TwinsUK: The UK adult twin registry update. *Twin Research and Human Genetics, 22*, 523–529. https://doi.org/10.1017/thg.2019.65 (accessed on 17th June 2025).

47. Virolainen, S. J., VonHandorf, A., Viel, K. C. M. F., Weirauch, M. T., & Kottyan, L. C. (2022). Gene–environment interactions and their impact on human health. *Genes and Immunity, 24*, 1–11. https://doi.org/10.1038/s41435-022-00192-6 (accessed on 17th June 2025).

48. Wells, P. M., Adebayo, A., Bowyer, R. C. E., Freidin, M. B., Finckh, A., Strowig, T., Lesker, T. R., et al. (2020). Associations between gut microbiota and genetic risk for rheumatoid arthritis in the absence of disease: A cross-sectional study. *The Lancet Rheumatology, 2*, e418–e427. https://doi.org/10.1016/s2665-9913(20)30064-3 (accessed on 17th June 2025).

49. Yépez, D., Grandes, X. A., Manjunatha, R. T., Habib, S., & Sangaraju, S. L. (2022). Fibromyalgia and depression: A literature review of their shared aspects. *Cureus*. https://doi.org/10.7759/cureus.24909 (accessed on 17th June 2025).

TISSUES IN HEALTH AND DISEASE

7

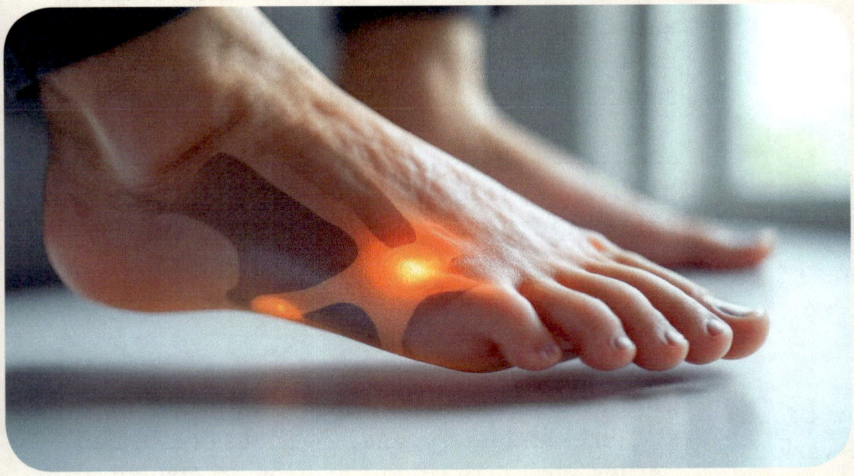

Introduction

The example of tissues in health and disease, as an introduction to the specialty of rheumatology, illustrates the intricate relationship between genetic predispositions and environmental influences in the development of autoimmune disease. Autoimmune diseases , such as rheumatoid arthritis (RA) and primary Sjögrens syndrome (PSS), demonstrate how specific genetic factors may predispose to disabling diseases. New research has produced convincing evidence for FCGR3A-FCGR3B haplotype association with RA development, thus leaving open the prospect of a disease-susceptibility marker (Mackie et al., 2005). This finding highlights the significance of a complete appreciation of the manner in which these genetic variations impinge on the pathological mechanisms in joint tissues. In addition, the wider implications of such research extend beyond specific diseases, as the identical genetic mechanisms may operate in the heterogeneous autoantibody-associated rheumatic conditions, paving the way for gene-directed therapeutic measures (Staunton et al., 2013).

LEARNING OBJECTIVES

After studying this chapter, you will be able to:

1. Identify types of tissues that are encountered in rheumatology;
2. Describe the pathophysiology of rheumatological diseases;
3. Explain the clinical presentation of tissue disorders.

7.1. Types of Tissues Involved in Rheumatology

Learning Outcome

1. Identify tissue characteristics of connective tissue;
2. Understand cartilage and cartilage's function in joint health;
3. Describe synovial tissue function and pathology;
4. Highlight muscle tissue in rheumatological diseases;
5. Discuss vascular tissue and inflammation;
6. Describe nerve tissue and perception of pain;
7. Know epithelial tissue in joint health;
8. Highlight bone tissue and relevance to rheumatology;
9. Discuss tissue interactions between tissue types.

The field of rheumatology involves a broad scope of tissues that are involved in various functions in health and disease. Connective tissues, particularly those of joints, are of primary interest, as they are targets for diseases , such as rheumatoid arthritis and systemic lupus erythematosus. Cartilage, ligaments, and synovial membranes maintain joint function; their inflammation or degeneration can lead to large-scale dysfunction and pain. Besides this, involvement of immune organs , such as the spleen and the lymph nodes, is crucial in the pathogenesis of autoimmune diseases, where the immune system targets the body's own cells. This is demonstrated in the association of some genetic determinants, e.g., the FcγR haplotype, with diseases like rheumatoid arthritis and primary Sjögrens syndrome, which highlights the complex interaction of environmental precipitants and gene predispositions in these rheumatic conditions (Mackie et al., 2005; Staunton et al., 2013). These tissue types are important to identify in order to have certain therapies (Figure 7.1).

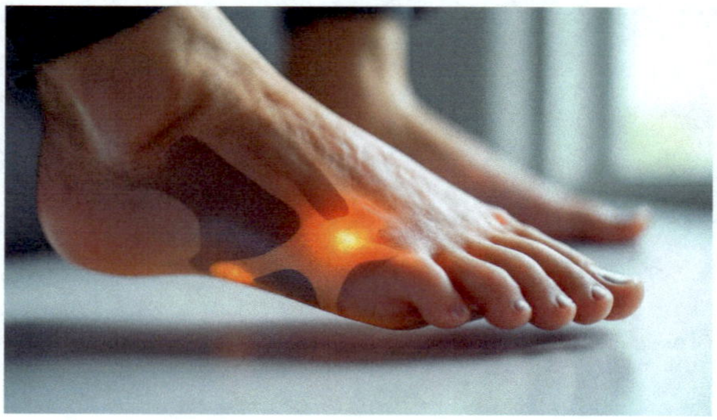

Figure 7.1. Cartilage, synovial membranes, and ligaments are integral to joint function; their degeneration or inflammation can lead to significant dysfunction and pain.

Source: https://images.byword.ai/HxRmwWsfBhTvUyZMOiyYSc3pkwU9hEKQAXBsmZb2Ah24J22JA-output.jpg.

7.1.1. Connective Tissue Characteristics

Connective tissue is the framework that stabilizes and interconnects various organs and tissues within the body to provide structural support and facilitate cells to interact with one another. High in extracellular matrix components like fibers and ground substances, connective tissues can be broadly classified into loose, dense, adipose, cartilage, bone, and blood. Each is bestowed with certain properties that make it suitable for certain functions within the musculoskeletal system, like mechanical support and metabolic function. In rheumatological conditions, the characteristics of connective tissues are significant, as in juvenile idiopathic arthritis, where the reliability of scoring systems like Juvenile Arthritis Disease Activity Score (JADAS) is examined to assess disease activity and severity in children (Adib et al., 2012). Moreover, the inability to measure connective tissue-associated pathology, for example, interstitial lung disease in connective tissue disorders, emphasizes the importance of harmonized outcome measures (Antoniou et al., 2013). In general, understanding the nature of connective tissue is important to be able to evaluate pathologies that occur in rheumatology.

7.1.2. Cartilage and Its Role in Joint Health

Cartilage plays a central role in joint health as an essential cushioning material between bones that enhances frictionless motion and stress absorption under exercise. Integrity of this unique connective tissue is not only essential for joint function in normal situations but also for the prevention of degenerative ailments , such as osteoarthritis (OA). In addition, as explored in recent criticism, alterations in nutrition may offer a fascinating avenue for the prevention of the onset or advancement of OA, with the suggestion that specific micronutrients and phytochemicals may enhance cartilage quality and protect joints against degeneration (Bao et al., 2014).

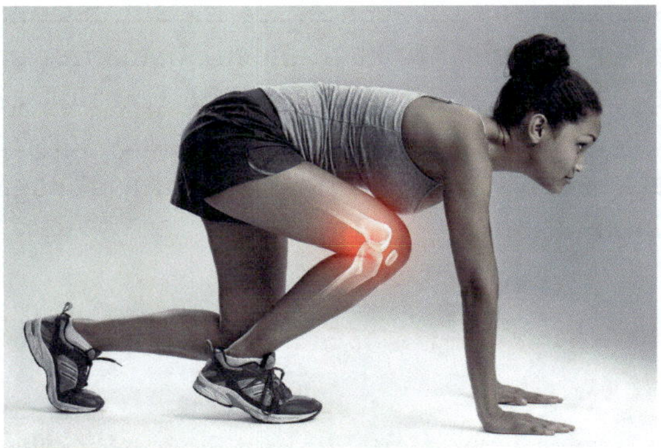

Figure 7.2. Cartilage plays a pivotal role in maintaining joint health, serving as a critical cushion between bones that facilitates smooth movement and absorbs shock during physical activity.

Source: https://www.racesmart.com/wp-content/uploads/2020/05/joint-health-nutrition.jpg.

Further, while gout directly affects joint health through the deposit of urate crystals, managing gout involves an understanding of cartilage's role in inflammatory processes within the joint, pointing to the interconnectedness of diverse joint tissues (Finucci et al., 2015). Thus, cartilage health maintained through dietary practices, exercise, and lifestyle choices emerges as a most significant way of improving overall joint health (Figure 7.2).

7.1.3. Synovial Tissue Function and Pathology

Synovial tissue plays a core role in joint function by secreting synovial fluid, which lubricates articulating surfaces and supplies nutrients to avascular cartilage. But when there is inflammation, as in rheumatoid arthritis, the tissue is hyperplastic and is involved in pathogenic mechanisms. The remodeling of the synovial tissue can lead to cartilage and bone damage and result in pain and mobility impairment. Data are demonstrating that some genetic polymorphisms, for instance, the FCGR3A-FCGR3B haplotype, play a role in susceptibility to inflammatory rheumatic diseases and strengthen the multifactorial nature of synovial pathology in these diseases (Mackie et al., 2005). Moreover, in osteoarthritis, pathological changes in synovial tissue are not always accompanied by pain intensity, complicating the treatment method (Aigner et al., 2014). It is crucial to the appreciation of the bi-functional role of synovial tissue in disease and health for the development of site-directed therapeutic interventions in rheumatology.

7.1.4. Muscle Tissue Involvement in Rheumatological Diseases

Involvement of muscle tissue in rheumatological disorders plays a significant pathophysiologic role in most such diseases and typically results in significant morbidity and impaired quality of life. Conditions , such as polymyositis and dermatomyositis show the autoaggressive effect of autoimmune mechanisms on muscle tissue, leading to inflammation and weakness of the muscles. Moreover, muscle involvement can be isolated but, in combination, also be accompanied by other systemic findings, thereby complicating diagnosis and treatment. Today's emphasis on multidisciplinary diagnoses of rheumatological disorders supports the role of such specialists as rheumatologists working together with other professionals to assess muscle tissue involvement accurately, particularly when symptoms of muscles become the first indicator of a latent autoimmune disease (Carnevale et al., 2019). As emphasized in the literature, a detailed understanding of musculoskeletal examinations is highly important for effective management of rheumatological diseases, including their muscular aspects. This integration of muscle tissue assessment into rheumatological management is critical to optimizing patient care (Figure 7.3).

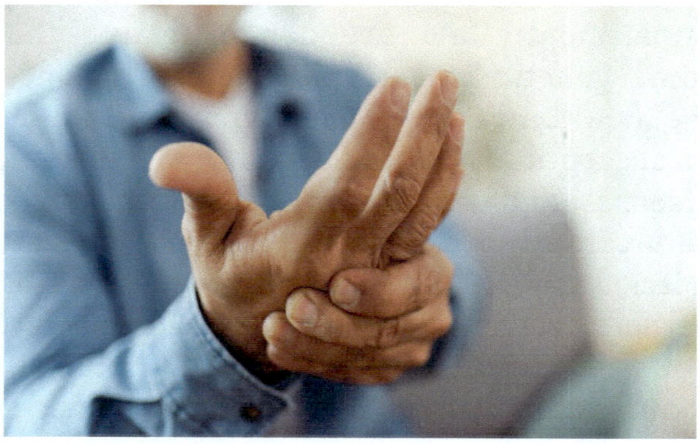

Figure 7.3. Muscle tissue involvement plays a critical role in the pathophysiology of various rheumatological diseases, often contributing to significant morbidity and impaired quality of life.

Source: https://jnj-content-lab2.brightspotcdn.com/dims4/default/fa64da9/2147483647/strip/true/crop/1920x1080+0+0/resize/1440x810!/quality/90/?url=https%3A%2F%2Fjnj-production-jnj.s3.us-east-1.amazonaws.com%2Fbrightspot%2F18%2Fc0%2F5567046e4ac1a4b2a92a3635dfd7%2Fwhat-is-a-rheumatic-disease-1024.png.

7.1.5. Vascular Tissue and Inflammation

The intricate relationship between vascular tissue and inflammation is one of special interest in rheumatology, particularly in diseases like rheumatoid arthritis (RA). During the early stages of RA, neovascularization is a significant factor in synovial chronic inflammation. Ultrasound assessments have proven to be essential in correlating synovial blood flow with RA clinical activity, demonstrating its effectiveness in quantifying vascular changes during inflammation (Koch et al., 2015). More specifically, further research has demonstrated that some genetic factors, such as those with FCGR3A and FCGR3B haplotypes, may influence susceptibility to RA by modifying inflammatory reactions through vascular regulation (Mackie et al., 2005). This interaction of vascular tissue dynamics and inflammation describes rheumatoid disease pathophysiology and places vascularity at the center of inflammation. A greater insight into such mechanisms not only adds to our understanding of RA but also indicates the potential for specifically targeted therapeutic maneuvers that can abrogate inflammation.

7.1.6. Nerve Tissue and Pain Perception

The intricate relationship between nerve tissue and pain perception is particularly pertinent in rheumatological disorders, where chronic pain is a prevalent symptom that has the tendency to bring patients to see their doctors. An understanding of the role of nervous tissue and how it feels pain is crucial in the effective treatment of diseases , such as rheumatoid arthritis, which typically consists of several aspects of osteoarticular pain that is not only multiform but also complex. As Molfetta et al. (2022) point out, such pain is processed by several nociceptive factors, leading to divergent clinical manifestations requiring particular therapeutic approaches. Besides, the role of comprehensive musculoskeletal examinations, is imperative in accurate diagnosis and management of these conditions, hence enhancing the patient care experience in general. Lastly, the role of understanding nerve tissue and pain perception is important to establish effective ways of alleviating symptoms and improving quality of life in those suffering from rheumatological disease (Figure 7.4).

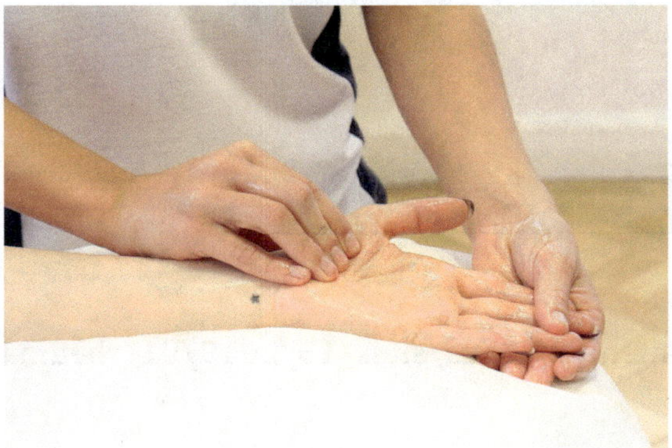

Figure 7.4. The intricate relationship between nerve tissue and pain perception is particularly significant in the context of rheumatological diseases, where chronic pain is a prevalent symptom that often drives patients to seek medical attention.

Source:.https://www.physio.co.uk/images/rheumatoid-arthritis/rheumatoid-arthritis1.jpg

7.1.7. Epithelial Tissue in Joint Health

Epithelial tissue plays a vital part in joint health, particularly in the case of its function within the synovial membrane surrounding joints. This synovial epithelial structure is responsible for the synthesis of synovial fluid, which lubricates the joint and enables the smooth movement. Any alteration of epithelial cell function will cause alterations in the composition of the synovial fluid and produce inflammatory conditions , such as RA and primary Sjögrens syndrome (PSS). Research has indicated that genetic factors, particularly with Fc gamma receptor polymorphisms, have an impact on epithelial cell function and hence joint health (Mackie et al., 2005).

Moreover, the function of innate immune cells , such as invariant natural killer T cells, also validates the complex interaction within the joint environment, highlighting how the wellness of the epithelium is pivotal to immune regulation and joint homeostasis (Barbera et al., 2019). Consequently, the integrity and function of epithelial tissue are of greatest significance in the prevention of musculoskeletal disease and the health of musculoskeletal tissues.

7.1.8. Bone Tissue and Its Relationship to Rheumatology

The bone tissue and rheumatology association illustrates the importance of a field of knowledge related to the pathophysiology of several rheumatic diseases. The bone is commonly involved in RA, where chronic inflammation leads to greater bone resorption and loss of bone density. The role of osteoclasts and osteoblasts is critical in this procedure since they regulate the remodeling of bones owing to inflammatory cytokines.

Moreover, similar to tendinopathy, wherein a realignment of the tendon matrix is linked with loading conditions (McCormick et al., 2008), bone tissue remodels in accordance with mechanical stress, which may develop into arthritis-related bone deformities. In addition, genetic predisposition, for example, specific haplotypes , such as FCGR3A-FCGR3B, has been involved in autoimmune conditions, pointing to a complex interaction of genes and bone condition (Mackie et al., 2005). This information is important for the creation of targeted drugs in rheumatology (Figure 7.5).

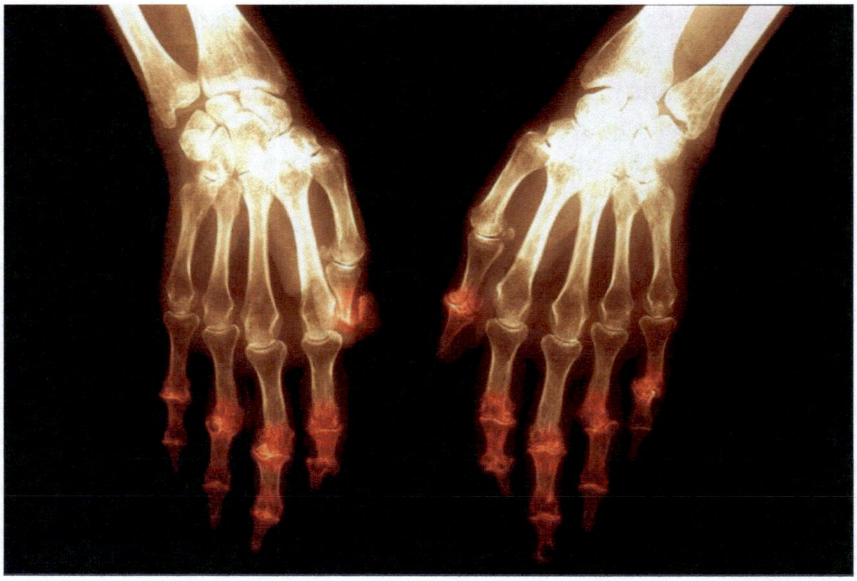

Figure 7.5. Bone tissue.

Source: https://www.rheumatologyadvisor.com/wp-content/uploads/sites/18/2019/01/rheumatoidpolyarthritismi01_1515906-860x573.jpg.

7.1.9. Interactions between Different Tissue Types

In rheumatology, the intricacies of interaction between various types of tissues are very relevant in delineating disease mechanisms and response to treatment. The synovial tissue enveloping joints, for instance, illustrates significant interaction with the surrounding cartilage and bone in the setting of rheumatoid arthritis. The inflammatory responses of synovial cells are involved in cartilage degradation and exacerbation of joint trauma, a process highlighted in models of examining biological mechanisms of rheumatoid arthritis (Chaplain et al., 2019). Similarly, lupus nephritis is a complex interplay between renal tissues and immune cells given that single-cell RNA sequencing has identified heterogeneous leukocyte subsets that invade the kidney, reflecting cross-connect between the renal microenvironment and the immune system. Such interactions not only inform us of the pathology of these diseases but also guide the formulation of targeted therapies to restore tissue homeostasis and function (Arazi et al., 2019).

Test Your Knowledge

1. How are tendons and ligaments drawn into enthesitis and spondyloarthropathies?
2. What are the cartilage histologic changes that develop in osteoarthritis as it advances?

7.2. Pathophysiology of Rheumatological Diseases

Learning Outcome

1. Understand mechanisms of autoimmune response;
2. Describe the function of cytokines in tissue injury;
3. Describe inflammatory pathways in rheumatology;
4. Be aware of genetic susceptibility to tissue disease;
5. Be aware of environmental stimuli influencing tissue health;
6. Discuss the effect of chronic inflammation on the tissue;
7. Describe tissue remodeling in rheumatological diseases;
8. Understand systemic manifestations of local tissue disease;
9. Recognize diagnostic markers associated with tissue pathology.

The pathophysiology of rheumatological diseases involves an intricate relationship of genetic, environmental, and immunological determinants that impair normal tissue homeostasis. Underlying such disorders is the hyperimmune response, which has a tendency to lead to tissue damage and inflammation. For instance, in conditions like rheumatoid arthritis, the synovial tissue hyperplasias with a consequent growth of pannus into cartilage and bone. Progress in diagnostic techniques during the last few years, such as the application of laser Doppler flowmetry and fluorescence spectroscopy, has enhanced the ability to assess microcirculatory disturbances in patients with rheumatism, with significant information about disease mechanisms and progression (Dremin et al., 2019). Similarly, HIV-induced arthritis pathogenesis is an example of how viral infections may induce inflammatory reactions, resulting in destruction of the joints, although they are generally self-limiting (Kasjmir et al., 2009). Knowledge of these processes is vital in order to devise targeted treatments that can reverse the ruinous impact of such diseases on joint and tissue well-being.

7.2.1. Mechanisms of Autoimmune Response

The mechanisms involved in autoimmune responses are multidimensional, exemplifying a complex interaction between environmental stimuli and genetic involvement. Genetic predisposition, such as specific haplotypes correlated with Fc gamma receptors, has also been identified as a causative factor for the susceptibility of autoimmune diseases like RA and primary Sjögrens syndrome, where increased homozygosity for certain haplotypes correlates with disease occurrence (Mackie et al., 2005).

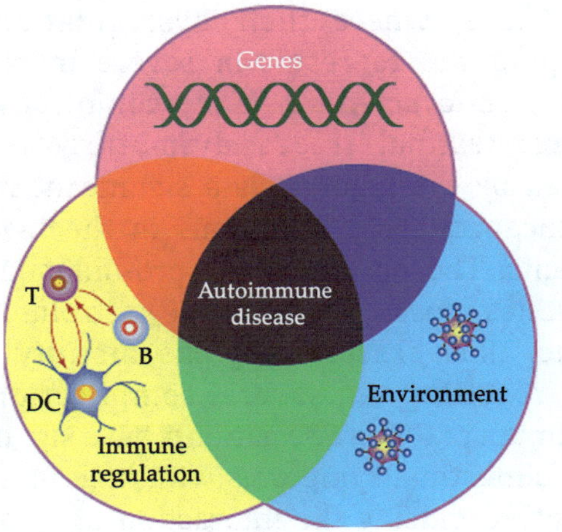

Figure 7.6. The mechanisms underlying autoimmune responses are multifaceted, reflecting a complex interplay between genetic predispositions and environmental influences.

Source: https://media.springernature.com/full/springer-static/image/art%3A10.1038%2Fni0901-759/MediaObjects/41590_2001_Article_BFni0901759_Fig1_HTML.gif.

Neither can the role of the microbiota be excluded; shifts in bacterial populations at mucosal sites influence immune regulation. These microbial populations establish a delicate equilibrium between tolerance and inflammation, with dysbiosis having the potential to stimulate autoimmune reactions through compromising gut permeability and promoting entry of pathogens (D'Amelio et al., 2018). Consequently, both genetic and microbial factors constitute the central components of the autoimmune reaction, determining the rheumatologic illness pathophysiology and highlighting integrative approaches in unraveling these complex disorders (Figure 7.6).

7.2.2. Role of Cytokines in Tissue Damage

Cytokines are pivotal to the pathogenesis of tissue damage, particularly in rheumatological conditions, where their dysregulation has the potential to result in severe morbidity. In systemic sclerosis (SSc) conditions, the gastrointestinal tract's dysmotility is also caused by cytokines. It is a significant reason for incapacitating symptoms in the involved patients. The production of pro-inflammatory cytokines causes fibrosis in the gastrointestinal tissue, thus exacerbating the motility issue and resulting in severe complications. A maximum of 8% of SSc patients have significant gastrointestinal symptoms with high mortality rates; recognizing the interaction of cytokines in these mechanisms is particularly important. Recent research indicates that autoantibodies against muscarinic receptors potentially mediate cytokine action, revealing potential therapeutic targets for modulating cytokine engagement to reduce symptoms. Thus, cytokines not merely broker tissue injury but also provide a promise of new approaches to therapy in rheumatology (Staunton et al., 2013 ; Kumar et al., 2017).

7.2.3. Inflammatory Pathways in Rheumatology

It is in the intricate play of inflammatory pathways at the center of the knowledge on the pathophysiology of rheumatic disease, particularly RA. This autoimmune disease is primarily induced by an abnormal immune system reaction, as genetic backgrounds converge with environmental triggers, causing sustained inflammation of joint tissue. Research has revealed significant correlations between particular genetic haplotypes, such as the FCGR3A-FCGR3B 158V-NA2, and RA susceptibility, indicating the role of Fc gamma receptors in modulating inflammatory mechanisms (Mackie et al., 2005). In addition, the systemic effects of inflammatory mechanisms also have a tendency to occur in peripheral tissues, for example, in the feet, where disabling pain and burden may result. The recognition of the pervasive reach of inflammatory mechanisms emphasizes the need for comprehensive healthcare approaches encompassing both the immunologic and symptomatic mechanisms of rheumatic disease to improve patient outcomes (Chapman et al., 2010) (Figure 7.7).

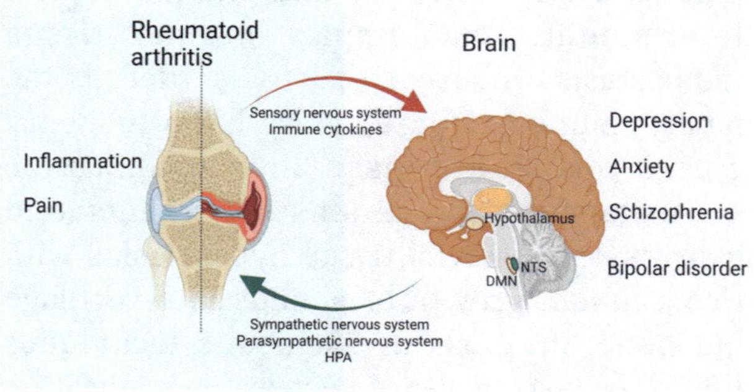

Figure 7.7. The intricate interplay of inflammatory pathways is central to understanding the pathophysiology of rheumatic diseases, particularly rheumatoid arthritis (RA).

Source: https://pub.mdpi-res.com/ijms/ijms-23-08158/article_deploy/html/images/ijms-23-08158-g001.png?1658664821.

7.2.4. Genetic Predispositions to Tissue Diseases

Examination of genetic vulnerabilities to tissue diseases, and more particularly in the realm of rheumatology, highlights the intricate interaction among genetic elements and autoimmune diseases. Research has identified that some alleles of the Human Leukocyte Antigen (HLA) are highly associated with diseases , such as Juvenile Idiopathic Arthritis (JIA), wherein HLA-DRB1 haplotype variation is associated with risk elevation and autoantibody status in patients, considerably influencing disease onset and severity (Saleh, 2024). Additionally, gut microbiome-RA interaction suggests that microbial flora and diet may also influence disease progression, showcasing the complex nature of environmental and genetic interactions (Antczak et al., 2024). Explaining such genetic predispositions not only tells us more about tissue pathologies of rheumatologic disorders but also points to the potential of individualized therapeutic strategies that aim at repairing such debilitating diseases.

7.2.5. Environmental Triggers Affecting Tissue Health

Environmental factors are crucial in determining the health of tissue, particularly in the case of rheumatologic diseases , such as RA and Systemic Lupus Erythematosus (SLE). Immune response dysregulation, typically activated by external stressors, leads to chronic inflammation and subsequent deterioration of joint tissues. Scientific studies have revealed that certain cytokines, such as APRIL and TSLP, not only function in immune signaling but also act as biomarkers of the severity of RA and SLE, indicating their therapeutic target potential (Alivernini et al., 2018). Further, the burden of these autoimmune diseases supports the need for effective diagnostics and treatment protocols, which may be addressed by understanding such environmental triggers (Weldon, 2014). In such regard, tackling the interplay between environmental exposure and tissue well-being is important in developing targeted therapies as well as improving patient outcomes in rheumatology (Figure 7.8).

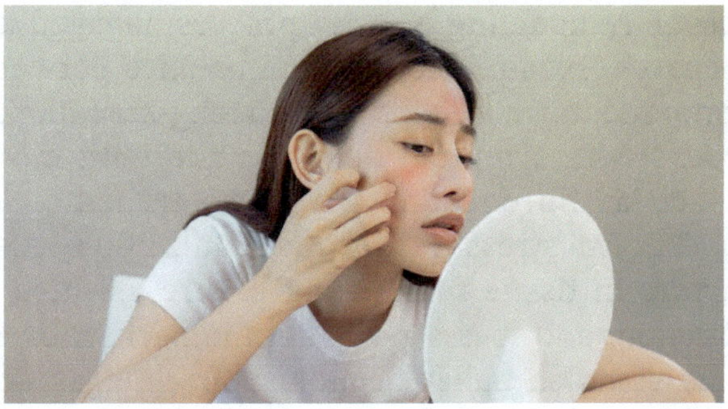

Figure 7.8. The dysregulation of immune responses, often triggered by external stressors, leads to chronic inflammation and subsequent destruction of joint tissues.

Source: https://www.heal-medical.com/media/images/service/%E7%B4%85%E6%96%91%E7%8B%BC%E7%98%A1.jpg.

7.2.6. Impact of Chronic Inflammation on Tissues

The impact of chronic inflammation on tissue structure and function, particularly in the context of rheumatic diseases, is immense. In the context of conditions , such as systemic lupus erythematosus, inflammation may lead to diverse sequelae , such as oral disease, for instance, an increased risk of periodontitis and dental caries due to the composition of saliva and immune change (Brown et al., 2018). Similarly, in rheumatoid arthritis, inflammation causes a cascade of tissue damage that is not merely confined to joints but spreads to systemic tissues, as evidenced in the association of certain genetic haplotypes with autoantibody formation (Mackie et al., 2005). The persistent inflammatory milieu not only perpetuates the cycle of tissue damage but also arrests the natural healing processes, ultimately leading to chronic pain and loss of function. Explanation of the mechanisms is behind the design of therapy regimens to decrease the deleterious impact of chronic inflammation of tissue and enhance patient outcomes in rheumatology.

7.2.7. Tissue Remodeling in Rheumatological Conditions

Tissue remodeling is a key process engaged in the pathophysiology of numerous rheumatological diseases, exemplified by an imbalance between synthesis and degradation of extracellular matrix components. In tendinopathy, a long-standing tendon disorder, disrupted matrix remodeling activity tracks with symptom development, with increased levels of type III collagen and other markers , such as fibronectin, marking a transition toward a reparative response under conditions of mechanical stress (McCormick et al., 2008). Also, SSc suggests the role of angiogenic and angiostatic factors in tissue remodeling, where elevated levels of endostatin correlate negatively with renal function, and it is a potential biomarker for SSc-related renal vasculopathy (Afeltra et al., 2017). This complex ballet of molecular changes does much to elucidate how tissue remodeling leads to adaptation and disease in rheumatological disease and how more study is required to define therapeutic targets (Figure 7.9).

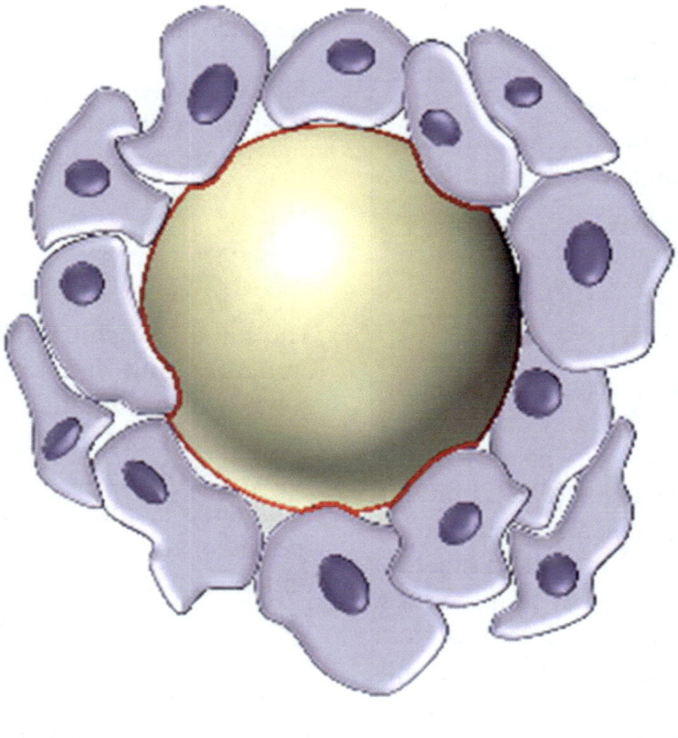

Figure 7.9. Tissue remodeling serves as a critical process in the pathophysiology of various rheumatological conditions, characterized by an imbalance between the synthesis and degradation of extracellular matrix components.

Source: https://www.mdpi.com/ijms/ijms-19-03028/article_deploy/html/images/ijms-19-03028-g005.png.

7.2.8. Systemic Effects of Localized Tissue Disease

Systemic effects of localized diseases, such as RA and juvenile localized scleroderma (LS), highlight the intricate relationship between local pathology and overall physiological considerations. RA, being predominantly an inflammatory arthritis, can have severe systemic implications, including cardiovascular diseases and high mortality, through chronic damage and inflammation (Diaconu et al., 2018). Similarly, juvenile LS, although localized, is riddled with risks of severe morbidity, often complicated by delayed diagnoses and treatments that can impede optimal management and cause permanent damage (Ardalan et al., 2023). These images emphasize the significance of early intervention and a clear vision for how local diseases can come about systemically. As rheumatology practice continues to evolve, recognizing the confluence of local tissue disease and systemic health is crucial for developing targeted therapy that addresses local signs and symptoms while excluding systemic complications that can have a profound effect on patient quality of life.

7.2.9. Diagnostic Markers related to Tissue Pathology

Identification and application of diagnostic markers linked to tissue pathology have become more prominent in the practice of rheumatology, particularly because they are utilized in the description of the underlying mechanisms of the disease. Diagnostic markers serve the purpose of providing critical information concerning the inflammatory processes that characterize conditions like autoimmune myopathies, where inflammation is targeted at muscle tissues (Benveniste et al., 2019). To this end, new biomarkers are examined in order to enhance diagnostic accuracy and therapeutic decision-making in the face of present shortcomings regarding validation in large cohorts. In addition, the link between systemic autoimmune disease and secondary effects, such as sensorineural hearing loss, reiterates the challenge of determining tissue pathology's impact on several organ systems (Ralli et al., 2018). As scientists explore further into these diagnostic markers, they hold the potential for individualized treatment pathways in rheumatological disorders that translate into improved patient outcomes and expand our understanding of tissue pathology in health and disease (Figure 7.10).

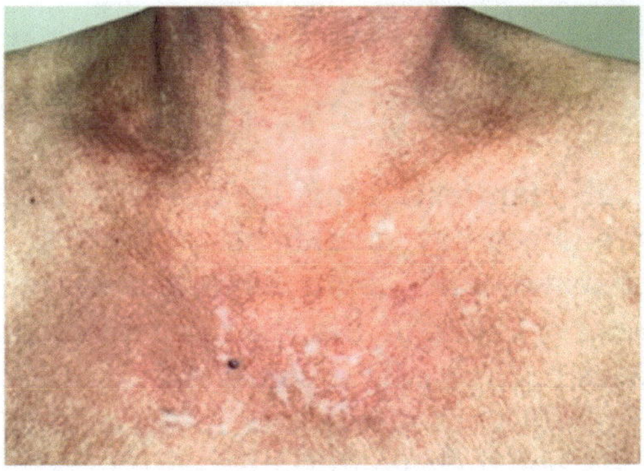

Figure 7.10. Diagnostic markers can provide essential insights into the inflammatory processes characterizing conditions , such as autoimmune myopathies, where inflammation affects muscle tissues.

Source: https://www.tandfonline.com/cms/asset/53b081cf-99d8-45af-90fe-89d8f178f857/ilab_a_2000584_f0005_c.jpg.

Test Your Knowledge

1. What mechanisms lead to fibrosis in systemic sclerosis?
2. How is cartilage breakdown mediated in osteoarthritis?

7.3. Clinical Manifestations of Tissue Disorders

Learning Outcome

1. Recognize rheumatoid arthritis signs;
2. Describe manifestations of osteoarthritis;
3. Emphasize gout and its effect on joint tissues;
4. Comprehend systemic lupus erythematosus and tissue involvement;
5. Describe scleroderma and impact on connective tissues;
6. Describe psoriatic arthritis and skin-tissue relationship;
7. Comprehend fibromyalgia and relation to muscle tissue;
8. Study ankylosing spondylitis and spinal tissue changes;
9. Recognize diagnostic challenges in identifying tissue disorders.

Clinical manifestations of tissue disorders in rheumatology could be numerous and multifaceted and could significantly impact patients' quality of life. In connective tissue diseases (CTDs), pain is common and disabling, particularly with conditions , such as SSc and SLE. Under such conditions, musculoskeletal pain is likely to manifest as arthralgia, myalgia, or even chronic widespread pain and thus poses difficulty in diagnosis and management (Atzeni et al., 2015). Immune-mediated disease can also involve the auditory system and cause sensorineural hearing loss, which is sudden or progressive, usually bilaterally asymmetric (Ralli et al., 2018). This symptomatology can overlap with other inner ear disorders, hence making it challenging to identify the clinical picture (Ralli et al., 2018). Therefore, correctly identifying and interpreting these manifestations are crucial in order to provide proper treatment modalities and enhance overall patient well-being under tissue disorders in rheumatology.

7.3.1. Symptoms of Rheumatoid Arthritis (RA)

RA is a chronic inflammatory disease with a variety of incapacitating symptoms that drastically impact patients' quality of life. The most typical symptoms are long-term joint pain, stiffness, and swelling of the hands and feet, which can lead to deformation over time. Additionally, systemic features like weakness, fever, and weight loss complicate the clinical presentation and further aggravate physical disability. Importantly, research observes the incidence of foot issues among patients with RA, requiring rearfoot deformity-associated symptoms to be extremely common and often overlooked in clinical assessments (Burns et al., 2013). Not only do these symptoms undermine mobility, but also interconnectivity in daily functioning, thereby emphasizing the value of comprehensive care approaches. Enhanced access to specialist foot care treatment, in combination with the recognition of the wider implications of the disease, is crucial for maximizing outcomes and managing the intricate symptoms associated with rheumatoid arthritis (Staunton et al., 2013) (Figure 7.11).

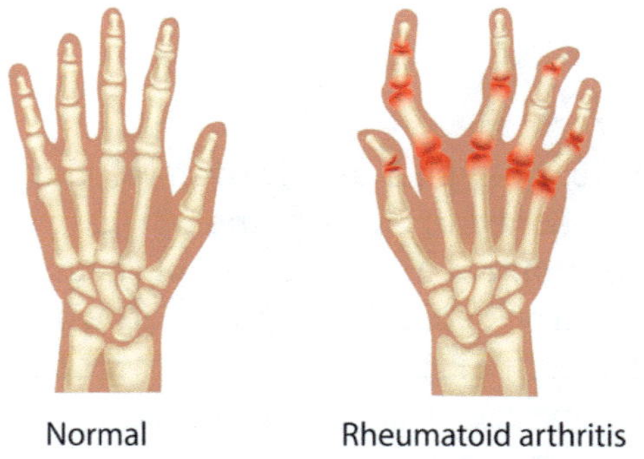

Figure 7.11. Rheumatoid arthritis (RA) is a chronic inflammatory disease characterized by a range of debilitating symptoms that significantly affect patients' quality of life.

Source: https://www.birlahospital.com/wp-content/uploads/2024/03/Rheumatoid-Arthritis.webp.

7.3.2. Manifestations of Osteoarthritis

Osteoarthritis, characterized by degeneration of the articular cartilage and underlying bone, is clinically and radiographically manifest through a broad spectrum of clinical and radiographic manifestations that ultimately influence a patient's quality of life. These include some of the frequent presentations , such as pain and stiffness in the joint, particularly after rest, and swelling and limited range of motion due to synovial inflammation and subchondral bone alterations. Patients also report crepitus or grating on joint movement, indicative of cartilage wear and bone friction. Radiological assessments reveal osteophytes, joint space narrowing, and subchondral sclerosis, supportive of the chronicity of the condition. Functional impairment and disability follow this, contributing to the psychosocial burden borne by the affected. Familiarity with these clinical presentations is critical for the creation of effective management programs and outcomes for individuals suffering from this prevalent condition (Mackie et al., 2005; Finucci et al., 2015).

7.3.3. Gout and Its Effects on Joint Tissues

Joint tissue effects of gout are considerable, directed by deposition of monosodium urate crystals, which cause extreme inflammation in involved joints. It creates a variety of symptoms ranging from acute inflammation and swelling during flare-ups to chronic degeneration of joint tissues if left untreated. The disease goes through several stages, like asymptomatic hyperuricemia and chronic tophaceous gout, each of which presents with unique challenges to joint function and health (Finucci et al., 2015). Research indicates that musculoskeletal ultrasound has the capacity to identify gout-associated abnormalities and enable early diagnosis and intervention (Finucci et al., 2015). More recent publications also emphasize the importance of pursuing additional research on gout's epidemiology and clinical management, contributing significantly to patient care and understanding tissue-pathological processes underlying the disease. Hence, gout treatment is imperative for preserving joint integrity and overall rheumatological health (Figure 7.12).

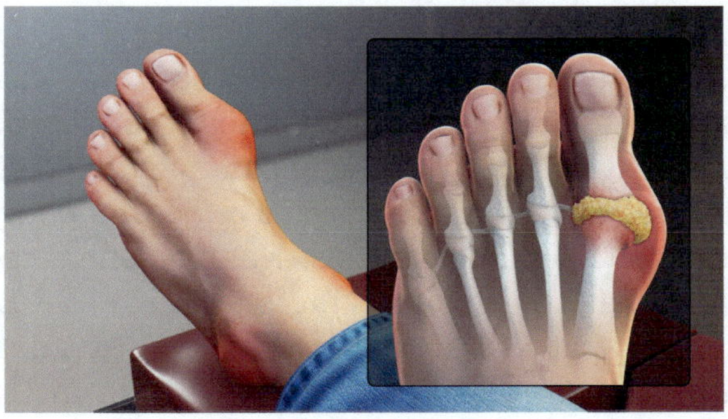

Figure 7.12. The impact of gout on joint tissues is profound, primarily driven by the deposition of monosodium urate crystals, which provoke intense inflammation within affected joints.

Source: https://upload.wikimedia.org/wikipedia/commons/0/0b/Gout_Signs_and_Symptoms.jpg.

7.3.4. Systemic Lupus Erythematosus (SLE) and Tissue Involvement

SLE is a complex autoimmune illness with wide tissue involvement involving many organ systems. One of the fascinating aspects of SLE is its impact on oral health; patients usually develop dental problems , such as increased. Incidence of periodontitis, dental caries, and fungal infections , such as lichen planus and angular cheilitis, which may result from impaired immune responses and reduced salivary flow (Brown et al., 2018). Moreover, SLE can impact hearing, as it has been correlated with hearing loss and vestibular manifestations due to autoimmune destruction of the inner ear structures and deposition of immune complexes in vascular structures (Stadio et al., 2017). This intricate tissue interaction mirrors the requirement for clinicians to adopt a comprehensive perspective when dealing with SLE patients, such that systemic and local manifestations are fully understood and addressed in clinical management.

7.3.5. Scleroderma and Its Impact on Connective Tissues

The autoimmune illness scleroderma, also known as SSc, has a significant effect on connective tissues, leading to pathophysiological changes that are characterized by vasculopathy, inflammation, and fibrosis. Notably, enhanced transforming growth factor-beta (TGF-ß) signaling pathways result in fibroblast activation, resulting in excess collagen deposition in the skin and internal organs , such as the lungs and heart.

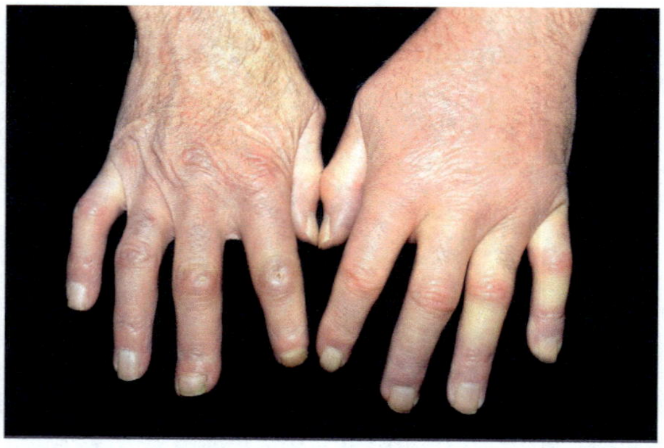

Figure 7.13. The autoimmune disorder scleroderma, also known as systemic sclerosis (SSc), significantly affects connective tissues, leading to pathophysiological changes characterized by vasculopathy, inflammation, and fibrosis.

Source: https://www.rarediseaseadvisor.com/wp-content/uploads/sites/25/2023/05/scleroderma.Ssc_SS_SS21241250-1.jpg.

Experiments evidence that peroxisome proliferator-activated receptor-gamma (PPAR-γ) nuclear receptor is reduced in SSc, suggesting that antifibrotic signaling is disrupted, enhancing tissue fibrosis and malfunction (Galli et al., 2010). Macrophages, a component of the immune response to disease, contribute to the complexity since they can perpetuate inflammation as well as induce fibrotic processes, thereby creating the relationship between the immune dysregulation and connective tissue pathology (Al-Adwi et al., 2022). Each of these interrelated mechanisms demonstrates the widespread participation of scleroderma in connective tissues, so it is essential to use certain interventions that can offset its noxious effects (Figure 7.13).

7.3.6. Psoriatic Arthritis (PsA) and Skin-tissue Interactions

The intricate interaction between PsA and skin-tissue interactions underscores the heterogeneity of this inflammatory disease. PsA usually occurs in association with psoriasis, indicating a close interaction between the musculoskeletal and skin apparatus, yet there is a variable correlation in individual patients between severity of skin lesions and joint inflammatory spread. This variability points to the need to better understand the root genotypic variability, particularly that involving the HLA region, which could provide insights into the mechanisms regulating such interactions (Chandran et al., 2021).

Current advancements in pharmacotherapies include various strategies targeting inflammatory pathways , such as TNF-α and IL-23/IL-17 axis, in attempts to control this complex spectrum of disease (Alivernini S et al., 2021). As the scientific journey continues, it is increasingly apparent that tailored treatments will play an important role in controlling the complex presentations, such that patient outcomes are enhanced through personalized medicine tailored to individualized soft tissue reactions.

7.3.7. Fibromyalgia (FM) and Its Relation to Muscle Tissue

FM is characterized by diffuse musculoskeletal pain, which commonly occurs with abnormalities of muscle tissue as well as central pain processing mechanisms. FM patients have been found to exhibit central sensitization commonly, which is a condition where central nervous system mechanisms increase pain perception, and the person experiences chronic pain and pain in the muscles (Cagnie et al., 2015). This sensitization is generally accompanied by cognitive dysfunction and reduced quality of life, unveiling the complex interrelationship between muscle tissue integrity and neurological function. Therapies like photobiomodulation therapy have been suggested as putative therapies, aiming to alleviate pain and improve muscle quality through enhanced mechanisms of tissue repair (Ledesma, 2022). Such notions stress the importance of integrated treatment approaches exerting influence on both muscle pathology and central nervous system engagement for correction of the intricate symptomatology in fibromyalgia. Understanding these interactions is crucial for the promotion of therapeutic outcomes in rheumatological practice (Figure 7.14).

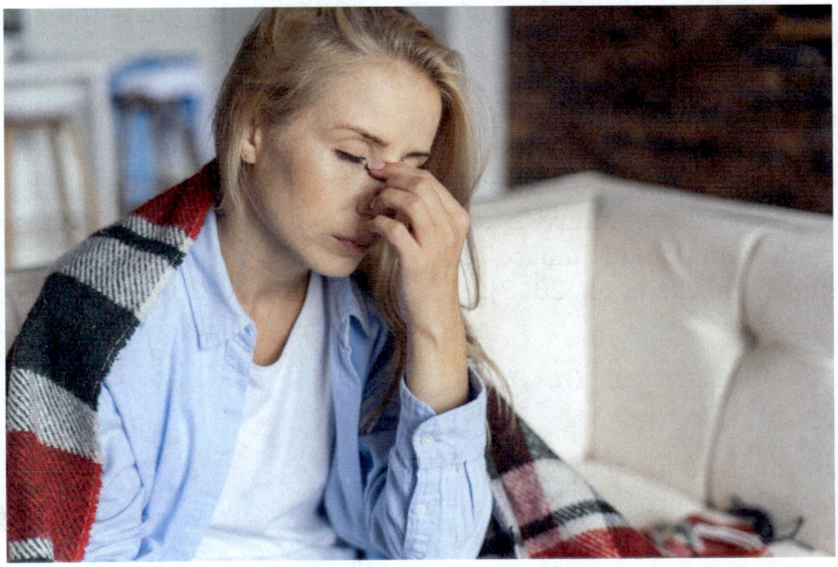

Figure 7.14. Fibromyalgia (FM) is characterized by widespread musculoskeletal pain, which is often linked to abnormalities in muscle tissue and central pain processing mechanisms.

Source: https://coastalhealth.com/wp-content/uploads/2022/11/Fibro-scaled.jpg.

7.3.8. Ankylosing Spondylitis (AS) and Spinal Tissue Changes

Test Your Knowledge

1. How does epigenetic regulation modulate environmental effects on gene expression in autoimmunity?
2. What is the role of the gut microbiome as an environmental mediator in genetically predisposed individuals?

AS is characterized by deep spinal tissue changes, which are mostly mediated through inflammation but also selectively in the entheses, or points of tendon and ligament attachment to bone. This inflammation leads to severe structural alterations, with the development of syndesmophytes, which ultimately result in bony ankylosis of the vertebrae, a hallmark of the condition. The pathogenetic processes of such spinal tissue changes are not yet well understood, with the onset and chronicity of inflammation not being well characterized. Evidence identifies that therapeutic agents targeting specific pathways, such as tumor necrosis factor-α and interleukin-17, have proven to be helpful in resolving symptoms of AS, highlighting the contribution of these inflammatory mediators to the disease (Furst et al., 2019). Moreover, evidence-based treatment protocols have evolved to indicate the necessity of an integrated approach to address the heterogeneous manifestations and impacts of AS on spinal health (Boehncke et al., 2008).

7.3.9. Diagnostic Challenges in Identifying Tissue Disorders

Tissue disorder diagnosis is an abundance of diagnostic challenges, particularly in the case of rheumatology, where the co-occurrence of symptoms makes clinical evaluations challenging. The majority of the connective tissue disorders have non-specific signs , such as fatigue, pain in the joints, and mood swings that may mask the underlying pathology. In addition, Joint Hypermobility and Postural Tachycardia Syndrome are common conditions that co-exist, hence making diagnosis tricky and leading to potential mismanagement of the patient's care. These issues of the system indicate the need for heightened awareness of interaction between psychological and physiological processes, for example, patients with Joint Hypermobility who will exhibit both tissue fragility as well as heightened anxiety, thereby escalating their clinical presentation (Aktas et al., 2015). Furthermore, the clinical heterogeneity of presentation among different patients necessitates a multidimensional and delicate approach to diagnosis, paying regard to patient-specific symptomology while integrating both biochemical and structural evaluation of tissue integrity (Staunton et al., 2013) (Figure 7.15).

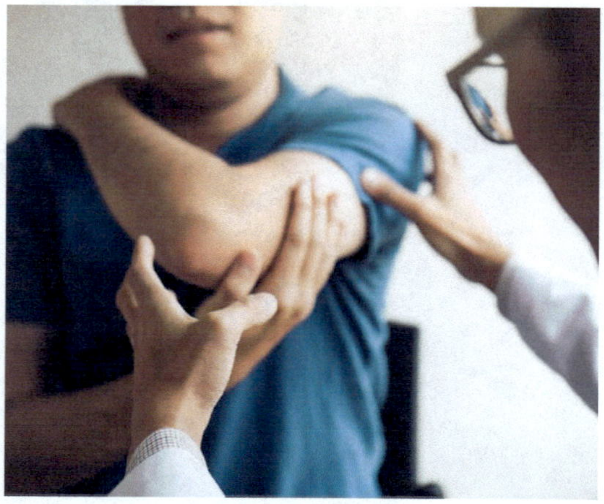

Figure 7.15. The identification of tissue disorders presents a multitude of diagnostic challenges, particularly within the realm of rheumatology, where overlapping symptoms complicate clinical evaluations.

Source: https://dranoofsrheumacare.com/images/treatments/fibromyalgia.jpg

Test Your Knowledge

1. What are the alterations observed in a joint in severe osteoarthritis (e.g., Heberden's nodes)?
2. How does fibrosis affect organ systems in systemic sclerosis?

Summary

The review of tissue investigation in health and disease in rheumatology emphasizes the intricate interrelationship between genetic, environmental, and autoimmune etiologies of conditions like RA and PSS. As observed in current studies, the association of some haplotypes, such as FCGR3A-FCGR3B 158V-NA2, with raised risk for RA indicates the prospects of genetic markers that can cause early diagnosis and tailored therapies (Mackie et al., 2005). Moreover, the identification of pathogenic mechanisms, such as the role of IFN-γ in macrophage activation syndrome, elucidates the intricacy of autoimmune mechanisms and their implications for patients (Bracaglia et al., 2018). Lastly, gaining insight into such relationships can more effectively enable therapeutic intervention and enhance the quality of life in rheumatic disease patients and emphasizing the need for additional research in this evolving field.

The intricate interaction between genetic susceptibility and autoimmune diseases , such as RA and PSS, emphasizes important areas for understanding tissue pathology in rheumatology. Recent research emphasizes a significant association of the FCGR3A-FCGR3B haplotype with susceptibility to RA, once again reflecting the importance of genetic influences in disease onset and progression. Homozygosity for the FCGR3A-FCGR3B 158V-NA2 haplotype has been found to be a critical risk factor, and the odds ratio has indicated a higher susceptibility within affected cohorts. This confirms earlier findings and suggests a shared pathological mechanism in heterogeneous autoimmune. diseases, as depicted in PSS comparisons. These results suggest the necessity of interdisciplinary research to reveal the complexities of autoimmune disease, ultimately improving therapeutic programs and patient management in rheumatology (Mackie et al., 2005; Staunton et al., 2013).

KEY TERMS FROM THIS CHAPTER

- Rheumatology
- Systemic lupus erythematosus
- Ligaments
- Immune organs
- Fibers
- Blood
- Micronutrients
- Pain intensity
- Disease-susceptibility marker
- Cartilage
- Synovial membranes
- Lymph nodes
- Bone
- Osteoarthritis
- Phytochemicals
- Vascular tissue

Critical Thinking Questions

1. **Which of the following types of tissues is mainly involved in contraction and movement within the body?**
   a. Epithelial tissue
   b. Connective tissue
   c. Nervous tissue
   d. Muscle tissue
2. **Which tissue type lines the body surfaces and cavities and is specialized for secretion and absorption?**
   a. Connective tissue
   b. Epithelial tissue
   c. Muscle tissue
   d. Adipose tissue
3. **Which connective tissue cell is primarily responsible for producing collagen and extracellular matrix?**
   a. Osteoblast
   b. Macrophage
   c. Fibroblast
   d. Chondrocyte
4. **In which tissue type would you most likely find intercalated discs?**
   a. Smooth muscle
   b. Skeletal muscle
   c. Cardiac muscle
   d. Epithelial tissue
5. **Which of the following tissues has the greatest capacity for regeneration after injury?**
   a. Cardiac muscle
   b. Nervous tissue
   c. Epithelial tissue
   d. Cartilage

Short Answer Questions

1. What are the most important tissue types that get affected in rheumatologic diseases?
2. How does synovial tissue contribute to inflammatory arthritis , such as rheumatoid arthritis?
3. What is the immunopathological basis of rheumatoid arthritis?
4. How does autoimmunity cause tissue injury in systemic lupus erythematosus?
5. What are the classic joint manifestations of rheumatoid arthritis (e.g., synovitis, deformities)?
6. How does muscle weakness manifest itself in inflammatory myopathies , such as polymyositis?

Answers to Critical Thinking Questions

1. (d); 2. (b); 3. (c); 4. (c); 5. (c)

References

1. Kumar, S., Singh, J., Rattan, S., DiMarino, A. J., Cohen, S., & Jimenez, S. A. (2017). Review article: pathogenesis and clinical manifestations of gastrointestinal involvement in systemic sclerosis. *Alimentary pharmacology & therapeutics*, *45*(7), 883–898. https://doi.org/10.1111/apt.13963(accessed on 17th June 2025).
2. Arazi, A., Rao, D. A., Berthier, C. C., Davidson, A., Liu, Y., Hoover, P. J., Chicoine, A., Eisenhaure, T. M., Jonsson, A. H., Li, S., Lieb, D. J., Zhang, F., Slowikowski, K., Browne, E. P., Noma, A., Sutherby, D., Steelman, S., Smilek, D. E., Tosta, P., Apruzzese, W., ... Accelerating Medicines Partnership in SLE network (2019). The immune cell landscape in kidneys of patients with lupus nephritis. *Nature immunology*, *20*(7), 902–914. https://doi.org/10.1038/s41590-019-0398-x (accessed on 17th June 2025).
3. Alivernini, S., Tolusso, B., Ferraccioli, G., Gremese, E., Kurowska-Stolarska, M., & McInnes, I. B. (2018). Driving chronicity in rheumatoid arthritis: perpetuating role of myeloid cells. *Clinical and experimental immunology*, *193*(1), 13–23. https://doi.org/10.1111/cei.13098 (accessed on 17th June 2025).
4. Ralli, M., D'Aguanno, V., Di Stadio, A., De Virgilio, A., Croce, A., Longo, L., Greco, A., & de Vincentiis, M. (2018). Audiovestibular Symptoms in Systemic Autoimmune Diseases. *Journal of immunology research*, *2018*, 5798103. https://doi.org/10.1155/2018/5798103 (accessed on 17th June 2025).
5. Adib, N., Aletaha, D., Bazso, A., Beresford, M. W., Consolaro, A., Baildam, E. M., McErlane, F., et al. (2012). Validity of a three-variable juvenile arthritis disease activity score in children with new-onset juvenile idiopathic arthritis. https://core.ac.uk/download/9652749.pdf (accessed on 17th June 2025).
6. Afeltra, A., Vittoria, M., Amoroso, A., Barbano, B., Cianci, R., et al. (2017). Angiogenic and angiostatic factors in renal scleroderma-associated vasculopathy. https://core.ac.uk/download/98348297.pdf (accessed on 17th June 2025).
7. Aigner, T., Kuttapitiya, A., Balanescu, A. R., Bannuru, R. R., Chou, R., da Costa, B. R., Danielsson, L., et al. (2014). Future directions for the management of pain in osteoarthritis. https://core.ac.uk/download/29469467.pdf (accessed on 17th June 2025).
8. Aktas, I., Al-Rawi, M., Anderson, J., Owens, A. P., Arunkalaivanan, A. S., Baeza-Velasco, C., Bagai, A., et al. (2015). Neurovisceral phenotypes in the expression of psychiatric symptoms. https://core.ac.uk/download/30611025.pdf (accessed on 17th June 2025).
9. Al-Adwi, Y., Burgess, J. K., Denton, C. P., Mulder, C. J., et al. (2022). Macrophages as determinants and regulators of fibrosis in systemic sclerosis. https://core.ac.uk/download/534955143.pdf (accessed on 17th June 2025).
10. Alivernini, S., Boncompagni, C., Bortoluzzi, A., Giorgi, C., Govoni, M., Missiroli, S., Patergnani, S., et al. (2021). From bed to bench and back: TNF-α, IL-23/IL-17A, and JAK-dependent inflammation in the pathogenesis of psoriatic synovitis. https://core.ac.uk/download/532388694.pdf (accessed on 17th June 2025).
11. Antczak, J., Bocianiak, B., Fenrych, U., Hamerska, K., et al. (2024). The importance of diet, intestinal microbiome and physical activity in rheumatoid arthritis (RA)–Review. https://core.ac.uk/download/613694736.pdf (accessed on 17th June 2025).

12. Antoniou, K., Baughman, R. P., Brown, K. K., Castelino, F. V., et al. (2013). Connective tissue disease related interstitial lung diseases and idiopathic pulmonary fibrosis: Provisional core sets of domains and instruments for use in clinical trials. https://core.ac.uk/download/77004246.pdf (accessed on 17th June 2025).

13. Ardalan, K., Childhood Arthritis, Rheumatology Research Alliance (CARRA) Scleroderma Workgroup, Chira, P., Ferry, B., et al. (2023). Barriers to care in juvenile localized and systemic scleroderma: An exploratory survey study of caregivers' perspectives. https://core.ac.uk/download/643777244.pdf (accessed on 17th June 2025).

14. Atzeni, F., Bazzichi, L., Casale, R., Di Franco, M., et al. (2015). Pain in systemic connective tissue diseases. https://core.ac.uk/download/54524187.pdf (accessed on 17th June 2025).

15. Bao, Y., Cassidy, A., Clark, I. M., Davidson, R. K., et al. (2014). The potential for dietary factors to prevent or treat osteoarthritis. https://core.ac.uk/download/29105737.pdf (accessed on 17th June 2025).

16. Barbera, L. L., Ciccia, F., Guggino, G., Pizzo, M. L., Rizzo, C., & Sireci, G. (2019). Invariant NKT cells and rheumatic disease: Focus on primary Sjögren syndrome. https://core.ac.uk/download/287859163.pdf (accessed on 17th June 2025).

17. Mackie, S., Robinson, J. I., Barrett, J. H., Lawson, C. A., Martin, S., Haroon-Rashid, L., Cooper, D., Bowman, S. J., Pease, C. T., Conaghan, P. G., Green, M., Quinn, M., Isaacs, J. D., Emery, P., & Morgan, A. W. (2005). Association of *FCGR3A* and *FCGR3B* haplotypes with rheumatoid arthritis and primary Sjögren's syndrome. *Arthritis Research & Therapy*, *7*(Suppl 1), P121. https://doi.org/10.1186/ar1642(accessed on 17th June 2025).

18. Benveniste, O., Goebel, H. H., & Stenzel, W. (2019). Biomarkers in inflammatory myopathies–An expanded definition. https://core.ac.uk/download/225124825.pdf (accessed on 17th June 2025).

19. Boehncke, W. H., Fiorentino, D., FitzGerald, O., Gladman, D., et al. (2008). Treatment recommendations for psoriatic arthritis. https://core.ac.uk/download/14507405.pdf (accessed on 17th June 2025).

20. Bracaglia, C., Caiello, I., Chatel, L., De Min, C., et al. (2018). Neutralization of IFN-γ reverts clinical and laboratory features in a mouse model of macrophage activation syndrome. https://core.ac.uk/download/127587867.pdf (accessed on 17th June 2025).

21. Brown, B., Simms, M., & Smith, S. C. (2018). Would you recognize lupus? https://core.ac.uk/download/215483268.pdf (accessed on 17th June 2025).

22. Burns, J., du Toit, V., Gibson, K., Hendry, G., et al. (2013). "They just scraped off the calluses": A mixed methods exploration of foot care access and provision for people with rheumatoid arthritis in south-western Sydney, Australia. https://core.ac.uk/download/293876500.pdf (accessed on 17th June 2025).

23. Cagnie, B., Coppieters, I., De Pauw, R., Ickmans, K., et al. (2015). Cognitive performance is related to central sensitization and health-related quality of life in patients with chronic whiplash-associated disorders and fibromyalgia. https://core.ac.uk/download/55848160.pdf (accessed on 17th June 2025).

24. Carnevale, A., Casoni, G. L., Cavagna, L., Furini, F., et al. (2019). The role of the multidisciplinary evaluation of interstitial lung diseases: Systematic literature review of the current evidence

and future perspectives. https://core.ac.uk/download/275692836.pdf (accessed on 17th June 2025).

25. Chandran, V., Coates, L. C., de Wit, M., FitzGerald, O., et al. (2021). Psoriatic arthritis. https://core.ac.uk/download/511310726.pdf (accessed on 17th June 2025).

26. Chaplain, M. A. J., Eftimie, R., & Macfarlane, F. R. (2019). Quantitative predictive modelling approaches to understanding rheumatoid arthritis: A brief review. https://core.ac.uk/download/286356117.pdf (accessed on 17th June 2025).

27. Chapman, J., Dalbeth, N., Gow, P., Rome, K., et al. (2010). Podiatry services for patients with arthritis: An unmet need. https://core.ac.uk/download/1662153.pdf (accessed on 17th June 2025).

28. Molfetta, L., Saviola, G., Fornasari, D., Grossi, P. A., Corcione, A., & Frediani, B. (2022). Osteoarticular pain: therapeutic approach by paradigms. *European review for medical and pharmacological sciences, 26*(11), 4054–4068. https://doi.org/10.26355/eurrev_202206_28975(accessed on 17th June 2025).

29. D'Amelio, R., Picchianti-Diamanti, A., & Rosado, M. M. (2018). Infectious agents and inflammation. The role of microbiota in autoimmune arthritis. https://core.ac.uk/download/153366739.pdf (accessed on 17th June 2025).

30. Di Stadio, A., & Ralli, M. (2017). Systemic lupus erythematosus and hearing disorders: Literature review and meta-analysis of clinical and temporal bone findings. https://core.ac.uk/download/98349075.pdf (accessed on 17th June 2025).

31. Diaconu, C. C., Hainarosie, R., Iancu, M. A., Iftimie, G., et al. (2018). The importance of early arthritis in patients with rheumatoid arthritis. https://core.ac.uk/download/216809651.pdf (accessed on 17th June 2025).

32. Dremin, V. V., Dunaev, A. V., Goltsov, A., Makovik, T., et al. (2019). Multimodal optical diagnostics of the microhaemodynamics in upper and lower limbs. https://core.ac.uk/download/228178569.pdf (accessed on 17th June 2025).

33. Finucci, A., Iagnocco, A., Rutigliano, I. M., Scirocco, T., et al. (2015). Musculoskeletal ultrasonography in gout. https://core.ac.uk/download/74318651.pdf (accessed on 17th June 2025).

34. S. O, Staunton L, FitzGerald O, R. S. Biomarkers of Inflammatory Arthritis and Proteomics [Internet]. Genes and Autoimmunity - Intracellular Signaling and Microbiome Contribution. InTech; 2013. Available from: http://dx.doi.org/10.5772/54218(accessed on 17th June 2025).

35. Furst, D. E., & Louie, J. S. (2019). Targeting inflammatory pathways in axial spondylarthritis. https://core.ac.uk/download/323075924.pdf (accessed on 17th June 2025).

36. Galli, A., Kis, A., Milano, A., Ghosh, A. K., et al. (2010). PPARγ downregulation by TGF in fibroblast and impaired expression and function in systemic sclerosis: A novel mechanism for progressive fibrogenesis. https://core.ac.uk/download/12212146.pdf (accessed on 17th June 2025).

37. Kasjmir, Y. I., Setiyohadi, B., & Suarjana, I. N. (2009). Knee arthritis in an HIV positive patient–Not associated with antiretroviral therapy. https://media.neliti.com/media/publications/231035-knee-arthritis-in-an-hiv-positive-patien-f9b16518.pdf (accessed on 17th June 2025).

38. Koch, A. E., Marrelli, A., Mahto, A., Mould, A. W., Pitzalis, C., Pyne, D., et al. (2015). Angiogenic

gene expression and vascular density are reflected in ultrasonographic features of synovitis in early rheumatoid arthritis: An observational study. https://core.ac.uk/download/30697659.pdf (accessed on 17th June 2025).

39. McCormick, A., Drummond, A. H., Banes, A. J., Bamji, A. N., Corps, A. N., et al. (2008). Tendinopathy—from basic science to treatment. https://core.ac.uk/download/2756893.pdf (accessed on 17th June 2025).

40. Navarro Ledesma, S. (2022). Short- and long-term effects of whole-body photo biomodulation on pain, functionality, tissue quality, central sensitization and psychological factors in a population suffering from fibromyalgia: Protocol for a triple-blinded randomized clinical trial. https://core.ac.uk/download/493006654.pdf (accessed on 17th June 2025).

41. Saleh, R. (2024). Understanding juvenile idiopathic arthritis: A multidimensional approach. https://core.ac.uk/download/599460676.pdf (accessed on 17th June 2025).

42. Weldon, A. J. (2014). The use of surface cytokines as biomarkers in B-cell mediated autoimmune diseases. https://core.ac.uk/download/151739792.pdf (accessed on 17th June 2025).

LABORATORY INVESTIGATIONS

8

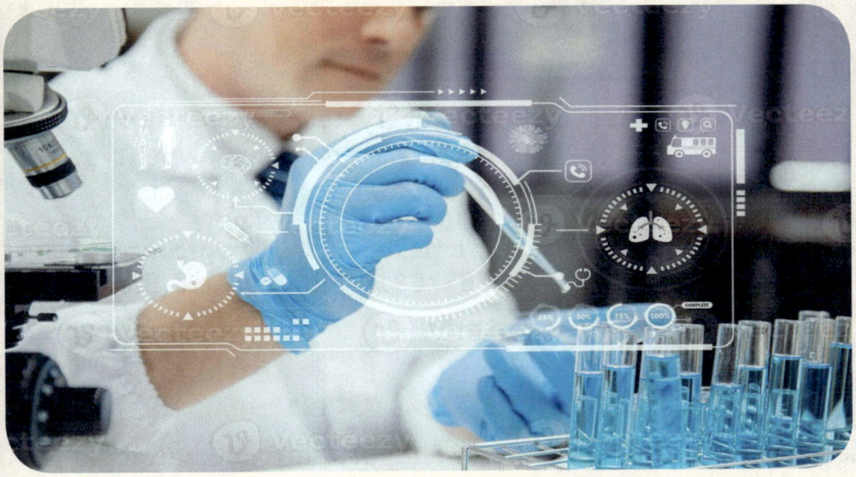

LEARNING OBJECTIVES

After studying this chapter, you will be able to:

1. Identify types of laboratory tests in rheumatology;
2. Explain laboratory result interpretation;
3. Relate laboratory technique advancements.

Introduction

Rheumatology entails a variety of complex diseases, and consequently, it necessitates the use of new laboratory studies in order to enhance diagnostic accuracy and efficacy of treatment. As the example with diseases , such as juvenile idiopathic inflammatory myopathies (IIMs) demonstrates, the rarity and heterogeneity of these diseases typically result in a huge knowledge deficit on the optimum management. For instance, the establishment of national registries and biobanks has been instrumental in promoting studies and clinical trials in such groups and has eventually improved outcomes for the affected children (Bohan et al., 2011). Similarly, the presence of urinary peptidomic biomarkers for diagnosing systemic lupus erythematosus (SLE) has highlighted the possibility of non-invasive methods for revolutionizing patient risk stratification and treatment (Burkly et al., 2018). Laboratory research, therefore, not only facilitates the identification of novel biomarkers but also paves the ways toward personalized treatment that is necessary in the new era of rheumatology.

8.1. Types of Laboratory Tests in Rheumatology

Learning Outcome

1. Understand the overview of blood tests;
2. Describe serological tests for autoantibodies;
3. Discuss complete blood count (CBC);
4. Emphasize erythrocyte sedimentation rate (ESR);
5. Describe C-reactive protein (CRP) testing;
6. Understand joint fluid analysis;
7. Recognize imaging studies and laboratory correlation;
8. Emphasize genetic testing in rheumatology;
9. Recognize emerging laboratory techniques.

Laboratory tests play a central role in the diagnosis and management of rheumatological diseases and are a heterogeneous group of techniques employed to quantify inflammation, autoimmunity, and target organ involvement. These are routinely used tests that encompass the quantification of serum markers, including rheumatoid factor and anti-citrullinated protein antibodies, which play a critical role in the diagnosis of rheumatoid arthritis.

Erythrocyte sedimentation rate (ESR) and C-reactive protein (CRP) also give quantitative measures of systemic inflammation, helping clinicians in assessing disease activity and response to treatment. More precise tests, including those conducted through registries associated with multidisciplinary networks, have emerged to enhance understanding of rare disorders , such as idiopathic inflammatory myopathies among children, as epitomized by the establishment of national biobanks in pediatric chronic inflammatory diseases (Bohan et al., 2011). Furthermore, the identification of marker indicators in electronic health records has also been found to be extremely useful in the context-based interpretation of disease progression, often appearing months before official diagnosis (Hansell et al., 2013) (Figure 8.1).

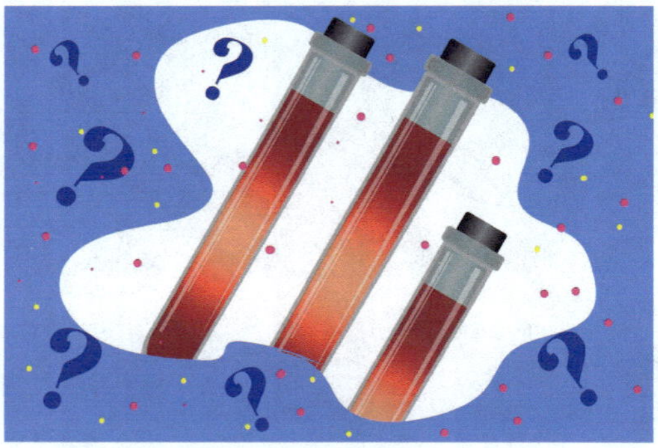

Figure 8.1. Laboratory tests play a crucial role in the diagnosis and management of rheumatological disorders.

Source: https://creakyjoints.org/wp-content/uploads/2019/03/0319_Fibromyalgia-Blood-Test.jpg.

8.1.1. Blood Tests Overview

Blood tests are important rheumatologic diagnostic tests that offer insight into autoimmune diseases , such as rheumatoid arthritis (RA) and primary Sjögren's syndrome (pSS) pathogenetic mechanisms. Blood tests typically check for various inflammatory markers and autoantibodies, yielding a comprehensive view of disease progression and disease activity. For instance, a study noted that lower serum levels of 25(OH) vitamin D correlated with increased RA activity, confirming the position of vitamin D in therapeutic efficacy and disease management (Barchetta et al., 2015). Similarly, the diagnostic criteria for pSS involving subjective symptoms and laboratory findings confirm the position of serum testing in the identification of glandular and extraglandular characteristics of the disease (Both et al., 2017). Therefore, blood tests not only facilitate early diagnosis but also direct treatment strategies, ultimately resulting in improved patient outcomes for rheumatology.

8.1.2. Serological Tests for Autoantibodies

Autoantibody serological tests are a valuable tool in the diagnosis and management of rheumatologic diseases, most notably systemic lupus erythematosus (SLE). These tests identify specific antibodies in the blood that may indicate an autoimmune response that can result in tissue damage and organ dysfunction. Notably, the presence of anti-C1q antibodies has also been linked with renal disease and disease activity in SLE patients, implying their utilization as disease monitoring markers (Makda, 2013). More significantly, even the diagnostic picture is changing, particularly in children, where timely diagnosis becomes important because of the high risk of progression to severe manifestations, including lupus nephritis (Lewandowski et al., 2016). The application of serological tests, combined with a systematized approach to the initial evaluation and multidisciplinary treatment, enhances clinical outcomes by enabling timely and personalized interventions for patients with rheumatic diseases (Figure 8.2).

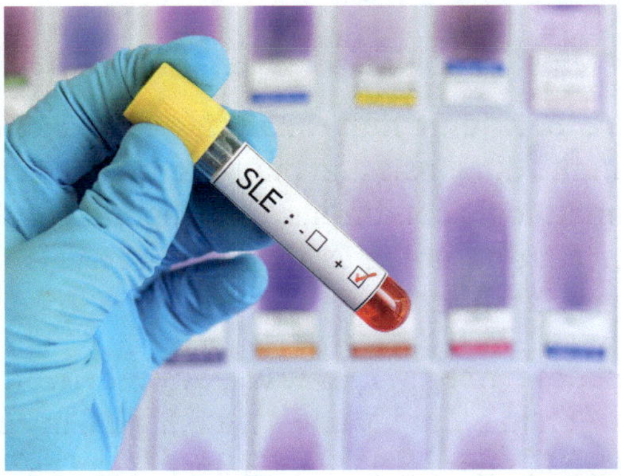

Figure 8.2. Serological tests for autoantibodies play a crucial role in the diagnosis and management of rheumatologic diseases, particularly systemic lupus erythematosus (SLE).

Source: https://www.medicalindependent.ie/wp-content/uploads/2022/01/iStock-512436346.jpg.

8.1.3. Complete Blood Count (CBC)

The CBC is a common laboratory examination in rheumatology that provides priceless information about the hematologic state of a patient, with substantial implications for both diagnosis and treatment of inflammatory diseases like RA. A CBC is a laboratory test to evaluate various elements of the blood, i.e., red cells, white cells, and platelets, thereby offering vital information regarding potential anemia or leukocytosis, which is prevalent in the context of active disease status. White blood cell elevation may indicate underlying infection or inflammation, and alterations in hemoglobin can indicate the extent of disease impact on the patient's overall condition. Studies have shown that serum levels of inflammatory indicators are correlated strongly with disease activity, further establishing the worth of the CBC and other tests, such as C-reactive protein and erythrocyte sedimentation rate, in the assessment of disease course and response to therapy (Hammoda et al., 2014). The CBC is thus still a cornerstone in the comprehensive evaluation of rheumatic diseases, guiding clinical decision-making (Puzanov et al., 2017).

8.1.4. Erythrocyte Sedimentation Rate (ESR)

From the variety of laboratory tests applied in rheumatology, the ESR is still a key marker to measure inflammation and disease activity in diseases , such as RA. The ESR measures the rate at which red blood cells sediment to the bottom of a test tube within an established time interval, indicating an acute as well as a chronic inflammatory process. Higher levels of ESR can indicate active disease and direct decision-making for therapy adjustments and follow-up response, particularly in early RA patients where early intervention is crucial for optimal long-term results. Clinicians must take other diagnostic findings into account, however, since the test is not disease-specific and can be influenced by age, gender, and comorbidities. Therefore, while ESR is a valuable tool, it emphasizes the subtlety of managing inflammatory arthritides and the requirement for careful patient evaluation (Berardicurti et al., 2017) (Figure 8.3).

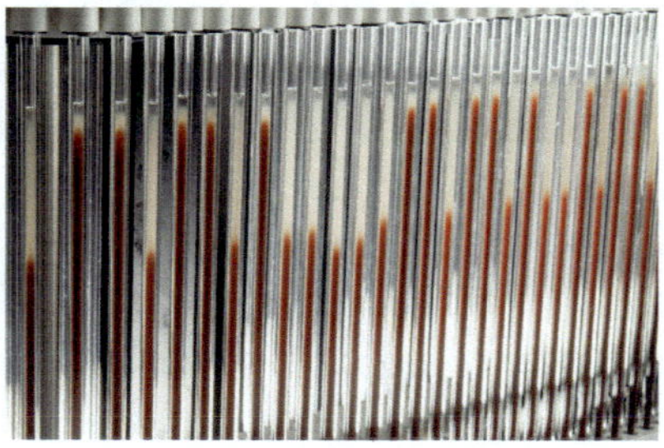

Figure 8.3. Erythrocyte sedimentation rate (ESR).

Source: https://upload.wikimedia.org/wikipedia/commons/9/9d/StaRRsed_pipet_array.jpg.

8.1.5. C-Reactive Protein (CRP) Testing

CRP testing has an invaluable role to play in rheumatology in its assessment of inflammatory response in various musculoskeletal conditions, particularly rheumatoid arthritis and psoriatic arthritis. Elevated CRP concentrations indicate acute and chronic inflammation, allowing clinicians to monitor disease activity and response to treatment. This biochemist marker is of high value as it correlates with the presence of proinflammatory cytokines, including interleukin-17A, which is involved in inflammatory disorder development (Conaghan et al., 2015). Additionally, hs-CRP has been reported to be predictive in postoperative outcomes after total knee arthroplasty in osteoarthritis patients with elevated hs-CRP, meaning that these patients will be at risk of poorer functional recovery (Smith, 2013). Therefore, CRP testing is both prognostic and diagnostic in enabling individualized therapeutic interventions in rheumatology treatment.

8.1.6. Joint Fluid Analysis

Joint fluid examination is crucial to the diagnosis and management of many rheumatologic conditions, offering insight into intrinsic pathologies based on synovial fluid examination. The fluid can be accessed by arthrocentesis and has the potential to be of value in offering insights into the presence of inflammatory mediators, crystals, and infection and to be of significant assistance in differentiating between the conditions of septic arthritis and gout. Advances in lab techniques in the last few years have accelerated our diagnostic armory, and methods like Raman spectroscopy have given us sophisticated data on crystal development and deposition, particularly CPPD ailments (Filippou et al., 2024).

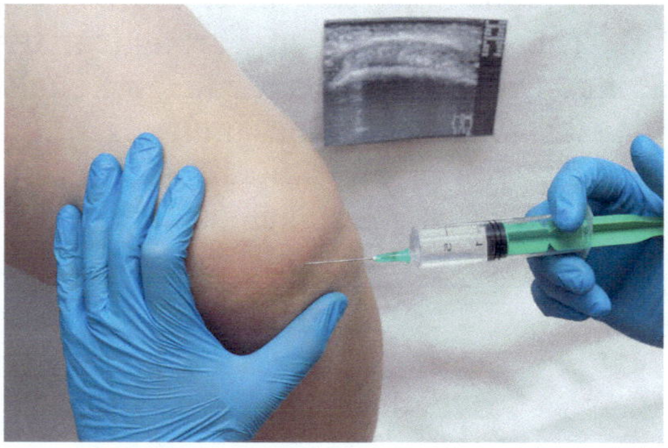

Figure 8.4. Joint fluid analysis plays a crucial role in the diagnosis and management of various rheumatologic conditions, offering insights into underlying pathologies through the evaluation of synovial fluid.

Source: https://www.verywellhealth.com/thmb/mhybIFjXz22ghCml68AN6YS8MsA=/2000x1333/filters:no_upscale():max_bytes(150000):strip_icc()/GettyImages-1174570027-d5ba663ef8bc4b5d823ede957a579100-82f2723256f1404284bb472a325bf177.jpg.

In addition, the relevance of joint fluid analysis is not just for adult rheumatoid arthritis but also for juvenile idiopathic arthritis (JIA), where analysis is able to direct therapeutic maneuvers and prognostic planning amidst the complexity of its etiology and heterogeneous presentation (Aji et al., 2024). Lastly, joint fluid analysis remains a useful resource in rheumatology, allowing individualized therapeutic strategies for patients (Figure 8.4).

8.1.7. Imaging Studies and Their Laboratory Correlation

Imaging studies play a vital role in the diagnostic and treatment setting of rheumatology, particularly when combined with laboratory findings. Techniques , such as ultrasonography (US) and magnetic resonance imaging (MRI) have been essential in detecting synovial inflammation that is typically occult on clinical examination alone. For instance, in juvenile idiopathic arthritis, US has proved helpful in the diagnosis of synovitis in more than one compartment of the wrist, thereby defining the targeted steroid injections and determining the response to treatment (Ravelli et al., 2012). In addition, the treatment strategies of spondyloarthritis put emphasis on establishing well-defined treatment objectives, e.g., achieving remission or low disease activity, necessitating frequent assessment by means of imaging (Baraliakos et al., 2013). The correlation of imaging tests with laboratory results enhances the validity of the diagnosis and impacts decision-making in clinical practice, leading to enhanced patient outcomes and therapeutic regimens in rheumatology.

8.1.8. Genetic Testing in Rheumatology

Advances in genetic testing have revolutionized rheumatology practice, with enhanced diagnostic sensitivity and patient-specific management. By identifying specific genetic markers observed in various rheumatic disorders, such as juvenile idiopathic arthritis and reactive arthritis, medical professionals can better understand disease susceptibility and disease progression. For instance, the incorporation of genetic data into the study of juvenile idiopathic inflammatory myopathies has enabled the establishment of a national registry, significantly enhancing the understanding of these complex diseases and facilitating clinical trials (Bohan et al., 2011). Besides, genetic testing in conditions , such as reactive arthritis, which is known to have common underlying genes , such as HLA-B27, enables clinicians to tailor treatment more effectively and be capable of predicting patient outcome (Cargnelutti et al., 2013). With ongoing advancement in the area, research and coordination are crucial to fully harness the potential of genetic testing for improving results in rheumatic disease patients (Figure 8.5).

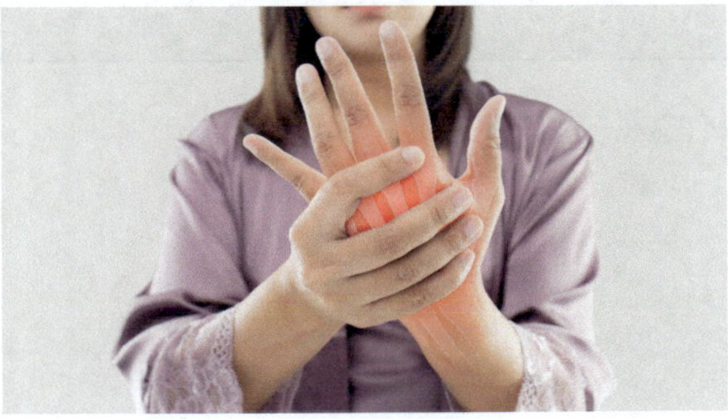

Figure 8.5. By identifying specific genetic markers associated with various rheumatic diseases, such as juvenile idiopathic arthritis and reactive arthritis, clinicians can better understand disease predisposition and progression.

Source: https://d35oenyzp35321.cloudfront.net/inflammatory_arthritis_00bdac4789.jpg.

8.1.9. Emerging Laboratory Techniques

With the advancement of rheumatology, new laboratory techniques can potentially transform disease management and patient outcomes. New methods , such as state-of-the-art imaging, biomarker measurement, and high-throughput sequencing, are providing unprecedented insights into the pathophysiology of rheumatic diseases. For instance, new composite indices for measuring disease activity in such diseases as RA underscore the importance of early intervention in treatment as a window of opportunity for improving long-term outcomes in patients. Also, using these methods makes it possible to individualize therapies to patient profiles and therefore optimize therapeutic efficiency and limit probable side effects. Furthermore, with the integration of sophisticated technologies, not only do rheumatologists optimize diagnostic accuracy, but they also identify responsive channels of therapy at an earlier stage in the disease process. The interactive dance of these technologies continues to shape the future of rheumatology laboratory research in a deepening transformation toward precision medicine.

Test Your Knowledge

1. What laboratory markers are increased in systemic inflammation (e.g., ESR, CRP)?
2. How is synovial fluid analysis used in evaluating joint disease?

8.2. Interpretation of Laboratory Results

Learning Outcome

1. Value normal vs. abnormal results;
2. Explain the specificity and sensitivity of tests;
3. Identify factors that affect test results;
4. Correlate with clinical symptoms;
5. Describe the role of laboratory standards;
6. Learn case studies in result interpretation;
7. Learn common misinterpretations;
8. Know the importance of follow-up testing;
9. Discuss a multidisciplinary approach to interpretation.

Laboratory result interpretation is of critical significance in diagnosing and managing rheumatological disorders, as these tests can reveal underlying pathology that is not evident on clinical assessment. For instance, in granulomatous myositis, physicians need to carefully scrutinize laboratory results , such as hypercalcemia, which may be a sign of any associated diseases , such as sarcoidosis. As illustrated through the history of a 16-year-old female patient who had initially come in with severe hypercalcemia and renal insufficiency but no typical symptoms, laboratory tests eventually resulted in a diagnosis following unproductive workups in the past that were extensive and revealed subtle myositis changes and biopsy-proven granulomas (Eutsler et al., 2016). In addition, other studies demonstrate high comorbidities in rheumatologic patients; for instance, the prevalence of cardiovascular disease in osteoarthritis patients necessitates putting laboratory findings into a broader clinical context, relating systemic health to rheumatological assessments (Hall et al., 2015).

8.2.1. Normal Versus Abnormal Results

In the practice of rheumatology, normal versus abnormal laboratory results must be distinguished in order to sound diagnosis and therapeutic efficacy. For instance, microalbuminuria in patients with systemic sclerosis is an indicator of renal involvement at an early stage, wherein 20% of patients have abnormal albumin/creatinine levels, which highlights its prognostic importance in the disease (Eid et al., 2012). Also, the presence of macrophage activation syndrome (MAS) in Still's disease could manifest concerning laboratory findings , such as elevated serum ferritin and hypoalbuminemia, which are essential to establish disease severity and complications (Al-Maghlouth et al., 2023). These fine interpretations of lab findings are used to underscore the importance of careful analysis in clinical practice, where small deviations from normal values are crucial to indicating important changes in disease progression and informing management strategies for rheumatologic diseases (Figure 8.6).

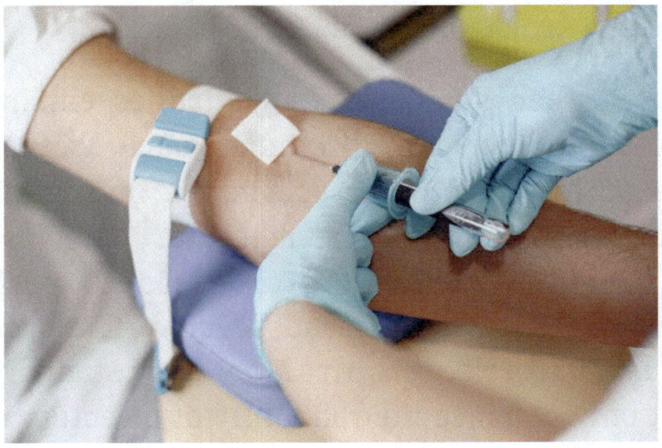

Figure 8.6. In the realm of rheumatology, distinguishing between normal and abnormal laboratory results is critical for accurate diagnosis and treatment efficacy.

Source: https://phuketmedicalclinic.com/wp-content/uploads/2024/07/laboratory-test-1.jpg.

8.2.2. Specificity and Sensitivity of Tests

In the realm of rheumatology, the specificity and sensitivity of diagnostic tests are crucial for effective disease management and patient outcomes. For instance, a recent study indicated the significance of urinary peptidomic biomarkers in SLE patients, where a biomarker panel exhibited 83% sensitivity and 73% specificity to distinguish SLE from healthy subjects for early diagnosis, crucial for timely intervention (Burkly et al., 2018). Further, in the case of RA, advanced diagnostic techniques emphasize the importance of establishing early arthritis to prevent permanent damage to joints; effective treatment heavily relies on accurate testing to ensure individuals are administered appropriate treatments, either by means of traditional DMARDs or biologic therapies (Diaconu et al., 2018). Thus, specificity and sensitivity testing in such tests not only enhances diagnostic ability but also has treatment protocol and clinical outcome implications for rheumatological disorders.

8.2.3. Factors Affecting Test Results

Many factors in the field of rheumatology can have considerable influence over test results, influencing diagnosis and the outcome of treatment. One of such major factors is the level of vitamin D, and it has been shown to exert immunomodulatory activity in conditions , such as RA.

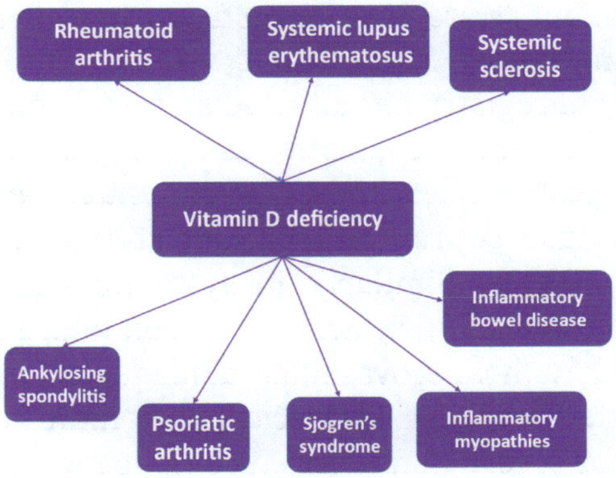

Figure 8.7. One crucial aspect is the level of vitamin D, which has been shown to have immunomodulatory effects in conditions , such as rheumatoid arthritis (RA).

Source: https://pub.mdpi-res.com/biomolecules/biomolecules-13-00709/article_deploy/html/images/biomolecules-13-00709-g001.png?1682067142.

It has been demonstrated that hypovitaminosis D patients experience augmented disease activity and diminished frequency of remission when compared to vitamin D level normal patients, and it is therefore plausible that serum 25(OH) vitamin D will serve as a predictive marker for RA patient disease progression (Barchetta et al., 2015). Also, the association between osteoarthritis (OA) and cardiovascular disease (CVD) shows how comorbid illnesses will make test interpretations more difficult because OA patients have significantly higher rates of heart failure and ischemic heart disease (Hall et al., 2015). It is important to know these various factors while doing appropriate assessments during lab testing in rheumatology (Figure 8.7).

8.2.4. Correlation with Clinical Symptoms

Laboratory correlation with clinical manifestations of rheumatological diseases is the key to correct diagnosis, as well as correct treatment strategies. For instance, in idiopathic inflammatory myopathies of childhood, a national registry has allowed an invaluable link between clinical evaluation and the gathering of biological samples, improving our understanding of disease course and patient status (Bohan et al., 2011). Similarly, in systemic sclerosis, serum levels of uric acid have been found to be linked with microvascular damage, indicating elevated levels of uric acid as an indicator of disease severity and related complications, such as renal impairment (Amoroso et al., 2016). These examples demonstrate the significance of integrative laboratory investigations in accounting for the clinical presentation of rheumatological disorders. Through critical analysis of laboratory findings in conjunction with clinical presentation, clinicians can more effectively track disease, tailor interventions, and finally deliver better quality care to patients with these complex conditions.

8.2.5. Role of Laboratory Standards

Setting good laboratory standards is of major importance in the complex nature of practice in rheumatology in order to make good diagnostic and therapeutic yields. These standards enable the accuracy and consistency of laboratory tests, which are crucial to the treatment and diagnosis of autoimmune diseases. For instance, research has found that learning resources, developed in line with suggested laboratory standards, significantly improve the learning curve for medical practitioners, enabling them to understand difficult diagnostics in rheumatology better (Armstrong et al., 2005).

Further, standardized guidelines enhance the validity of clinical studies, such as those measuring serum uric acid levels in systemic sclerosis patients, where laboratory standards need to be adhered to in a bid to verify correlations with disease severity (Amoroso et al., 2016). Hence, strict laboratory standards not only enhance the reliability of investigative results but also help advance rheumatological research, which ultimately reaps dividends in terms of improved patient care and treatment models (Figure 8.8).

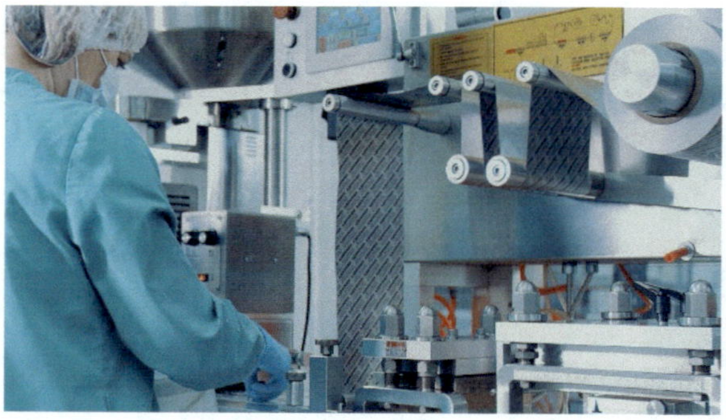

Figure 8.8. In the intricate field of rheumatology, the establishment of robust laboratory standards is vital for ensuring reliable diagnostic and therapeutic outcomes.

Source: https://d2jx2rerrg6sh3.cloudfront.net/images/Article_Images/ImageForArticle_25632_17346171581002484.jpg.

8.2.6. Case Studies in Result Interpretation

Laboratory test interpretation in rheumatology is often based on sensitive case studies portraying the interaction between different conditions. One such case is a systematic review, which concluded that patients with OA had significantly higher rates of CVD, with nearly 38.4% of them suffering from the condition, emphasizing the extreme necessity of integrated clinical approaches (Hall et al., 2015). This association requires keen interpretive skills to separate underlying pathophysiological processes shared by OA and CVD, suggesting a multifaceted rather than linear association. Alternatively, conditions like Takayasu arteritis (TA) have different interpretative challenges, especially in the pediatric environment, in which the disease is multifaceted. The clinical presentation and treatment response in children and disease activity assessment need strict case analyses to execute proper management plans (Al-Obaidi et al., 2015). Strict case studies are thus crucial instruments for maximizing diagnostic and treatment approaches in rheumatology, eventually having a positive outcome for patients.

8.2.7. Common Misinterpretations

Common misinterpretations frequently arise in rheumatology with regard to laboratory investigations, which usually render significant clinical implications. One such applicable misconception is the application of non-specific markers , such as CRP or ESR, that indicate inflammation but have no direct relationship with the severity of rheumatological conditions. Furthermore, high-tech imaging techniques, as important as they are, can also give false readings. For instance, the use of highly advanced imaging modalities like MRI in pediatric musculoskeletal infections emphasizes the necessity of individualized protocols to improve diagnostic performance, while standard protocols are not efficient for every disease (Alavi, 2022). Moreover, the complexities of the complement system, particularly in systemic lupus erythematosus, illustrate how genetics and variations in immunological responses can complicate diagnosis as well as treatment protocols (Yu et al., 2016). Therefore, ongoing education and sensitization are critical in evading such misinterpretation (Figure 8.9).

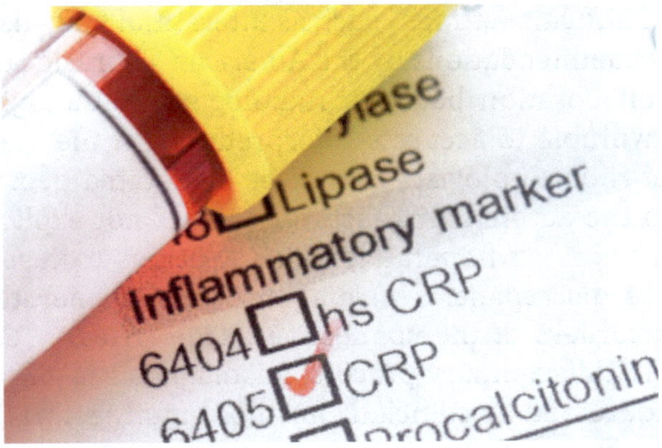

Figure 8.9. One pertinent misunderstanding is the reliance on non-specific markers , such as C-reactive protein (CRP) or erythrocyte sedimentation rate (ESR), which can indicate inflammation but do not specifically correlate with the severity of rheumatic diseases.

Source: https://s3.ap-south-1.amazonaws.com/m3india-app-dev/ckeditor/content/crp-1549023954.jpg.

8.2.8. Importance of Follow-Up Testing

Follow-up testing in rheumatology is significant as it serves a number of important roles that assist in successful patient care. This process not only makes it easy to ascertain the efficacy of treatment but also plays a critical role in the early identification of complications due to ongoing treatments, such as immune-related adverse events in patients on immunotherapy. For instance, the late onset and prolonged course of these immune-mediated adverse effects mandate prompt follow-up to avoid treatment-related death, an outcome that can occur in up to 2% of patients (Puzanov et al., 2017). On top of this, conditions , such as Kawasaki disease demonstrate the value of close follow-up; otherwise, severe long-term cardiovascular sequelae can be missed by clinicians, potentially leading to worse patient outcomes when patients transition to adult care (Brogan et al., 2020). Therefore, the worth of follow-up investigation cannot be overstressed as it is the cornerstone of complete and active rheumatological management.

8.2.9. Multidisciplinary Approach to Interpretation

Multidisciplinary collaboration is essential for enhancing the accuracy of diagnosis in rheumatology in difficult settings , such as interstitial lung disease caused by autoimmune diseases. As per current recommendations by the American Thoracic Society and other well-established organizations, team collaboration between radiologists, pathologists, and rheumatologists provides an environment favorable to accurate interpretation of the diagnostic criteria. During such consultations, the role of rheumatologists cannot be overstated because they can provide important information related to the autoimmune factor that does not explicitly come to light. Such collaboration becomes even more of an imperative when it comes to cases of joint hypermobility assessment, wherein there are discrepancies in diagnosis, thus generating misconceptions about the underlying heritable disorders of the connective tissue (HDCT) (Carnevale et al., 2019). By stimulating an organized multidisciplinary process, misdiagnosis is minimized and patient needs may be more appropriately addressed by clinicians for those multifactorial rheumatologic patients (Dolan et al., 2009) (Figure 8.10).

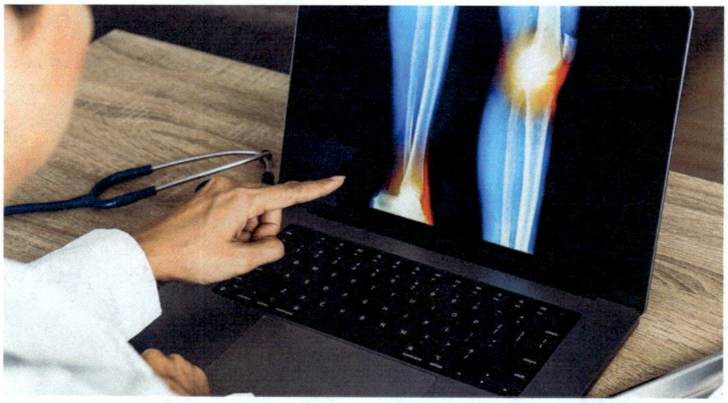

Figure 8.10. The integration of a multidisciplinary approach is essential for enhancing diagnostic accuracy in rheumatology, particularly in complex cases , such as interstitial lung disease associated with autoimmune disorders.

Source: https://assets.isu.pub/document-structure/241220163851-4e3dfd61db7ee89767cefd5174c2c45a/v1/593cf348a19f9d6ac595b69ca6710257.jpeg.

Test Your Knowledge

1. When is a positive rheumatoid factor non-specific?
2. How can autoantibody profiles discriminate between mixed connective tissue disease and other CTDs?

8.3. Advances in Laboratory Techniques

Learning Outcome

1. Appreciate advances in technology in testing;
2. Discuss automation in the laboratory;
3. Explain biomarker development;
4. Learn advances in imaging methodology;
5. Describe point-of-care testing;
6. Emphasize the incorporation of artificial intelligence;
7. Learn future developments in laboratory tests;
8. Know the impact of research on clinical practice;
9. Discuss ethical concerns in new technologies.

The evolution of laboratory procedures has transformed the landscape of rheumatology by enhancing the diagnosis and the rate of treatment success. Some of the new developments in the field involve targeted molecular imaging, which has been a landmark in distinguishing the intrinsic pathophysiologic processes of diseases like RA and spondyloarthritis (SpA). For instance, E-selectin targeted optical imaging demonstrates the potential to quantify disease activity and define the effect of novel therapies, promising a future of precision medicine in rheumatology (Gompels, 2010). Concurrently with these advancements, the beginning of treatment objectives by means of systematic reviews has formed the basis of SpA management, with an emphasis on joint patient-clinician decision-making towards a shared goal to achieve remission or low disease activity (Baraliakos et al., 2013).

With further advancements in these, they have the potential to make therapeutic strategies more specific and improve patient care in the constantly evolving scenario of rheumatology.

8.3.1. Technological Innovations in Testing

The rheumatology landscape is undergoing a transformation fundamentally due to the advent of testing technology that enhances diagnosis and patient outcomes. Advances in areas , such as biomarker discovery and the utilization of high-throughput screening approaches have made it possible to recognize autoimmune diseases at an earlier stage, thus early intervention is possible. Additionally, cloud-sharing platforms of data and analysis enable clinicians to view real-time complete patient histories and test results, thereby facilitating collaborative decision-making by healthcare teams.

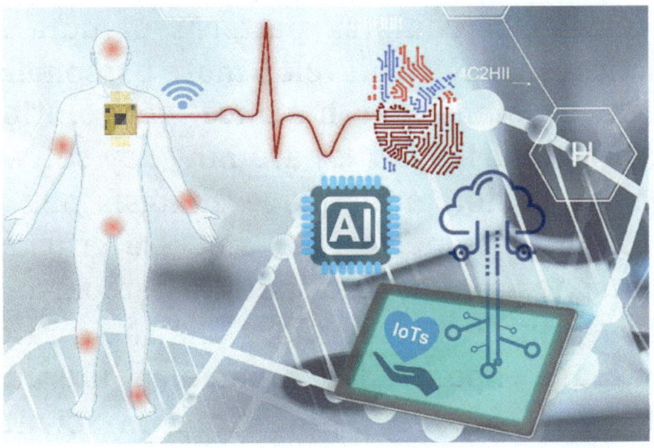

Figure 8.11. Advancements , such as biomarker discovery and high-throughput screening techniques have revolutionized the ability to identify autoimmune diseases at earlier stages, thus facilitating timely intervention.

Source: https://pub.mdpi-res.com/biosensors/biosensors-14-00356/article_deploy/html/images/biosensors-14-00356-ag.png?1721826654.

Further, overlay mapping techniques, cited in recent studies, provide strategic intelligence by illustrating the migration of developing biotechnology in biomedical testing, particularly rheumatology. This follows the need for constant adjustment and addition of innovative practices in hospital settings, as outlined by hospital roles in medical innovation literature (Thune & Mina,

2016). Ultimately, these innovations are what will be crucial in building a more responsive and effective healthcare system in response to the complexity of rheumatological diseases (Hopkins et al., 2014) (Figure 8.11).

8.3.2. Role of Automation in Laboratories

The integration of automation into laboratories has revolutionized rheumatology research and practice in clinical settings, particularly with regard to managing large data sets and improving diagnostic precision. Automation software, including machine learning models and advanced imaging equipment, enables the processing of complex patterns of data and patient responses to develop more personalized treatment plans. For instance, convolutional neural networks (CNNs) are now key software used for radiological image analysis and the detection of some lesions that are crucial in the diagnosis of conditions like osteoarthritis and sacroiliitis. Furthermore, the rapid rate of knowledge expansion in biomedical literature, with over 750,000 publications in scientific literature in 2007 alone being a case in point, emphasizes the need for automatic systems to process and integrate information, as traditional methods cannot cope (Burke et al., 2009; Hügle, 2024). By automating processes, treatment impacts are increased and clinicians are empowered to make data-driven decisions, essentially taking the quality of care in rheumatology to the next level.

8.3.3. Development of Biomarkers

Biomarker development plays a pivotal role in enhancing laboratory research in rheumatology since it provides helpful tools in early diagnosis, disease activity monitoring, and tailoring treatment regimens. For instance, multicenter registries and biobanks, as used in pediatric idiopathic inflammatory myopathies, enhance our understanding of rare inflammatory conditions by providing standard data collection and sample accessibility to researchers (Bohan et al., 2011). Similarly, in the case of systemic lupus erythematosus, high-level biomarker panels through urinary peptidomic profiling have been employed to distinguish between disease status effectively, thereby improving patient risk stratification and more effective drug interventions (Burkly et al., 2018). Such advancement underscores not only the potential of personalized medicine in rheumatology but also the ongoing requirement for synergistic research to facilitate biomarker discovery and use, ultimately influencing patient outcomes in these multidimensional diseases (Figure 8.12).

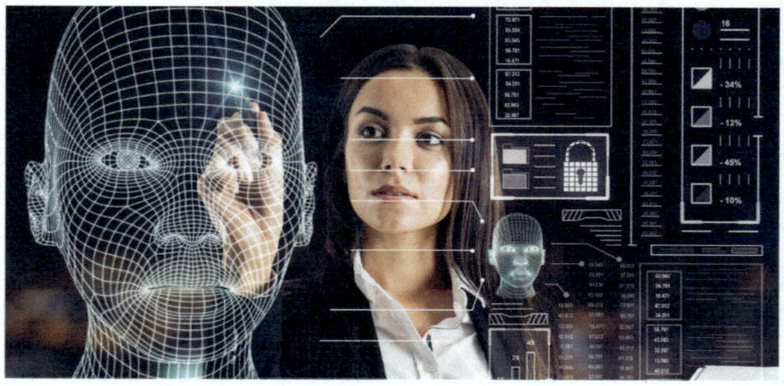

Figure 8.12. The development of biomarkers plays a crucial role in advancing laboratory investigations in rheumatology, as they provide invaluable tools for early diagnosis, monitoring disease progression, and tailoring treatment strategies.

Source: https://sonraianalytics.com/wp-content/uploads/2022/10/AI-in-biomarkers.jpg.

8.3.4. Advances in Imaging Techniques

Recent advances in imaging technologies have optimally enhanced the diagnostic and therapeutic approach in rheumatology, particularly for conditions like RA and spondyloarthritis. Emerging technologies , such as near-infrared (NIR) fluorescent imaging, have emerged as comprehensive tools, which permit the visualization of new molecular targets *in vivo*, thereby reducing tissue autofluorescence and enhancing diagnostic effectiveness. For instance, E-selectin, an inflammatory mechanism biomarker in RA, has been successfully dynamically imaged using this new technique, whereby disease activity and treatment response can be more fully appreciated (Gompels, 2010). Furthermore, the ever-increasing development of imaging modalities that align targets of treatment, like remission or low disease activity in spondyloarthritis through a treat-to-target strategy, underscores the imperative role of such innovation in ensuring optimal patient outcomes (Baraliakos et al., 2013). The provision of advanced imaging modalities, thus, not only supports diagnosis but also informs management strategies for rheumatological diseases.

8.3.5. Point-of-Care Testing (POCT)

The integration of POCT in rheumatology significantly enhances patient management for patients with autoimmune diseases, enabling timely and informed clinical decisions. POCT offers immediate turnaround times, which facilitate rapid adjustment of treatment regimens, particularly for disorders with episodic signs and symptoms, such as rheumatoid arthritis. Through direct measurement of biomarkers at the point of care, clinicians are able to evaluate disease activity and response to treatment more efficiently. For example, studies have shown that self-efficacy issues among patients are handled by improving patients' compliance with health recommendations, particularly in autoimmune conditions (Rasker et al., 1993). In cases like lupus nephritis, too, individualized decision aids improving POCT have been shown to reduce decisional conflict for immunosuppressive therapy, hence empowering the patient and giving them vital information regarding their treatment options (Alarcón et al., 2019). All in all, POCT not only hastens clinical workflow but also enhances patient involvement in their care (Figure 8.13).

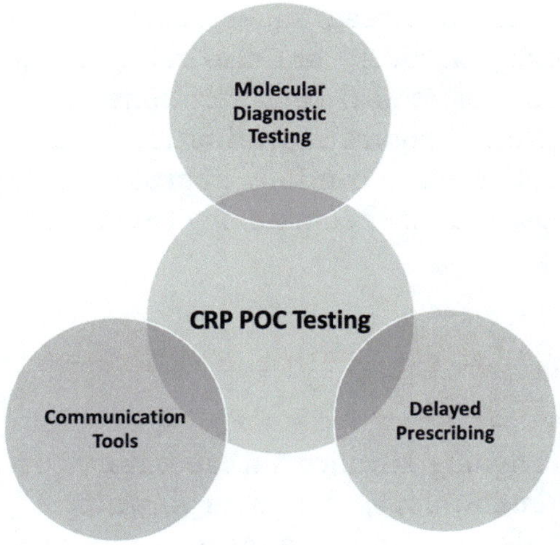

Figure 8.13. The integration of point-of-care testing (POCT) in rheumatology significantly enhances the management of patients with autoimmune diseases, enabling timely and informed clinical decisions.

Source: https://www.mdpi.com/diagnostics/diagnostics-13-00320/article_deploy/html/images/diagnostics-13-00320-g003.png.

8.3.6. Integration of Artificial Intelligence (AI)

The use of AI in rheumatology is a research paradigm shift as well as in clinical practice, significantly enhancing laboratory investigations. By employing machine learning algorithms, researchers can efficiently classify numerous rheumatic conditions and make accurate predictions related to therapeutic reactions from within different sets of information, including radiographic images and clinical findings (Hügle et al., 2024). The use of this technology is to detect disease patterns unique to the patient, thus encouraging more personalized treatment. Moreover, AI-driven digital biomarkers are able to facilitate real-time monitoring of disease progression and treatment efficacy to improve the engagement and management of patients outside of traditional clinical settings (Hügle, 2024). With the development of AI, it not only promises to streamline research processes and drug discovery but also raises challenges in terms of ethical considerations as well as demanding rigorous validation, making it imperative for a cautious approach to tap its full potential in rheumatology (Benavent et al., 2025).

8.3.7. Future Trends in Laboratory Investigations

With ongoing advances in laboratory research in rheumatology, the incorporation of new technologies and techniques is likely to be decisive in enhancing the accuracy of diagnosis and the outcomes of treatment. The implementation of EHRs is a major trend since they enable the detection of indicator markers in early onset cases of RA, thereby enabling early and accurate diagnosis (Hansell et al., 2013).

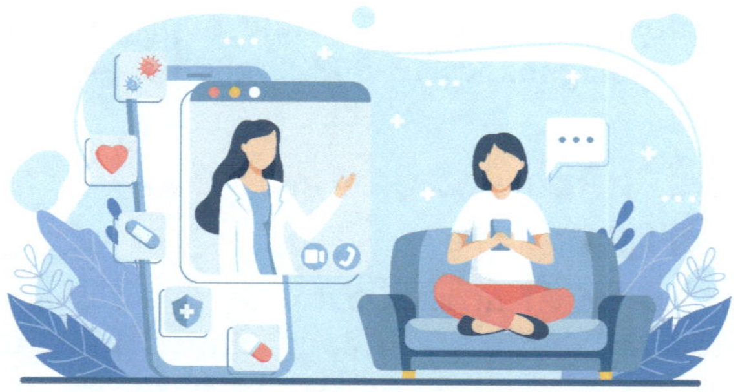

Figure 8.14. As laboratory investigations in rheumatology continue to evolve, the integration of advanced technologies and methodologies is expected to play a crucial role in enhancing diagnostic accuracy and treatment outcomes.

Source: https://www.the-rheumatologist.org/wp-content/uploads/2025/01/AdobeStock_602863099.png.

Moreover, patient decision aids, particularly in conditions like lupus, are being built to reduce decisional conflict and improve patient understanding of treatment options among different populations (Alarcón et al., 2019). These advances, coupled with growing emphasis on personalized medicine, can transform laboratory research, leading to improved management options and improved patient outcomes in rheumatology. While the specialty embraces these innovations, it also needs to overcome the data integration and patient engagement issues to have its maximum impact (Figure 8.14).

8.3.8. Impact of Research on Clinical Practice

Research has an extremely significant role to play in shaping the methodologies adopted in clinical practice, particularly rheumatology. Through a better understanding of disease processes, laboratory research not only enhances diagnosis and disease management, such as fibromyalgia syndrome (FM), but also emphasizes early detection and treatment. Early diagnosis and proper and prompt treatments contribute positively to the history of FM with positive impacts on clinical, psychological, social and economic levels. Diagnostic delay and access difficulty to new therapy are still widespread, with an important influence on patients' quality of life. Thus, the formation of protocols, like the Diagnostic-Therapeutic Care Pathway (DTCP), has the objective of simplifying patient care through the unification of different healthcare professionals to treat chronic diseases from a complete perspective. These innovations show the imperative role of research in developing clinical practices and subsequently improving patient outcomes (Sarzi-Puttini et al., 2021).

8.3.9. Ethical Considerations in New Technologies

The use of new technologies in rheumatology, through teleconsultation and machine learning, poses natural ethical problems to be treated with caution. With digital biomarkers increasingly coming to the fore, their use in clinical trials must be very strictly regulated so that patient data and privacy are not compromised, thereby balancing clinical efficacy with ethical accountability. The COVID-19 pandemic accelerated the shift toward remote consultations, which, while beneficial in enhancing accessibility and data management, introduced challenges , such as the potential for misdiagnosis due to inadequate training or technical issues, as highlighted by Abdulla et al. (2024). Furthermore, the application of machine learning algorithms requires transparency in decision-making processes to foster trust among patients who may be apprehensive about algorithm-driven care. An interdisciplinary approach that puts significant emphasis on moral consideration in the use of these technologies is required to optimize patient gain and mitigate undesired effects, aligning rheumatology progress with the codes of ethical healthcare practice, as reviewed in Hügle (2024) (Figure 8.15).

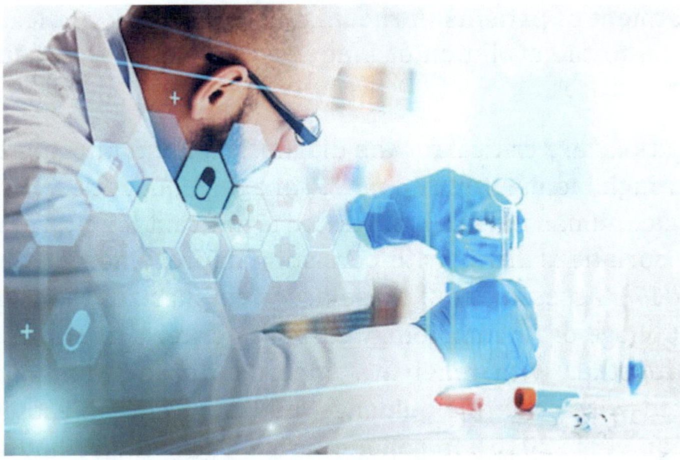

Figure 8.15. The advent of new technologies in rheumatology, specifically through machine learning and teleconsultation, inherently raises ethical concerns that must be carefully navigated.

Source: https://images.forbesindia.com/blog/wp-content/uploads/2022/07/Why-technological-advancement-is-the-key-to-unlocking-a-robust-healthcare-system-in-India.jpg?im=Resize,width=500,aspect=fit,type=normal.

Test Your Knowledge

1. How is next-generation sequencing utilized to identify genetic predispositions in rheumatology?
2. What are the advantages of automated immunofluorescence for ANA screening?

Summary

These laboratory investigation advances in rheumatology not only enhance our understanding of disease mechanisms but also provide avenues for improved patient management strategies. Development of a multicenter registry and biobank for juvenile idiopathic inflammatory myopathies is a vivid exemplification of the critical significance of collaborative research within this field that facilitates evidence-based treatment protocols where previously there existed a significant lack of data (Bohan et al., 2011). Besides, the biochemical research of serum concentration of uric acid in systemic sclerosis patients consolidates the intricate interaction between inflammation, endothelial function, and disease severity, and offers possible biomarkers for clinical assessment (Amoroso et al., 2016). Such findings reinforce the need to establish connections between clinical practice and laboratory research, as the present studies offer useful information with the ability to revolutionize the treatment of patients in rheumatology. Last but not least, constant investment in research will be critical to the evolution of innovative approaches to addressing the challenges presented by rheumatic diseases.

Laboratory investigations are critical for the diagnosis and monitoring of numerous rheumatic diseases, particularly through biomarkers and newer imaging modalities. For instance, clinical trials comparing drugs like secukinumab have demonstrated significant long-term efficacy and tolerability in patients with active psoriatic arthritis with persisting improvement in clinical responses at 104 weeks (Delicha et al., 2017). Assessment of these drugs emphasizes the use of multiple endpoints , such as the American College of Rheumatology response criteria, that provide a robust reflection of patients' responses together with relief in symptoms. In addition, support funding by drug companies, albeit granted with scientific guidance, questions the objectivity of results and their meaning to practice (Dean et al., 2016). In general terms, such studies not only enhance treatment protocols but also attach greater emphasis to the necessity of continuous monitoring in therapeutic efficiency in rheumatology.

KEY TERMS FROM THIS CHAPTER

- Juvenile idiopathic inflammatory myopathies
- Urinary peptidomic biomarkers
- Erythrocyte sedimentation rate (ESR)
- Red cells
- Platelets
- Hemoglobin
- Joint fluid examination
- Sarcoidosis
- Elevated serum ferritin
- Management
- Laboratory research
- C-reactive protein (CRP)
- White cells
- Anemia
- Serum levels
- Ultrasonography
- Macrophage activation syndrome (MAS)
- Hypoalbuminemia

Critical Thinking Questions

1. **What is the most specific antibody for the diagnosis of systemic lupus erythematosus (SLE)?**
   a. Anti-Ro (SSA)
   b. Antinuclear antibody (ANA)
   c. Anti-dsDNA
   d. Rheumatoid factor (RF)
2. **A positive anti-CCP (cyclic citrullinated peptide) test is most suggestive of which rheumatic disease?**
   a. Systemic lupus erythematosus
   b. Rheumatoid arthritis
   c. Sjögren's syndrome
   d. Polymyositis
3. **Which of the following tests is most commonly used as a screening test for autoimmune connective tissue diseases?**
   a. Anti-Smith antibody
   b. ANA (antinuclear antibody)
   c. C-reactive protein (CRP)
   d. Serum uric acid
4. **Which acute-phase protein is generally elevated during active inflammation and mirrored in rheumatologic disease?**
   a. Hemoglobin
   b. C-reactive protein (CRP)
   c. Creatine kinase
   d. Glucose
5. **The dry-eyed, dry-mouthed patient with a positive anti-Ro/SSA is most likely to have:**
   a. Rheumatoid arthritis
   b. SLE
   c. Sjögren's syndrome
   d. Gout

Short Answer Questions

1. What are the most common serologic tests used in autoimmune rheumatic diseases?
2. What is the method for testing for the antinuclear antibody (ANA) and what does a positive test mean?
3. How should a weakly positive result from an ANA be interpreted in an asymptomatic patient?
4. What are the advantages of employing ELISA over older methods of autoantibody detection?
5. What are the limitations of a positive ANA test as a diagnostic tool in autoimmune diseases?
6. Why might seronegative results present in obviously symptomatic autoimmune patients?

Answers to Critical Thinking Questions

1. (c); 2. (b); 3. (b); 4. (b); 5. (c)

References

1. Puzanov, I., Diab, A., Abdallah, K., Bingham, C. O., 3rd, Brogdon, C., Dadu, R., Hamad, L., Kim, S., Lacouture, M. E., LeBoeuf, N. R., Lenihan, D., Onofrei, C., Shannon, V., Sharma, R., Silk, A. W., Skondra, D., Suarez-Almazor, M. E., Wang, Y., Wiley, K., Kaufman, H. L., ... Society for Immunotherapy of Cancer Toxicity Management Working Group (2017). Managing toxicities associated with immune checkpoint inhibitors: consensus recommendations from the Society for Immunotherapy of Cancer (SITC) Toxicity Management Working Group. *Journal for immunotherapy of cancer*, *5*(1), 95. https://doi.org/10.1186/s40425-017-0300-z(accessed on 17th June 2025).
2. Abdulla, F. M., Alawar, D. T., Alfehaidi, A. S., Alrashid, S., et al. (2024). An outline on the global insights of implementation and challenges in primary healthcare telemedicine. https://core.ac.uk/download/603896239.pdf (accessed on 17th June 2025).
3. Sarzi-Puttini, P., Giorgi, V., Atzeni, F., Gorla, R., Kosek, E., Choy, E. H., Bazzichi, L., Häuser, W., Ablin, J. N., Aloush, V., Buskila, D., Amital, H., Da Silva, J. A. P., Perrot, S., Morlion, B., Polati, E., Schweiger, V., Coaccioli, S., Varrassi, G., Di Franco, M., ... Batticciotto, A. (2021). Diagnostic and therapeutic care pathway for fibromyalgia. *Clinical and experimental rheumatology*, *39 Suppl 130*(3), 120–127. https://doi.org/10.55563/clinexprheumatol/zcp5hz(accessed on 17th June 2025).
4. Abramov, Y., Almeida, F. G., Berghmans, B., Bo, K., et al. (2016). An International Urogynecological Association (IUGA)/International Continence Society (ICS) joint report on the terminology for the conservative and nonpharmacological management of female pelvic floor dysfunction. https://core.ac.uk/download/293861075.pdf (accessed on 17th June 2025).
5. Abril, A., Bachta, A., Balint, P., Barraclough, D., et al. (2017). 2015 recommendations for the management of polymyalgia rheumatica: A European League Against Rheumatism/American College of Rheumatology collaborative initiative. https://core.ac.uk/download/95616356.pdf (accessed on 17th June 2025).
6. Ahluwalia, V., Aydin, S. Z., Barber, C. E. H., Barnabe, C., et al. (2022). Best practices for virtual care: A consensus statement from the Canadian Rheumatology Association. https://core.ac.uk/download/534387636.pdf (accessed on 17th June 2025).
7. Aji, N., Alshareefy, Y., et al. (2024). Advancements and progress in juvenile idiopathic arthritis: A review of pathophysiology and treatment. https://core.ac.uk/download/603360608.pdf (accessed on 17th June 2025).
8. Alarcón, G. S., Barton, J. L., Caro, B., Chatham, W., et al. (2019). Individualized decision aid for diverse women with lupus nephritis (IDEA-WON): A randomized controlled trial. https://core.ac.uk/download/323072808.pdf (accessed on 17th June 2025).
9. Alavi, A. (2022). Novel MRI techniques in the diagnosis of musculoskeletal infection in children. https://core.ac.uk/download/590558522.pdf (accessed on 17th June 2025).
10. Aletaha, D., Bijlsma, J. W. J., Bombardier, C., Bykerk, V., et al. (2010). Multinational evidence-based recommendations on how to investigate and follow-up undifferentiated peripheral inflammatory arthritis: Integrating systematic literature research and expert opinion of a broad international panel of rheumatologists in the 3E Initiative. https://core.ac.uk/download/pdf/8499431.pdf (accessed on 17th June 2025).

11. Al-Maghlouth, I., Ali, H. H., Alibaz-Oner, F., Asfina, K. N., Balistreri, A., Bartoloni, E., Bindoli, S., et al. (2023). Clinical and laboratory features associated with macrophage activation syndrome in Still's disease: Data from the international AIDA Network Still's Disease Registry. https://core.ac.uk/download/593048300.pdf (accessed on 17th June 2025).

12. Al-Obaidi, M., Brogan, P. A., Dolezalova, P., Eleftheriou, D., et al. (2015). Takayasu arteritis in childhood: Retrospective experience from a tertiary referral center in the United Kingdom. https://core.ac.uk/download/29415232.pdf (accessed on 17th June 2025).

13. Amoroso, A., Barbano, B., Barilaro, G., Cianci, R., et al. (2016). Serum uric acid as a marker of microvascular damage in systemic sclerosis patients. https://core.ac.uk/download/74319192.pdf (accessed on 17th June 2025).

14. Ansari, A., Chang, C., Gershwin, M. E., Ortiz, B. L., et al. (2016). The Zika outbreak of the 21st century. https://core.ac.uk/download/323068480.pdf (accessed on 17th June 2025).

15. Araujo-Pradere, E., Bilitza, D., Dandenault, P. B., Hernández Pajares, M., et al. (2019). Critical issues in ionospheric data quality and implications for scientific studies. https://core.ac.uk/download/286456048.pdf (accessed on 17th June 2025).

16. Armstrong, R., Hall, W., Maier, P., Ng, M., et al. (2005). JointZone: Users' view of an adaptive online learning resource for rheumatology. *(No DOI or full link provided to verify publication details.)*

17. Baraliakos, X., Betteridge, N., Braun, J., Burgos-Vargas, R., et al. (2013). Treating spondylarthritis, including ankylosing spondylitis and psoriatic arthritis, to target: Recommendations of an international task force. https://core.ac.uk/download/55764870.pdf (accessed on 17th June 2025).

18. Barchetta, I., Cavallo, M. G., Ceccarelli, F., Di Franco, M., et al. (2015). Hypovitaminosis D in recent onset rheumatoid arthritis is predictive of reduced response to treatment and increased disease activity: A 12-month follow-up study. https://core.ac.uk/download/54518317.pdf (accessed on 17th June 2025).

19. Basu, N., Goni, M., Murray, A. D., Waiter, G., et al. (2018). Neural indicators of fatigue in chronic diseases: A systematic review of MRI studies. https://core.ac.uk/download/159067075.pdf (accessed on 17th June 2025).

20. Benavent, D., & Sequí Sabater, J. M. (2025). Artificial intelligence in rheumatology research: What is it good for? https://core.ac.uk/download/643237088.pdf (accessed on 17th June 2025).

21. Berardicurti, O., Carubbi, F., Ciccia, F., Cipriani, P., et al. (2017). Prevalence of type 2 diabetes and impaired fasting glucose in patients affected by rheumatoid arthritis. https://core.ac.uk/download/127501932.pdf (accessed on 17th June 2025).

22. Bichile, L., Chopra, A., Handa, R., Narsimulu, G., et al. (2011). A randomized controlled exploratory evaluation of standardized Ayurvedic formulations in symptomatic osteoarthritis knees: A Government of India NMITLI Project. https://core.ac.uk/download/pdf/8470002.pdf (accessed on 17th June 2025).

23. Bohan, B., Brown, G., Chinoy, H., Christen-Zaech, S., Pilkington, C. A., et al. (2011). A national registry for juvenile dermatomyositis and other pediatric idiopathic inflammatory myopathies: 10 years' experience; the Juvenile Dermatomyositis National (UK and Ireland) Cohort

Biomarker Study and Repository for Idiopathic Inflammatory Myopathies. https://core.ac.uk/download/10413.pdf (accessed on 17th June 2025).

24. Both, T., van Daele, P. L. A., Dalm, V. A. S. H., Hagen, M., et al. (2017). Reviewing primary Sjögren's syndrome: Beyond the dryness–From pathophysiology to diagnosis and treatment. https://core.ac.uk/download/154414050.pdf (accessed on 17th June 2025).
25. Brogan, P., Burns, J. C., Cornish, J., Diwakar, V., et al. (2020). Lifetime cardiovascular management of patients with previous Kawasaki disease. https://core.ac.uk/download/323066717.pdf (accessed on 17th June 2025).
26. Buchbinder, R., Calderone, A., Celermajer, D., Chin, J., et al. (2016). Multicenter randomized placebo-controlled trial of oral anticoagulation with apixaban in systemic sclerosis-related pulmonary arterial hypertension: The SPHInX study protocol. https://core.ac.uk/download/83638220.pdf (accessed on 17th June 2025).
27. Burke, S., Dahlke, C., Hagler, H., Herb, J., et al. (2009). Ontology-based knowledge representation of experiment metadata in biological data mining. https://core.ac.uk/download/131216239.pdf (accessed on 17th June 2025).
28. Cargnelutti, E., & Di Genaro, M. S. (2013). Reactive arthritis: From clinical features to pathogenesis. https://core.ac.uk/download/52480361.pdf (accessed on 17th June 2025).
29. Carnevale, A., Casoni, G. L., Cavagna, L., Furini, F., et al. (2019). The role of the multidisciplinary evaluation of interstitial lung diseases: Systematic literature review of the current evidence and future perspectives. https://core.ac.uk/download/275692836.pdf (accessed on 17th June 2025).
30. Conaghan, P. G., Gottlieb, A. B., Kavanaugh, A., Kirkham, B., et al. (2015). Secukinumab, a human anti-interleukin-17A monoclonal antibody, in patients with psoriatic arthritis (FUTURE 2): A randomized, double-blind, placebo-controlled, phase 3 trial. https://core.ac.uk/download/42365516.pdf (accessed on 17th June 2025).
31. Corato, A., Doganci, A., Knueppel, A., Kojima, A., Mqadmi, A., Saxena, A., Zanella, A., et al. (2016). Characterization of the immunophenotype of dogs with primary immune-mediated hemolytic anemia. https://core.ac.uk/download/76980975.pdf (accessed on 17th June 2025).
32. De Souza, L. H., Frank, A. O., & Frank, C. A. (2004). Neck pain and disability: A cross-sectional survey of the demographic and clinical characteristics of neck pain seen in a rheumatology clinic. https://core.ac.uk/download/333427.pdf (accessed on 17th June 2025).
33. Dean, L. E., Gibson, J., Hunter, J., Jones, G. T., et al. (2016). Scotland Registry for Ankylosing Spondylitis (SIRAS)–Protocol. https://core.ac.uk/download/42130456.pdf (accessed on 17th June 2025).
34. Delicha, E. M., Gottlieb, A. B., Kajekar, R., Kirkham, B., et al. (2017). Secukinumab sustains improvement in signs and symptoms of psoriatic arthritis: 2-year results from the phase 3 FUTURE 2 study. https://core.ac.uk/download/111557556.pdf (accessed on 17th June 2025).
35. Diaconu, C. C., Hainarosie, R., Iancu, M. A., Iftimie, M., et al. (2018). The importance of early arthritis in patients with rheumatoid arthritis. https://core.ac.uk/download/216809651.pdf (accessed on 17th June 2025).
36. Dolan, A. L., Loeys, B. L., Munns, C., Sillence, D., Rikken-Bultman, D. G., et al. (2009). The differential diagnosis of children with joint hypermobility: A review of the literature. https://

core.ac.uk/download/pdf/8249814.pdf (accessed on 17th June 2025).

37. Eid, D. A., Hussien, S. A., Kamal, M. M., Sayed, A., et al. (2012). Evaluation of microalbuminuria in patients with systemic sclerosis as an indicator of early renal damage and increased morbidity. https://core.ac.uk/download/pdf/82519997.pdf (accessed on 17th June 2025).

38. Eutsler, E., Ferguson, C., Kitcharoensakkul, M., Orandi, A., et al. (2016). Sarcoidosis presenting as granulomatous myositis in a 16-year-old adolescent. https://core.ac.uk/download/80495063.pdf (accessed on 17th June 2025).

39. Fahmy, N., Mohamed, S., Mohamed, S., Morshedy, S., et al. (2019). Effect of self-care guideline on quality of life among pregnant women with systemic lupus erythematosus. https://core.ac.uk/download/524771838.pdf (accessed on 17th June 2025).

40. Filippou, G., Lombardi, G., Maroni, P., Niessink, R., et al. (2024). Calcium pyrophosphate crystal formation and deposition: Where do we stand and what does the future hold? https://core.ac.uk/download/636759731.pdf (accessed on 17th June 2025).

41. Gompels, L. (2010). *In vivo* fluorescence imaging of E-selectin: Quantitative detection of endothelial activation in arthritis. https://core.ac.uk/download/1589084.pdf (accessed on 17th June 2025).

42. Hall, A. J., Mamas, M. A., Myint, P. K., Smith, S. C., et al. (2015). Association between osteoarthritis and cardiovascular disease: Systematic review and meta-analysis. https://core.ac.uk/download/41991643.pdf (accessed on 17th June 2025).

43. Hammoda, G. E., Korah, T. E., Mousa, W., Soliman, A., et al. (2014). Significance of serum levels of angiopoietin-2 and its relationship to Doppler ultrasonographic findings in rheumatoid arthritis patients. https://core.ac.uk/download/pdf/82564415.pdf (accessed on 17th June 2025).

44. Hansell, A., Tate, A. R., Nicholson, A., Lovis, C., Edwards, C. J., et al. (2013). Optimizing use of electronic health records to describe the presentation of rheumatoid arthritis in primary care: A strategy for developing code lists. https://core.ac.uk/download/9837008.pdf (accessed on 17th June 2025).

45. Hopkins, M., Leydersdorff, L., Rafols, I., Rotolo, D., et al. (2014). Scientometric mapping as a strategic intelligence tool for the governance of emerging technologies. https://core.ac.uk/download/30608389.pdf (accessed on 17th June 2025).

46. Hügle, T. (2024). Advancing rheumatology care through machine learning. https://core.ac.uk/download/611826872.pdf (accessed on 17th June 2025).

47. Lewandowski, L. B., Scott, C., & Spittal, G. W. (2016). A clinical update on pediatric lupus. https://core.ac.uk/download/478308768.pdf (accessed on 17th June 2025).

48. Makda, M. A. (2013). The prevalence of anti-C1q antibodies in Black South Africans with systemic lupus erythematosus and their clinical significance. https://core.ac.uk/download/39671407.pdf (accessed on 17th June 2025).

49. Rasker, J. J., Seydel, E., Taal, E., Wiegman, O., et al. (1993). Health status, adherence with health recommendations, self-efficacy and social support in patients with rheumatoid arthritis. https://core.ac.uk/download/pdf/11456304.pdf (accessed on 17th June 2025).

50. Ravelli, A., Shahin, A. A., Fasth, A., Karmazyn, B., Bloom, B. J., Ansell, B. M., Job-Deslandre, C., et al. (2012). Ultrasonography and color Doppler in juvenile idiopathic arthritis: Diagnosis

and follow-up of ultrasound-guided steroid injection in the wrist region. A descriptive interventional study. https://core.ac.uk/download/pdf/8726668.pdf (accessed on 17th June 2025).

51. Smith, J. W. (2013). *Doctor of Philosophy* [Doctoral dissertation]. https://core.ac.uk/download/276264519.pdf (accessed on 17th June 2025).

52. Yu, C. Y., Spencer, C. H., Hauptmann, G., Atkinson, J. P., Lintner, K. E., Hebert, L. A., Yang, Y., et al. (2016). Early components of the complement classical activation pathway in human systemic autoimmune diseases. https://core.ac.uk/download/pdf/82878724.pdf (accessed on 17th June 2025).

IMAGING IN RHEUMATOLOGY

9

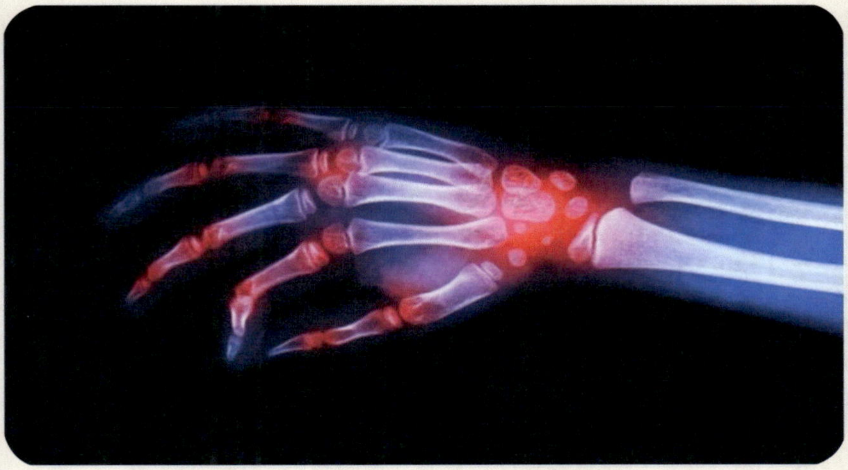

Introduction

There has been a long way to go for rheumatology with the application of various imaging technologies that enhance the diagnosis and management of autoimmune diseases. Imaging tools , such as ultrasound, magnetic resonance imaging (MRI), and nailfold videocapillaroscopy have transformed the ability to assess diseases like osteoarthritis and systemic sclerosis. Nailfold videocapillaroscopy, specifically, allows an individual to examine in precise detail microvascular alterations that can precede disease symptoms, thus making it a superior marker of systemic sclerosis development (Pizzorni et al., 2016). At the same time, a combination of ultrasound and MRI produces accurate cartilage thickness measurements, facilitating extensive treatment evaluations in osteoarthritis (Barbulescu et al., 2019). As these imaging modalities continue to evolve, they offer clinicians valuable information regarding disease activity and treatment response, pointing towards the integration of advanced imaging modalities into everyday rheumatological practice.

LEARNING OBJECTIVES

After studying this chapter, you will be able to:

1. Enumerate types of imaging modalities used in rheumatology;
2. Explain imaging techniques and applications;
3. Appreciate the interpretation of imaging reports;
4. Discuss the limitations and drawbacks of imaging in rheumatology.

9.1. Types of Imaging Modalities in Rheumatology

Learning Outcome

1. Understand X-ray imaging;
2. Highlight ultrasound imaging;
3. Define magnetic resonance imaging (MRI);
4. Understand computed tomography (CT);
5. Define positron emission tomography (PET);
6. Define dual-energy X-ray absorptiometry (DEXA);
7. Highlight scintigraphy;
8. Understand new emerging imaging modalities.

Imaging modalities in rheumatology have critical roles in diagnosing and monitoring autoimmune and inflammatory illnesses. They are traditional radiography, ultrasonography, magnetic resonance imaging (MRI), and computed tomography (CT). Each modality has its own strengths; e.g., radiography helps assess damage to joints but might be insensitive to early changes in soft tissues. In contrast, ultrasonography provides real-time imaging, and therefore, the assessment of synovitis and other soft tissue alterations becomes easier, particularly in children (Backhaus et al., 2016). MRI also has a superior ability to detect alterations in bone marrow and soft tissues and therefore, continues to be paramount in diagnosing diseases like rheumatoid arthritis. Specifically, the use of ultrasonography in gout demonstrated its ability to identify monosodium urate crystal deposits with precision, enhancing clinical management and disease monitoring (Finucci et al., 2015). Together, these imaging techniques have an essential role in an integral diagnosis of rheumatic disease and its progression.

9.1.1. X-ray Imaging

X-ray imaging is a basic tool in rheumatology practice, particularly in bone and joint disease assessment. This modality is of critical importance in the diagnosis of diseases , such as rheumatoid arthritis and osteoarthritis by providing clear images of bone structure and position. Using conventional X-ray techniques, medical staff can observe joint space alteration, erosions, and osteophyte development, all significant disease activity indices. Current advancements, such as the implementation of photon-counting detectors (PCDs), have otherwise enhanced the performance of X-ray imaging, offering enhanced spatial resolution and lower image noise. Such developments allow for more efficient visualization of mineralized tissue and enable physicians to identify crystal deposits, which are essential in accurately diagnosing gout and other crystal-associated arthropathies (Becce et al., 2024). With advances in rheumatology, X-ray imaging remains a cornerstone technique in the management and understanding of musculoskeletal disorders (Figure 9.1).

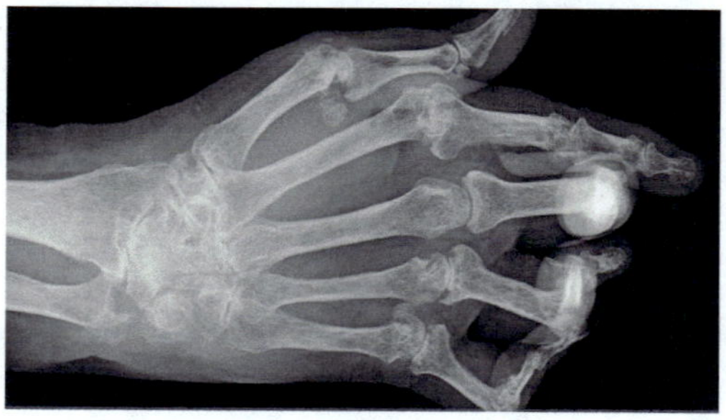

Figure 9.1. X-ray imaging plays a crucial role in the field of rheumatology, particularly for the assessment of bone and joint diseases.

Source: https://media.post.rvohealth.io/wp-content/uploads/sites/3/2024/10/slide1-rheumatoid-arthritis-radiology-X-ray-1296x728-1.jpg.

9.1.2. Ultrasound Imaging

Ultrasound imaging is increasingly a core tool in rheumatology, with numerous advantages to musculoskeletal and pulmonary disorder evaluation. Compared to traditional imaging modalities, ultrasound is non-invasive and free from ionizing radiation, making it particularly advantageous in patient populations that require to be reassessed on a repeated basis, such as those with Systemic Autoimmune Rheumatic Diseases (SARDs). In addition, its use is not only confined to joint assessment but also encompasses lung tests, where it has become more and more familiar to identify pulmonary complications of SARDs , such as interstitial lung disease and pleural lesions (Bruni et al., 2024). Notably, studies have established that ultrasound can indeed assess silent synovitis, allowing for better diagnostic effectiveness and enabling earlier interventions (Kisten et al., 2023). With this technology evolving further, its application in routine clinical practice has the potential to greatly advance disease surveillance, which in turn will lead to better patient outcomes in rheumatologic practice.

9.1.3. Magnetic Resonance Imaging (MRI)

In rheumatology, MRI has been an invaluable diagnostic tool, giving the clinician unique insight into joint pathology that may be lost with conventional imaging methods. With 90% sensitivity and 60% specificity reported, MRI is better at identifying early features of degenerative change and inflammation of conditions , such as rheumatoid arthritis (RA) (Buisman et al., 2016). With it, healthcare providers are able to visualize soft tissues and bone marrow edema, providing a clearer picture of disease activity and progression. Notably, MRI cost-effectiveness in inflammatory arthritis diagnosis has been highlighted in more recent studies, which state that MRI can be an effective add-on approach if used in conjunction with traditional diagnostic criteria, culminating in better patient outcomes (Buisman et al., 2016). Through ongoing efforts of rheumatologists to enhance diagnostic approaches, MRI as part of diagnostic algorithms is an essential advancement in that it places emphasis on its position as an essential agent in imaging for rheumatology (Figure 9.2).

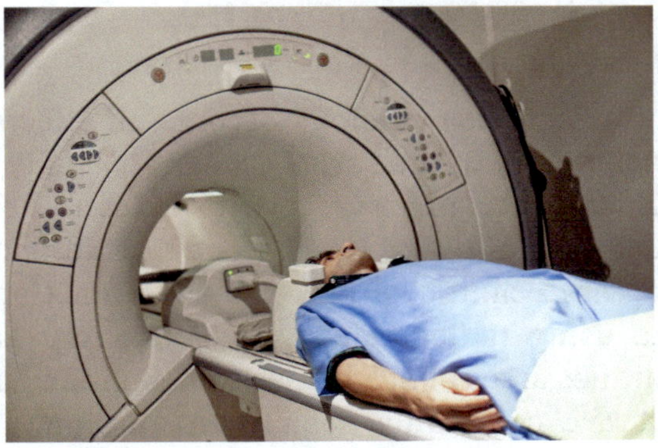

Figure 9.2. Magnetic resonance imaging (MRI).

Source: https://images.ctfassets.net/yixw23k2v6vo/spu_wysiwyg_fid43605_asset/c8d9dcfc3478e2919d84a5e463b8fcef/MRI_closed_machine-patient_scanner_bed_iStock-185097182.jpg.

9.1.4. Computed Tomography (CT)

CT has emerged as a core imaging modality in rheumatology, particularly in assessing conditions , such as idiopathic skeletal hyperostosis (DISH) and other spinal conditions. With the demonstration of high-resolution images of bone structures, CT enables clinicians to estimate vertebral bone mineral density (BMD) with precision, which is very important in diagnosing degenerative changes of conditions associated with rheumatological diseases. Studies have demonstrated that vertebral BMD alterations are significant predictors of disease severity, especially in DISH, where low BMD is the rule. In 59 Boxer dogs scanned by CT for vertebral BMD variation, results indicated a definite correlation between reduced BMD and DISH status, demonstrating the usefulness of CT in allowing for accurate determinations of spinal integrity (Decker et al., 2015; Maghraoui et al., 2015). Development and application of CT in clinical practice not only enhances diagnostic accuracy but also guides the therapeutic intervention, marking a significant advance in rheumatological imaging.

9.1.5. Positron Emission Tomography (PET)

PET has in rheumatology become an effective imaging tool, particularly through its ability to evaluate inflammatory activity in conditions affecting the joints. In contrast to traditional imaging techniques, PET provides functional data using radiolabeled glucose analogs and identifies areas of heightened metabolic activity that are commonly seen with autoimmune disorders.

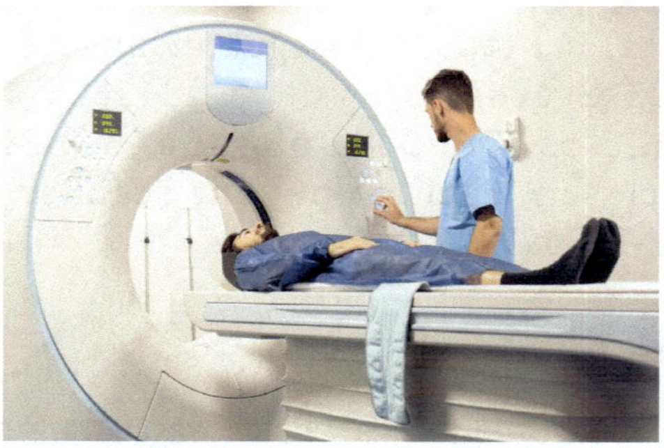

Figure 9.3. Positron Emission Tomography (PET) has emerged as a valuable imaging technique, particularly for its ability to evaluate inflammatory processes in joint diseases.

Source: https://img.lb.wbmdstatic.com/vim/live/webmd/consumer_assets/site_images/article_thumbnails/BigBead/pet-scan-positron-emission-tomography-bigbead/1800x1200-pet-scan-positron-emission-tomography-bigbead.jpg.

This unique ability allows for the detection of early inflammation, allowing for earlier interventions that enhance patient outcomes. The addition of PET to computed tomography (CT), thus creating PET/CT imaging, has also improved diagnostic capability and clinical decision support. Research underscores the value of this combined modality, which is described as being able to assess reactions to treatment and guide therapeutic choices in many types of rheumatic diseases and therefore represents an evolution from traditional paradigms of diagnosis to more interactive forms in the handling of these multisystem disorders (Al-Bulushi et al., 2013) (Figure 9.3).

9.1.6. Dual-Energy X-ray Absorptiometry (DEXA)

DEXA has been a key tool in the field of rheumatology, perhaps most prominently used to quantify BMD in patients with RA. DEXA is a noninvasive imaging tool that enables physicians to quantify changes in BMD over time, providing them with incredibly useful information regarding the skeletal health of those affected by inflammation. Evidence indicates significant loss of BMD among RA patients, as studies showed a precise drop in hand BMD compared to overall loss of BMD in the spine and hip after one year of antirheumatic treatment (Allaart et al., 2009). Moreover, the prevalence of rheumatoid cachexia, typically quantified in terms of DEXA scans, shows a high prevalence of low muscle mass among RA patients, emphasizing the broad-ranging contribution of this imaging modality to the comprehension of RA's multifaceted impacts (Espírito Santo et al., 2018). Thus, DEXA represents a key element in the strategic planning of rheumatic diseases, advancing patient care through evidence-based clinical decision-making.

9.1.7. Scintigraphy

In imaging methods, scintigraphy has been found to be helpful in quantification of inflammatory activity in rheumatology, particularly in diseases , such as RA. The technique is based on the use of radiotracers that bind themselves at sites of inflammation and thus enable quantitative assessments of disease activity, which can further assist the clinical evaluation of patients. Recent studies have found that scintigraphy, in conjunction with low-field magnetic resonance imaging (MRI), provides complementary information regarding joint pathology from increased visualization of synovial hypertrophy and other inflammatory changes (Palosaari, 2008). Of special interest is the high correlation between scintigraphy and MRI measurements to indicate its usefulness as an objective marker for monitoring inflammation and erosive damage longitudinally. Accordingly, scintigraphy constitutes part of maximizing treatment strategies in RA such that clinicians can identify patients who may require augmented treatment interventions depending on the intensity levels of their inflammatory activity (Backhaus et al., 2019) (Figure 9.4).

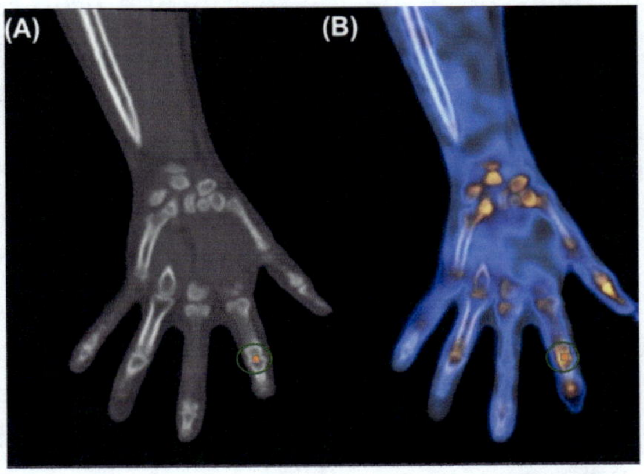

Figure 9.4. Scintigraphy has emerged as a valuable tool for assessing inflammatory activity in rheumatology, particularly in conditions , such as rheumatoid arthritis (RA).

Source: https://media.springernature.com/m685/springer-static/image/art%3A10.1038%2Fs41598-021-03874-9/MediaObjects/41598_2021_3874_Fig1_HTML.jpg.

9.1.8. Emerging Imaging Technologies

With the upcoming technology in rheumatology, novel imaging technologies play a key role in enhancing diagnostic accuracy and therapy protocols. Of these technologies, machine learning algorithms are notable for their capabilities in evaluating complex rheumatic diseases by analyzing different kinds of data, including imaging and laboratory results. For instance, convolutional neural networks (CNN) have proven useful in the identification and classification of lesions , such as erosions and sacroiliitis, which are priceless in disease prognosis and management (Hügle, 2024). Besides, the integration of artificial intelligence into imaging pipelines not only aids in the detection of pathological alterations but also determines clinical decisions, thereby achieving personalized patient care (Benavent et al., 2025). As such technologies develop, they constitute a revolutionary opportunity for the improvement of patient outcomes in rheumatology, highlighting a requirement for rigorous validation and ethical consideration in their application.

Test Your Knowledge

1. What is the role of ultrasound in musculoskeletal and rheumatologic examinations?
2. How does CT scanning assist in the diagnosis of rheumatic diseases?

9.2. Imaging Techniques and Their Applications

Learning Outcome

1. Know about imaging for joint examination;
2. Describe imaging for the evaluation of soft tissue;
3. Vigilance on imaging in the assessment of bones;
4. Imaging in inflammatory arthritis;
5. Imaging in osteoarthritis;
6. Imaging in systemic lupus erythematosus;
7. Imaging in scleroderma;
8. Imaging in gout;
9. Imaging in psoriatic arthritis.

Advances in imaging have injected a new level of sophistication into the field of rheumatology, offering subtle diagnostic and monitoring instruments for autoimmune disorders. Of these procedures, nailfold videocapillaroscopy is a valuable diagnostic tool for assessment of microvascular injury in conditions , such as systemic sclerosis (SSc). The procedure is non-invasive and allows physicians to observe peripheral capillary morphology, a necessity for classifying and scoring microangiopathy patterns that can be employed as novel markers of disease activity (Pizzorni et al., 2016). Furthermore, other imaging modalities, including laser Doppler and thermography, supplement the understanding of peripheral blood perfusion abnormalities prevalent in SSc. As the integration of imaging data into patient management becomes more sophisticated, the role of evidence-based medicine becomes elevated, and complete approaches to biomedical data integration are required (Anjum et al., 2007). Ultimately, these advances in imaging not only facilitate early diagnosis but also make personalized therapeutic interventions possible in rheumatology.

9.2.1. Imaging for Joint Evaluation

Within rheumatology, imaging technologies like musculoskeletal ultrasonography (US) and MRI have greatly altered joint condition assessment. Not only do these sophisticated methods allow for an assessment of cartilage thickness—a significant consideration in the case of osteoarthritis—relating to diseases, but they also report on changes in joint morphology over time.

For instance, a study documented that US precisely measured femoral hyaline cartilage thickness and demonstrated statistically significant differences pre- and post-treatment in patients on a specific therapeutic protocol, testifying to its value for tracking treatment (Barbulescu et al., 2019). Similarly, integrated imaging assessment in juvenile idiopathic arthritis has been important for the identification of disorders of the foot and ankle, while existing evidence remains sparse and often from small studies (Manca et al., 2009). Integration of multi-mode imaging techniques is thus central to enhancing diagnostic sensitivity as well as treatment efficacy in joint evaluation in rheumatology (Figure 9.5).

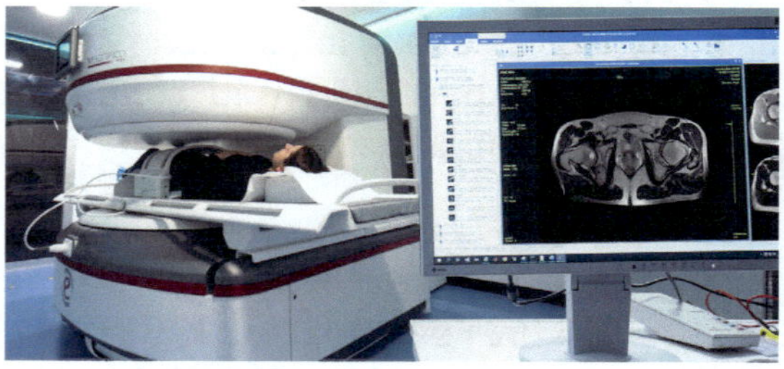

Figure 9.5. Imaging modalities , such as musculoskeletal ultrasonography (US) and magnetic resonance imaging (MRI) have revolutionized the evaluation of joint conditions.

Source: https://www2.esaote.com/fileadmin/GLOBAL/Magnetic_Resonance/Clinical_applications/Musculoskeletal_Imaging/esaote-hero-MSK.jpg.

9.2.2. Imaging for Soft Tissue Assessment

Successful soft tissue assessment is the cornerstone of diagnosis and management of a variety of inflammatory diseases in rheumatology. MRI in this regard is a valuable tool, particularly in the evaluation of psoriatic dactylitis, where MRI is able to show marked abnormalities in involved fingers. Evidence indicates that in such individuals, MRI reveals widespread soft-tissue edema and synovitis, which are suggestive of the extent of the inflammation not easily seen by clinical inspection alone (Chandramohan et al., 2008). Besides this, imaging techniques, including musculoskeletal ultrasound, are also proving to be important diagnostics for conditions like gout, characterized by precipitation of monosodium urate crystals. Imaging modalities enable early pathology detection and enhanced clinical monitoring, reinforcing their pivotal position in optimizing the outcome for patients in rheumatology (Finucci et al., 2015). Thus, imaging to assess soft tissues not only develops our understanding of musculoskeletal disease but also guides treatment.

9.2.3. Imaging for Bone Assessment

Bone assessment imaging plays a vital role in the early diagnosis and follow-up of rheumatology inflammatory diseases. Various imaging modalities, particularly MRI and US, provide useful information regarding bone and cartilage integrity. MRI is particularly beneficial in evaluating minor changes with conditions , such as psoriatic arthritis through imaging of synovitis and bone edema that might not be visible with clinical examination. For instance, research noted that MRI findings showed widespread abnormalities in dactylitic digits, significant in disease severity and treatment response (Chandramohan et al., 2008). Parallel to this, US has proven useful for cartilage thickness measurements, so the ability to monitor long-term disease change and therapy response has been significantly enhanced (Barbulescu et al., 2019). Both these imaging modalities not only facilitate precise bone health measurements but also guide therapy choices, which ultimately have a positive impact on patient outcomes in rheumatology (Figure 9.6).

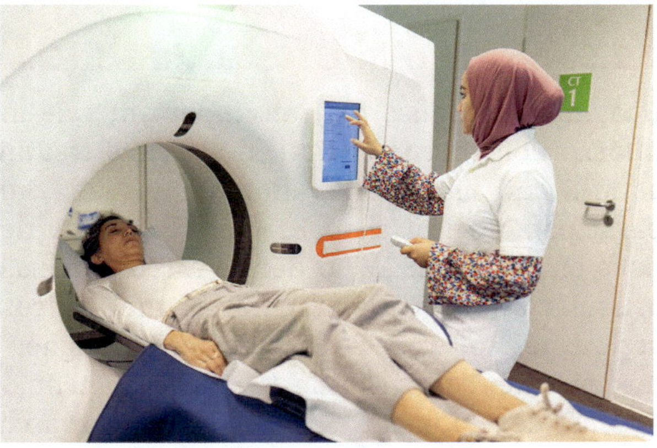

Figure 9.6. Imaging for bone assessment plays a crucial role in the early diagnosis and monitoring of inflammatory conditions in rheumatology.

Source: https://www.verywellhealth.com/thmb/W6TtRACS98Akd6IjkS7Iqp7iM3Y=/1500x0/filters:no_upscale():max_bytes(150000):strip_icc()/GettyImages-1440517462-6a2bc54d96aa47e98a9558ba9f8af5f7.jpg.

9.2.4. Imaging in Inflammatory Arthritis

The evolving image of imaging modality develops a central role in the diagnosis and management of inflammatory arthritis, providing clinicians improved tools to measure disease activity and joint health. Musculoskeletal ultrasound, in particular, has been found to be an effective modality for the identification of gout and calcium pyrophosphate crystal deposition disease (CPPD) abnormalities. For gout, ultrasound can identify monosodium urate crystals, thereby facilitating early interventions and improved patient outcomes (Finucci et al., 2015). In a similar vein, studies have established that ultrasound is more than 80% sensitive to detect CPPD crystals, replacing conventional radiographic methods (Chen et al., 2016). With further advancements in imaging technology, their utility in routine rheumatological practice will not only improve the accuracy of diagnosis but also allow patient-tailored treatment regimens, further establishing the importance of imaging in the entire ambit of rheumatology. By utilizing these instruments, healthcare providers can be in a position to deal with the complexities of treating inflammatory arthritis.

9.2.5. Imaging in Osteoarthritis (OA)

Imaging techniques play an important role in the earlier diagnosis and control of OA, providing information that is critical in effective treatment regimens. Higher-tech imaging methods , such as MRI and ultrasound, allow for visualization of the cartilaginous tissues and identification of early pathological changes that cannot be detected by ordinary radiography. The latest studies have employed LSCM to derive three-dimensional observations of wear particles generated from articular cartilage, demonstrating the intricate topography of surface texture with regard to the seriousness of wear conditions in OA (Aigner et al., 2012). This reveals the ability of quantitative measurement in defining the development of wear particle textures in comparison to disease process development. Besides, recent research emphasizes the necessity of relating these imaging advances to clinical samples to ensure an enhancement in diagnostic criteria and ultimately patient care in rheumatology (Adinolfi et al., 2016) (Figure 9.7).

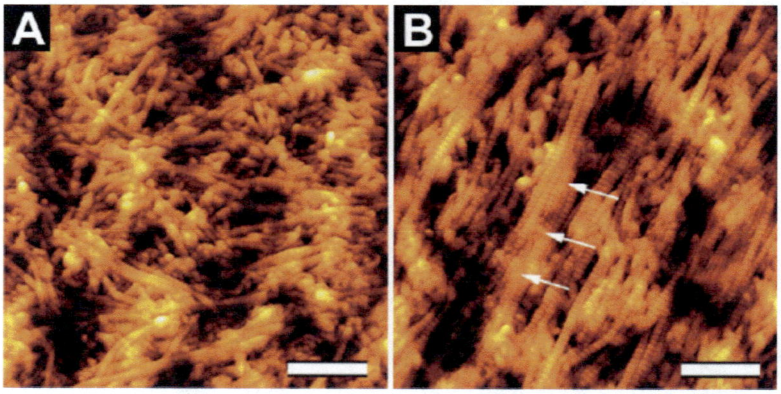

Figure 9.7. Laser scanning confocal microscopy (LSCM) to acquire three-dimensional images of wear particles generated from articular cartilage, revealing the intricate surface topography that correlates with the severity of wear conditions in OA.

Source: https://www.researchgate.net/publication/51030971/figure/fig1/AS:305960426983424@1449958058628/Surface-topography-of-normal-articular-cartilage-A-and-osteoarthritic-articular.png.

9.2.6. Imaging in Systemic Lupus Erythematosus (SLE)

Imaging in SLE has undergone a major transformation, particularly in assessing joint disease and erosive change. With the newer imaging technologies , such as US, the inherent prevalence of non-erosive arthritis in SLE has been highlighted, the requirement for biomarkers for the prediction of the onset of erosive disease. Surprisingly, the existence of anti-carbamylated protein antibodies (anti-CarP) has been found to be highly related to erosive damage and could potentially act as biomarkers for those at risk for more disabling joint manifestations (Alessandri et al., 2018). Apart from this, imaging techniques like perfusion brain single photon emission computed tomography (SPECT) have been encouraging not only in the diagnosis of SLE-related cerebral vasculitis but also in evaluating the therapeutic response, which allows clinicians to distinguish between responders and non-responders with high effectiveness (Maffione et al., 2015). These advancements underscore the very crucial aspect of overlapping between imaging and management planning in rheumatology.

9.2.7. Imaging in Scleroderma

In scleroderma, advanced imaging is pivotal in evaluating the multi-dimensional aspect of this complex autoimmune disease.

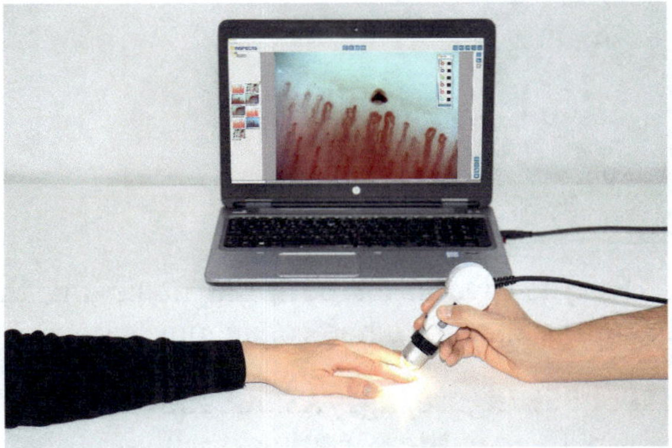

Figure 9.8. Nailfold videocapillaroscopy.

Source: https://www.inspect-is.com/wp-content/uploads/2022/06/video-Capillaroscopy.jpg.

Of greater significance, nailfold videocapillaroscopy is the best device to examine for microvascular abnormalities, which are essential to detect in diagnosing SSc since it defines capillary structure and detects patterns of microangiopathy that emerge years before other manifestations (Pizzorni et al., 2016). Additional echocardiographic advancements, such as three-dimensional echocardiography (3DE) and two-dimensional speckle tracking (2DSTE), provide valuable information on right ventricular (RV) function, particularly in patients without overt heart disease or pulmonary arterial hypertension (PAH) (Badano et al., 2015). Such imaging modalities not only improve diagnostic accuracy but also allow early intervention, hence improving patient outcomes in a disease process with gradual vascular compromise and pulmonary involvement. Thus, imaging remains a key feature in the total management of scleroderma (Figure 9.8).

9.2.8. Imaging in Gout

Imaging is a crucial agent in the diagnosis and management of gout, a prevalent inflammatory condition that includes monosodium urate crystal deposition in rheumatology. Musculoskeletal ultrasound has also been an extremely valuable modality, providing the ability to detect a variety of gout abnormalities that are frequently not diagnosed with standard imaging modalities. Being non-invasive, not only does it aid in the diagnosis of acute bouts, but it also makes it possible to maintain clinical monitoring during intercritical periods and in chronic tophaceous gout (Finucci et al., 2015). Additionally, although traditional crystal analysis and radiographic examination are still the reference standard for diagnosis, new technologies like dual-energy computed tomography (DECT) and sophisticated ultrasound techniques hold immense potential, providing improved sensitivity in detecting crystals and clearer resolution of joint pathology (Chen et al., 2016). Integration of these imaging modalities is therefore critical in improving diagnostic precision and management strategies in gout treatment.

9.2.9. Imaging in Psoriatic Arthritis

Imaging plays an important function in psoriatic arthritis (PsA) not merely in making a diagnosis but also in monitoring disease activity, especially considering the diseases heterogeneity. Radiographic techniques, particularly X-rays and MRI, enable clinicians to see joint erosions, enthesitis, and inflammation of the soft tissues characteristic of PsA. The identification of extra-articular manifestations , such as uveitis and inflammatory bowel disease (IBD), cannot be overestimated as they bear a direct influence on patient management strategies (Elewaut et al., 2009). Furthermore, changes in treatment objectives of PsA have led to proposed recommendations for remission or low disease activity, and therefore, regular follow-up assessment for disease determination and modulation of therapy strategies accordingly (Baraliakos et al., 2013). Thus, effective imaging modalities not only allow for early detection of skin and joint changes but are also integral to optimal patient management in the multidimensional approach to PsA (Figure 9.9).

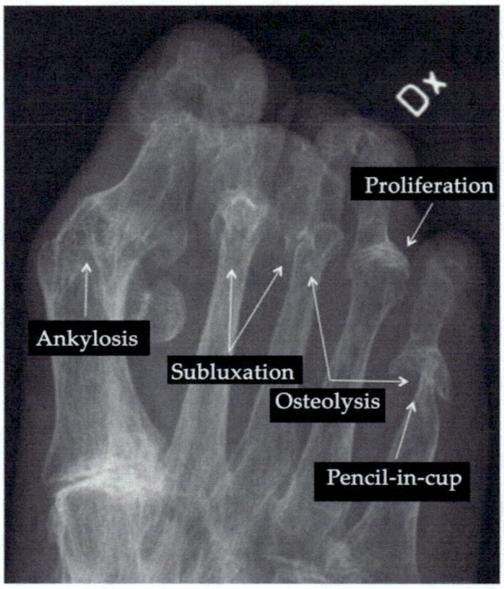

Figure 9.9. The role of imaging in psoriatic arthritis (PsA) is pivotal for both diagnosis and the monitoring of disease progression, especially considering the disease's heterogeneous nature.

Source: https://www.researchgate.net/publication/340960553/figure/fig1/AS:885153618472960@1588048476460/Radiography-of-a-66-year-old-female-patient-with-psoriatic-arthritis-mutilans-with-a.ppm.

Test Your Knowledge

1. What are common imaging findings in psoriatic arthritis?
2. How does ultrasound aid in the guidance of joint aspiration or injection in rheumatologic management?

9.3. Interpretation of Imaging Results

Learning Outcome

1. Understand imaging reports;
2. Discuss the role of radiologists in rheumatology;
3. Learn common imaging findings in rheumatologic diseases;
4. Differentiating between normal and abnormal findings;
5. Know limitations of imaging interpretation;
6. Explain the importance of clinical correlation;
7. Understand a multidisciplinary approach to imaging interpretation;
8. Discuss case studies in imaging interpretation;
9. Explain future directions in imaging interpretation.

Rheumatology imaging result interpretation is critical for diagnosis and follow-up of diseases , such as osteoarthritis and childhood arthritides. Advanced technologies like musculoskeletal US and MRI are highly informative about cartilage integrity and synovial inflammation. For instance, femoral hyaline cartilage thickness measurement by US has been found to have statistically significant results after treatment, thereby enhancing the measurement of treatment effectiveness (Barbulescu et al., 2019). Furthermore, the development of consensus-based standardized synovitis definitions guarantees consistent diagnosis of inflammatory conditions in children with proper therapeutic measures being implemented (Backhaus et al., 2016). These improvements highlight the team collaboration behind imaging interpretation, wherein radiologists, rheumatologists, and other clinicians collaborate to utilize imaging findings appropriately. Thus, the integration of new imaging modalities significantly improves the understanding and management of rheumatic diseases.

9.3.1. Understanding Imaging Reports

Imaging reports are extremely significant reports that are utilized to translate sophisticated diagnostic information into practical information, particularly in the specialty of rheumatology. They are not technical reports; they provide a comprehensive summary of findings with a potential to have a significant impact on patient management and therapeutic plans. For instance, advanced imaging techniques like photoacoustic imaging can delineate bone surfaces and demarcate the joint space, which are especially important for assessing rheumatoid arthritis disease progression and targeting inflammatory activities in the synovial membrane (Biswas et al., 2015). In addition, insight into the limitations of imaging, such as the low yield of gastrointestinal cancer in dermatomyositis patients revealed with endoscopic examinations, underscores the importance of clinical correlation and judicious interpretation of imaging reports (Gross et al., 2017). Thus, a high level of understanding of imaging reports enhances the clinician's role to synthesize imaging results with clinical data, leading to improved patient outcomes in rheumatology (Figure 9.10).

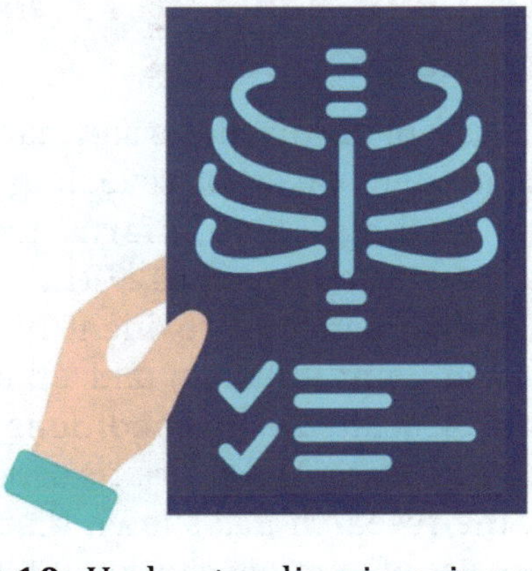

Figure 9.10. Understanding imaging reports.

Source: https://www.tranow.com/wp-content/uploads/2024/04/Imaging-Results-Clipart-820x460.jpg.

9.3.2. Role of Radiologists in Rheumatology

The role of the rheumatologist radiologist has significantly changed, especially with the advent of improved imaging technology that refines the diagnostic process. Not only do radiologists interpret imaging modalities like MRI and ultrasound, but they also interact intimately with the rheumatologist to customize individualized treatment plans for autoimmune and inflammatory conditions. For instance, radiologists in juvenile idiopathic arthritis (JIA) use sophisticated modalities , such as panoramic imaging (PAN) and cone beam computed tomography (CBCT) to assess temporomandibular joint (TMJ) involvement, which is of utmost significance for monitoring disease activity and optimizing interventions (Collin et al., 2023). Moreover, new technologies like artificial intelligence have the potential to improve diagnostic performance and reduce variability of readings, and hence patient outcomes (Beschi, 2023). Lastly, collaboration of radiologists with the rheumatology team will lead the way forward for enhancing patient care in a timely and accurate manner through imaging evaluations.

9.3.3. Common Imaging Findings in Rheumatologic Diseases

Imaging is part of the diagnosis and management of rheumatologic disease, revealing a range of classic findings that inform treatment. Required modalities , such as MRI and US, are part of routine imaging to identify synovial inflammation, joint effusion, and other classic alterations associated with conditions , such as rheumatoid arthritis and psoriatic arthritis. For instance, the research has shown that imaging characteristics of immune checkpoint inhibitor-induced arthritis are nearly identical to those of the usual arthropathies, such as widespread hand and wrist involvement in polymyalgia rheumatica-like presentations (Azuaga et al., 2022). The prevalence of osteoarthritis and other degenerative conditions also underscores the role of imaging in differentiating inflammatory and non-inflammatory joint diseases to the advantage of clinicians in administering specific treatments. Thus, it is crucial to identify these imaging findings to maximize the results of patients in rheumatology (Figure 9.11).

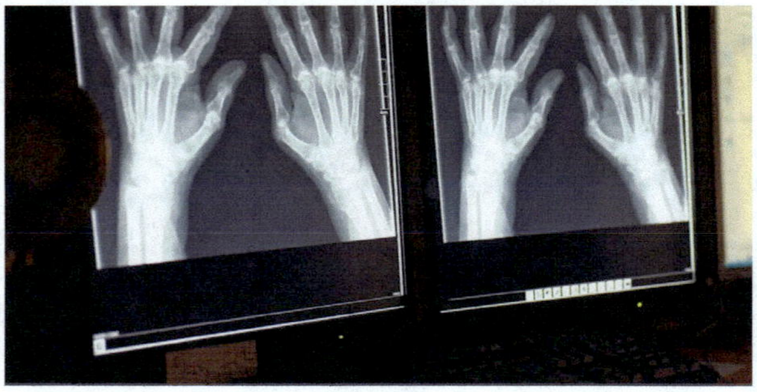

Figure 9.11. Imaging plays a crucial role in the diagnosis and management of rheumatologic diseases, revealing a range of common findings that inform treatment decisions.

Source: https://images.ctfassets.net/yixw23k2v6vo/4cjuQBoEgyxDcY1ejSfauN/f4970b5ac5677de04a2b0d195fcce29a/large-GettyImages-154947185-3000x2000.jpg?fm=webp&q=50&w=1200&h=600&fit=thumb.

9.3.4. Differentiating Between Normal and Abnormal Findings

It is crucial in imaging in rheumatology to distinguish normal from abnormal findings to make correct diagnoses and provide effective treatment. Rheumatological conditions typically present with insidious changes on imaging examinations that must be interpreted with care. For instance, autoimmune diseases of the major salivary glands, such as Sjögren's syndrome, have characteristic imaging findings that indicate pathological changes, namely inflammation and gland atrophy, which must be interpreted to avoid misdiagnosis (Vincentiis et al., 2017). Similarly, Charcot neuroarthropathy (CN) that complicates diabetes mellitus can manifest as an edematous foot on imaging, but the inflammatory context can be overlooked without a definable clinical template (Cachia et al., 2008). Rheumatologists thus must possess proficiency in deducing the association of clinical presentation and imaging findings, as the latter is critical in the early detection of conditions as well as improving patient outcomes with timely intervention.

9.3.5. Limitations of Imaging Interpretation

Imaging findings in rheumatology carry strong limitations to interpretation that can strongly influence diagnosis and treatment. For instance, standard imaging techniques cannot sensitively pick up on subtle muscle inflammation and fibrosis of myositis. While new modalities like T1 and T2 mapping in cardiovascular magnetic resonance provide increased sensitivity, their use in real-world clinical practice is currently hampered by the need for rigorous standardization and validation to be applied across broad populations of patients (Dancy, 2023).

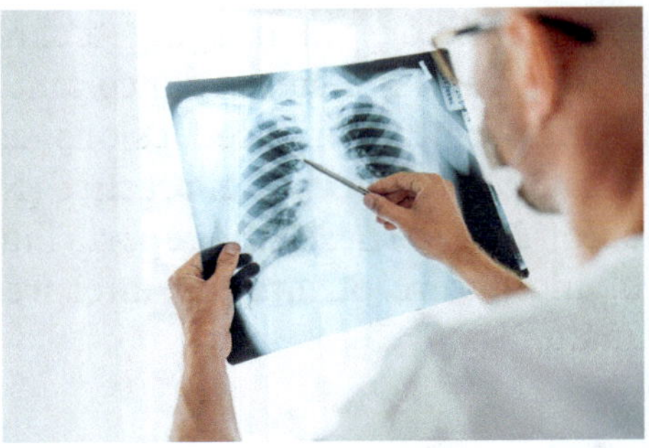

Figure 9.12. The interpretation of imaging results in rheumatology presents notable limitations that can significantly impact diagnosis and treatment outcomes.

Source: https://d2jx2rerrg6sh3.cloudfront.net/images/news/ImageForNews_777561_1713410847902402.jpg.

Further, heterogeneity in imaging protocols can produce differential results, and thus longitudinal data needed to document disease progression are more difficult to interpret (Bykov et al., 2017). These factors underscore the necessity of the introduction of a multidisciplinary solution that unites imaging findings with clinical evaluation and laboratory examinations. With continued development of the field, future research in the optimization of imaging modalities will be essential to overcome these limitations and enhance diagnostic quality in rheumatological management (Figure 9.12).

9.3.6. Importance of Clinical Correlation

In rheumatology, no aspect can be overemphasized more than the importance of clinical correlation in radiologic interpretation. The radiographic findings must be interpreted in the context of the overall clinical situation to enable correct diagnosis and proper management of the rheumatic condition. For instance, while imaging technologies , such as musculoskeletal ultrasound can reveal basic pathologies associated with illnesses like gout, patient history and clinical presentation are required for clarification and validation of the same (Finucci et al., 2015). Besides, having a thorough knowledge of the patient's complete medical history enhances the integration of heterogeneous sources of data, something vital to evidence-based medicine (Anjum et al., 2007). This clinical data-imaging integration not only optimizes diagnostic accuracy but also allows for tailored treatment strategies, and thus the key role of clinical correlation in optimizing patient outcomes in rheumatology cannot be overstated.

9.3.7. Multidisciplinary Approach to Imaging Interpretation

Multidisciplinary interpretation of imaging in

rheumatology is significantly improved through a multidisciplinary approach, which facilitates collaboration among multiple healthcare providers, for example, rheumatologists, radiologists, and podiatrists.

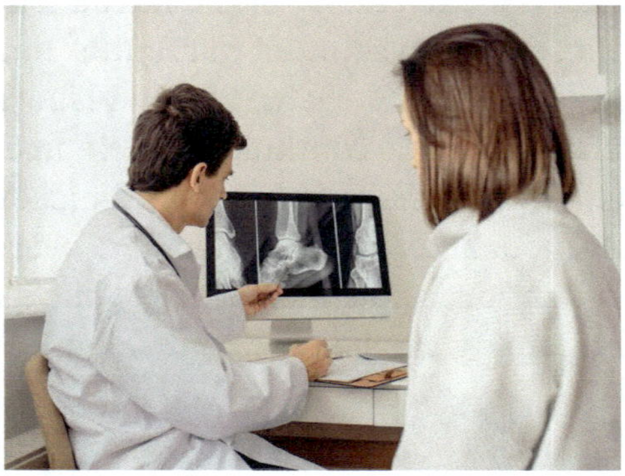

Figure 9.13. The interpretation of imaging in rheumatology benefits significantly from a multidisciplinary approach, which fosters collaboration among various healthcare professionals, including rheumatologists, radiologists, and podiatrists.

Source: https://www.inspirahealthnetwork.org/sites/default/files/styles/image_card_focal_point/public/2023-06/Orthopedic%20Surgeon%20Explaining%20X-Ray%20to%20Women.jpg?itok=xZ1rXWZQ.

This unifying model enhances diagnostic accuracy and treatment efficacy, as evidenced by studies chronicling the need for comprehensive assessments for conditions like juvenile idiopathic arthritis. A randomized controlled trial of integrated podiatric care for foot and ankle complaints in children with juvenile idiopathic arthritis demonstrates how multidisciplinary communication can be utilized to generate improved clinical outcomes; it highlights the need for coordinated care between specialties, both clinical evaluation and imaging modalities like ultrasonography (Manca et al., 2009). Furthermore, the use of musculoskeletal ultrasound within podiatry for diagnosis and therapy illustrates the expanding role of imaging in interdisciplinary settings and underscores the necessity for consistent training and competencies to enable effective communication and joint decision-making among specialists (Patience et al., 2018) (Figure 9.13).

9.3.8. Case Studies in Imaging Interpretation

Imaging has a significant role to play in the management and assessment of rheumatological diseases, and case studies are revealing regarding imaging modality interpretation. For instance, effectiveness of musculoskeletal US and MRI in quantifying cartilage thickness validates their applicability in monitoring and diagnosis of osteoarthritis. A study comparing a Symptomatic Slow Acting Drug for Osteoarthritis showed statistically significant increments in femoral hyaline cartilage thickness following treatment, which emphasizes the therapeutic potential of US as an important tool in monitoring disease progression and therapeutic evaluation (Barbulescu et al., 2019). Furthermore, application of cadaver models to assess US accuracy at identifying tendon injury pertinent to rheumatoid arthritis shows the advanced technology in imaging techniques. In this study, the high concordance among US findings and surgically induced lesions justified the application of US in clinical practice (Naredo & Iagnocco,, 2016). These case reports illustrate the evolving nature of imaging interpretation in rheumatology.

9.3.9. Future Directions in Imaging Interpretation

With the advancements in artificial intelligence (AI) and new imaging technologies, future imaging interpretation developments are poised to leverage these technologies. AI, particularly utilizing machine learning and deep learning algorithms, can potentially enhance diagnostic accuracy and efficiency of imaging interpretation to allow for more personalized treatment approaches to address individual patient needs (Asri et al., 2024). Moreover, novel modalities , such as muscle ultrasound (MUS) provide valuable information regarding muscle status in rheumatologic conditions. This imaging modality not just permits the detection of pathologies but also disease evolution follow-up, being sensitive, sometimes superior to plain MRI in certain contexts (van Alfen et al., 2024). The coming together of such novel approaches into everyday practice invites an advanced understanding of rheumatic disorders, promising a brighter future for imaging modalities and patient outcomes in rheumatology's tomorrow as well (Figure 9.14).

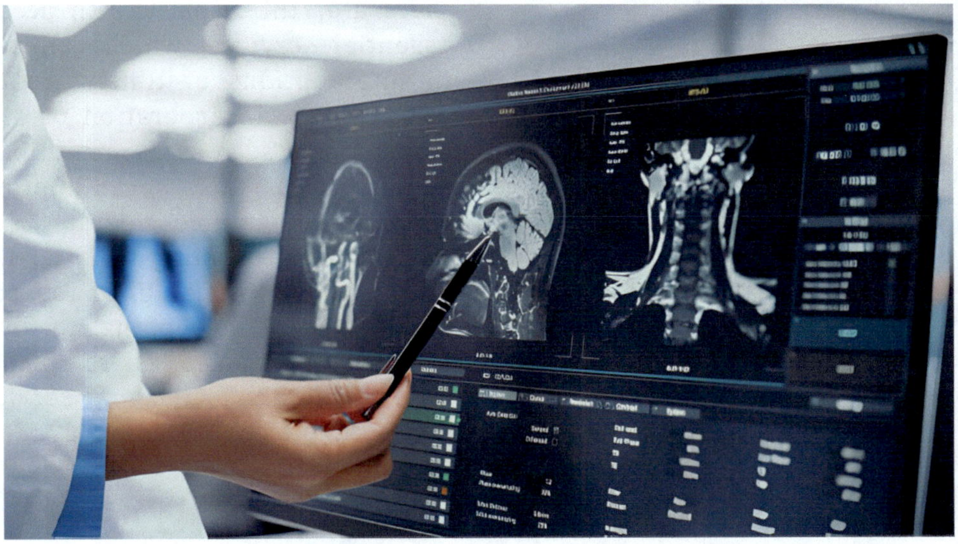

Figure 9.14. As the field of rheumatology evolves, the future directions in imaging interpretation are poised to leverage advancements in artificial intelligence (AI) and new imaging technologies.

Source: https://lakezurichopenmri.com/wp-content/uploads/2024/06/MRI-and-Artificial-Intelligence-The-Future-of-Diagnostics.jpg.

Test Your Knowledge

1. How is bone marrow edema on MRI interpreted in early inflammatory arthritis?
2. What are the characteristics that indicate active inflammation versus chronic damage on musculoskeletal ultrasound?

9.4. Challenges and Limitations of Imaging in Rheumatology

Learning Outcome

1. Discuss availability of imaging services;
2. Know cost factors of advanced imaging;
3. Focus on concerns of radiation exposure;
4. Discuss heterogeneity of imaging techniques;
5. Know the heterogeneity of interpretation by practitioners;
6. Identify patient-related factors that affect imaging quality;
7. Define limitations of the detection of early disease;
8. Discuss ethical issues in imaging;
9. Understand the future challenges of imaging technology.

Imaging techniques are extremely crucial in the diagnosis and treatment of rheumatologic disorders, but are plagued by deficiencies and challenges. A major concern is the variability in the diagnostic validity of different imaging modalities and sites of application. For instance, research indicates that while aggregating clinical data can enhance the validity of diagnoses , such as RA, the validity of an isolated RA diagnosis is merely moderate, particularly for seronegative diagnoses (Paltta, 2024). Also, polymyalgia rheumatica (PMR) misdiagnosis rates indicate the limitations of imaging in distinguishing between related inflammatory and non-inflammatory conditions, which could lead to mismanagement (Paltta, 2024). Moreover, the evolving immunotherapy profile, which is associated with unique immune-related adverse events, complicates imaging results and mandates a harmonized management strategy, thereby highlighting the necessity of multidisciplinary care.

9.4.1. Accessibility of Imaging Services

Availability of imaging services is critical to effective diagnosis and management of rheumatology, particularly in consideration of the autoimmune diseases. Despite the advancements achieved in imaging technologies, there are still disparities in accessing these essential services, which can cause delays in interventions of timely treatments. For example, the incorporation of digital health technologies, such as telehealth platforms and AI-imaging diagnostics, can improve access to sophisticated care considerably, especially for those patients coming from far-flung places. Through the provision of remote consultations and screenings, teleophthalmology is a model that may be transferred to rheumatology to improve access to imaging services through new technologies (Pfranjpe, 2023).

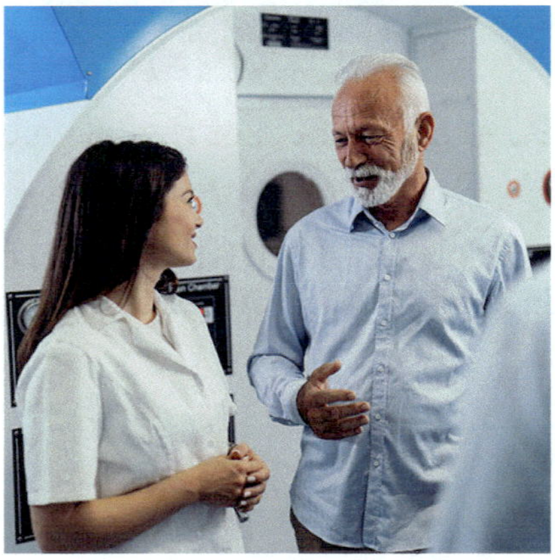

Figure 9.15. The accessibility of imaging services is critical for effective diagnosis and management in rheumatology, particularly given the complexity of autoimmune disorders.

Source: https://pure-medical.co.uk/wp-content/uploads/2021/09/Pure-Medical-Group-Hyper-Baric-Oxygen-Therapy-HBOT-2-Mobile.jpg.

Furthermore, examining the impact of health technology assessments (HTA) can provide an insight into how research funding contributes to improved access to healthcare and policy (Ligtvoet et al., 2008). Finally, equal access to imaging procedures is fundamental to enhancing the quality of care in rheumatology (Figure 9.15).

9.4.2. Cost Implications of Advanced Imaging

The integration of advanced imaging techniques in rheumatology, particularly in the diagnosis and treatment of osteoarthritis diseases, has significant cost implications that must be closely evaluated. While newer modalities , such as polarized-light methods, second-harmonic generation microscopy, and polarization-sensitive optical coherence tomography, hold the potential to enhance the effectiveness of treatment by enabling more precise measurements of articular cartilage, they also bear significant financial costs in the form of equipment and training (Matcher, 2009). These costs, in addition to maintenance requirements and even insurance coverage, can become a strain on the healthcare budget. Secondly, the additional cost burden could potentially fuel disparities in access to these technologies, particularly in the developing world. Hence, while clinical benefits stand unchallenged with advanced imaging, their cost-effectiveness must be scrutinized critically in the broader context of health resource planning and allocation for rheumatologic care.

9.4.3. Radiation Exposure Concerns

In rheumatology, imaging techniques have been used more extensively, with the application of high-resolution computed tomography (HRCT) in the diagnosis of diseases like systemic sclerosis-associated interstitial lung disease. Though HRCT is valuable in early diagnosis as well as follow-up, concerns regarding radiation exposure cannot be overlooked. The inherent risk of cumulative imaging should lead to serious consideration about how the advantages of diagnosis are balanced against potential harm. Experts recommend that while HRCT should be performed on initial diagnosis, its rate should be based on the patient risk profile and ideally limit repeats to biennial or yearly unless the clinical symptoms break. In recent years, improved low-radiation techniques and other technologies like lung ultrasound have emerged, potentially reducing exposure with the diagnostic efficacy maintained (Brown et al., 2022). Additionally, greater vigilance for imaging-related harm is needed, especially with lifelong implications in diseases like Kawasaki disease, where coronary complications require ongoing monitoring (Brogan et al., 2020) (Figure 9.16).

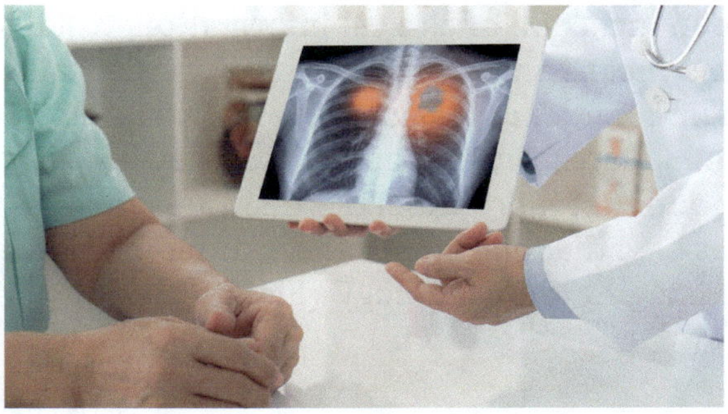

Figure 9.16. In the realm of rheumatology, the use of imaging techniques has escalated, particularly with high-resolution computed tomography (HRCT) for diagnosing conditions like systemic sclerosis-associated interstitial lung disease.

Source: https://lignosus.com/wp-content/uploads/2025/03/Untitled-design-4.png.

9.4.4. Variability in Imaging Techniques

The modality heterogeneity is significant in the constitution of the science of rheumatology, with each modality yielding complementary information about the multifactorial nature of various diseases. For instance, technological advancement in functional and morphological imaging has demonstrated that imaging of microvascular injury may be well correlated with disease progression in SSc and systemic vasculitis. The most recent studies have emphasized the importance of microcirculatory function measurement alongside morphological changes, as both elements can give the clinician information concerning organ involvement, i.e., pulmonary complications of SSc patients (Ruaro et al., 2022). Moreover, integration of newer imaging techniques , such as positron emission tomography integrated with computed tomography (PET/CT) has established its usefulness in the diagnosis of systemic vasculitides in the presence of heterogeneity of individual patient presentation and diagnostic delay (Taimen, 2021). This highlights the requirement for an individualized imaging approach to counteract the heterogeneity of rheumatological disease manifestations.

9.4.5. Interpretation Variability Among Practitioners

Inter-reader variability among clinicians significantly influences diagnostic validity in imaging in rheumatology, particularly with modalities like radiography and musculoskeletal ultrasound (MSUS). Evidence indicates that the integration of clinical information enhances imaging assessment accuracy since there is evidence from a study where radiograph interpretation improved from 70% to 78% upon inclusion of clinical information, while MRI rose slightly from 81%–82% (Braun et al., 2024). This means that contextual information aids radiologists in decision-making, thereby increasing their confidence levels. However, it has also been seen through one study that novice practitioners could match the diagnostic accuracy of experienced experts when interpreting MSUS, refuting the notion that more experience always provides the best outcome (Backhaus et al., 2010). Ultimately, it is best that one grasps these differences to standardize practice and improve diagnostic reliability in imaging rheumatology (Figure 9.17).

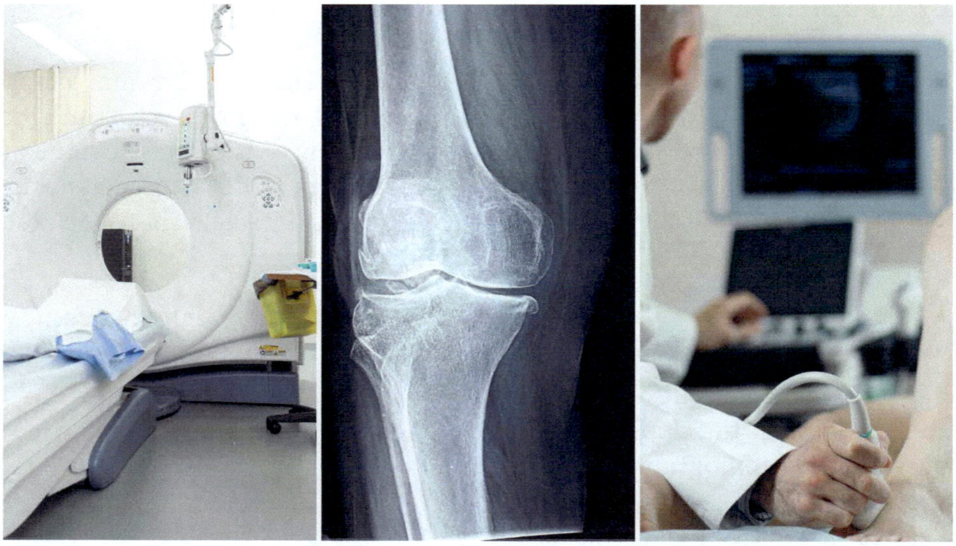

Figure 9.17. Interpretation variability among practitioners significantly impacts diagnostic accuracy in imaging for rheumatology, particularly with modalities like radiography and musculoskeletal ultrasound (MSUS).

Source: https://www.swflrheum.com/wp-content/uploads/2022/04/Difference-Musculoskeletal-Ultrasound-MRI-XRay.jpg.

9.4.6. Patient Factors Affecting Imaging Quality

Image quality in rheumatology can similarly be significantly determined by a variety of patient factors that are both psychosocial and physiological in nature. Compliance of patients, particularly in remaining still during the imaging process, remains a key factor toward enhancing image quality. This is especially true in MSUS, where the precision of images must be of utmost accuracy for effective evaluation and management of rheumatic diseases. Furthermore, the presence of comorbidities , such as hypertension or diabetes, increases the level of complexity of the imaging process because of changes in tissue characteristics and metabolism, leading to a poor image. Of equal concern is the emotional state of the patient; anxiety or discomfort will undermine cooperation, hence affecting the imaging experience and quality in general. Therefore, it is important that rheumatology physicians monitor these patient-specific factors to optimize imaging outcomes and improve disease management procedures effectively (Baraliakos et al., 2013; Naredo & Iagnocco,, 2016).

9.4.7. Limitations in Detecting Early Disease

A challenge of early disease detection in rheumatology is compounded by a variety of limitations of image modalities. The principal issue is the variability in interpreting ultrasounds, notably tendon damage in the case of diseases , such as RA. An instance is a study done on cadaver models, which showed the possibility for ultrasounds to well differentiate tendon lesions but differing interobserver agreement that reflected inconsistent diagnostic accuracy among rheumatologists (Naredo & Iagnocco,, 2016). Moreover, the usual preceding pelvic enthesitis complicates early diagnosis. In a retrospective study, pelvic enthesitis was detected in a high percentage of patients, but frequently remained undiagnosed in clinically asymptomatic patients (Baraliakos et al., 2015). Such blind spots bear witness to the limitation of relying entirely on imaging to identify the subtle nuances of incipient disease presentations, and the necessity for strengthening diagnostic criteria by combining both imaging techniques as well as clinical assessment (Figure 9.18).

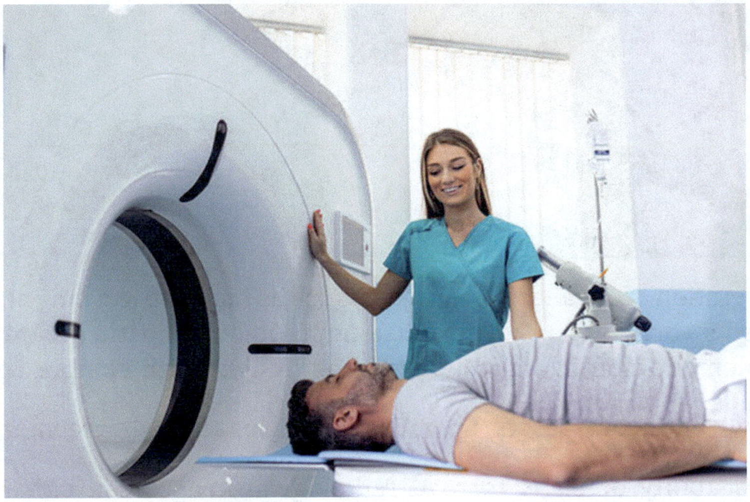

Figure 9.18. The challenge of detecting early disease in rheumatology is compounded by several limitations inherent in imaging techniques.

Source: https://preferredimagingcenters.com/wp-content/uploads/2025/01/blog-mri-fast.jpg.

9.4.8. Ethical Considerations in Imaging

Ethical considerations in imaging are beyond question paramount in rheumatology, particularly in the management of diseases like JIA. The use of sophisticated imaging techniques requires a stringent evaluation of the benefits and risks, particularly in vulnerable subjects like children and adolescents. Obtaining patient consent, valuing the impact of radiation exposure, and potential psychological effects are the foremost considerations of the ethical practice of imaging. Furthermore, as highlighted in recent studies, there is an urgent requirement for integrated care with holistic imaging modalities to improve patient outcomes without being oblivious to ethical guidelines. Evidence also suggests that multidisciplinary treatment approaches can enhance the assessment and management of foot and ankle disease in JIA, but these treatments must be balanced against ethical concerns regarding the efficacy and safety of imaging procedures employed to guide treatment (Manca et al., 2009; Hendry et al., 2013). Ethical concerns must still, therefore, remain the main focus for imaging practice in rheumatology.

9.4.9. Future Challenges in Imaging Technology

With the evolving imaging technology, the field of rheumatology has to deal with significant challenges that call for innovative solutions. The integration of advanced approaches, such as machine learning and digital biomarkers, is a two-edged sword; they can potentially provide improved diagnostic accuracy and precise therapy, but their functionality in clinical practice is afflicted with complexity.

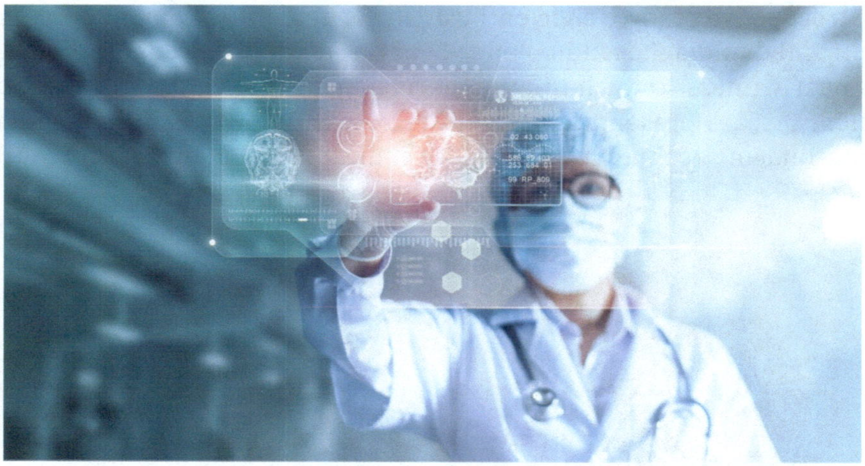

Figure 9.19. The integration of advanced techniques, such as machine learning and digital biomarkers, presents a dual-edged sword; while they promise improved diagnostic accuracy and personalized treatment, their implementation in clinical settings is fraught with complexity.

Source: https://www.aranca.com/assets/uploads/blogs/globalhealthcareemergban.jpg.

For instance, the ability of CNNs to read radiological images can enhance the diagnosis of conditions like erosions or sacroiliitis, but the requirement for high-quality, standardized data poses a major challenge in heterogeneous patient populations (Hügle, 2024). In addition, as noted in juvenile idiopathic arthritis, the complex etiology of diseases complicates the establishment of standard imaging protocols and biomarkers, thereby thwarting the availability of valid therapeutic outcomes and diagnostic criteria (Aji et al., 2024). Overcoming the aforementioned future challenges will require an integrated multidisciplinary approach to enable reliable integration of imaging technology into rheumatology practice (Figure 9.19).

Test Your Knowledge

1. What are the technical issues with musculoskeletal ultrasound?
2. How does over-reliance on imaging lead to rheumatological misdiagnosis?

Summary

Evolution in imaging modalities has greatly influenced the management of rheumatologic diseases, highlighting their all-important function in diagnosing and monitoring the success of treatment. Imaging modalities , such as US and MRI have also enhanced the accuracy of evaluating conditions , such as osteoarthritis and psoriatic arthritis. For example, a US-based study showed notable increases in cartilage thickness, which were positively correlated with treatment response, as seen by statistically significant changes in measurements during one year of follow-up (Barbulescu et al., 2019). Likewise, the use of MRI to determine psoriatic dactylitis showed widespread abnormalities, highlighting the pitfalls of clinical examination alone (Chandramohan et al., 2008). These imaging technologies not only provide accurate information regarding the progression of disease but also enable more customized treatment strategies, ultimately improving patient outcomes and helping to secure the importance of imaging in rheumatology.

In rheumatology, imaging techniques are of pivotal importance to the diagnosis and management follow-up of arthritic conditions like OA and RA. One of the key advances is the utilization of three-dimensional (3D) imaging techniques to quantify wear particles generated from articular cartilage, which are valuable sources of information regarding the extent of OA-related conditions. The novel method applies LSCM to analyze the surface topography of such wear particles, as highlighted in studies indicating that feature parameters may be responsible for significantly predicting texture evolution relative to OA development (Aigner et al., 2012). Besides, cadaver models have also been explored as effective surrogates for quantifying tendon injury in RA, with high intraobserver and interobserver correlation for grading of various tendon ruptures by ultrasound (Naredo & Iagnocco,, 2016). Combined, these advances demonstrate the pivotal position of imaging in enhancing understanding and management of rheumatologic illnesses.

KEY TERMS FROM THIS CHAPTER

- Radiography
- Bone marrow
- Clinical management
- X-ray imaging
- Joint assessment
- Pleural lesions
- Technology
- Computed tomography (CT)
- Soft tissues
- Photon-counting detectors (PCDs)
- Ionizing radiation
- Interstitial lung disease
- Silent synovitis
- Surveillance

Critical Thinking Questions

1. **Which imaging modality is most sensitive for early detection of bone erosions in rheumatoid arthritis?**
   a. X-ray
   b. CT scan
   c. Ultrasound
   d. MRI
2. **Which radiographic finding is most characteristic of osteoarthritis?**
   a. Periarticular osteopenia
   b. Joint space narrowing with marginal osteophytes
   c. Erosions at the MCP joints
   d. Bamboo spine
3. **"Bamboo spine" on spinal imaging is typically associated with:**
   a. Rheumatoid arthritis
   b. Psoriatic arthritis
   c. Ankylosing spondylitis
   d. Osteoarthritis
4. **Which imaging technique is most useful for evaluating soft tissue inflammation and joint effusions at the bedside?**
   a. MRI
   b. CT
   c. Ultrasound
   d. Bone scintigraphy
5. **Which imaging finding is characteristic of advanced rheumatoid arthritis?**
   a. Subchondral sclerosis
   b. Central joint erosions
   c. Marginal bone erosions and joint space narrowing
   d. Normal joint appearance

Short Answer Questions

1. What are the most commonly used imaging modalities in rheumatology practice?
2. How is X-ray distinct from MRI in the evaluation of joint pathology?
3. Through which mechanisms is ultrasound used to assess synovitis and tenosynovitis?
4. Which imaging modalities are used to detect early erosions in rheumatoid arthritis?
5. What are the characteristic X-ray findings of osteoarthritis versus rheumatoid arthritis?
6. How do radiologic features of ankylosing spondylitis evolve with disease progression?
7. What are the limitations of plain radiographs in early inflammatory arthritis?
8. Why might MRI findings be non-specific in autoimmune conditions?

Answers to Critical Thinking Questions

1. (d); 2. (b); 3. (c); 4. (c); 5. (c)

References

1. Puzanov, I., Diab, A., Abdallah, K., Bingham, C. O., 3rd, Brogdon, C., Dadu, R., Hamad, L., Kim, S., Lacouture, M. E., LeBoeuf, N, R., Lenihan, D., Onofrei, C., Shannon, V., Sharma, R., Silk, A. W., Skondra, D., Suarez-Almazor, M. E., Wang, Y., Wiley, K., Kaufman, H. L., ... Society for Immunotherapy of Cancer Toxicity Management Working Group (2017). Managing toxicities associated with immune checkpoint inhibitors: consensus recommendations from the Society for Immunotherapy of Cancer (SITC) Toxicity Management Working Group. *Journal for immunotherapy of cancer*, *5*(1), 95. https://doi.org/10.1186/s40425-017-0300-z(accessed on 17th June 2025).

2. Adinolfi, A., Bertoldi, I., Cimmino, M. A., Delle Sedie, A., et al. (2016). Ultrasound in the diagnosis of calcium pyrophosphate dihydrate deposition disease: A systematic literature review and a meta-analysis. https://core.ac.uk/download/74318650.pdf (accessed on 17th June 2025).

3. Aigner, T., Anamalay, S., Ballantine, J., Blunt, L., Buckland-Wright, C., Chan, K., Chiffre, L., et al. (2012). A new approach to numerical characterization of wear particle surfaces in three-dimensions for wear study. https://core.ac.uk/download/30732623.pdf (accessed on 17th June 2025).

4. Aji, N., Alshareefy, Y., et al. (2024). Advancements and progress in juvenile idiopathic arthritis: A review of pathophysiology and treatment. https://core.ac.uk/download/603360608.pdf (accessed on 17th June 2025).

5. Al-Bulushi, N. K., Bailey, D., & Mariani, G. (2013). The medical case for a positron emission tomography and X-ray computed tomography combined service in Oman. https://core.ac.uk/download/480857427.pdf (accessed on 17th June 2025).

6. Alessandri, C., Ceccarelli, F., Cipriano, E., Colasanti, T., et al. (2018). Anti-carbamylated protein antibodies as a new biomarker of erosive joint damage in systemic lupus erythematosus. https://core.ac.uk/download/159269169.pdf (accessed on 17th June 2025).

7. Allaart, C. F., Bois, M. H. W. de, Bouwstra, J. K., Breedveld, F. C., et al. (2009). Changes in hand and generalized bone mineral density in patients with recent-onset rheumatoid arthritis. https://core.ac.uk/download/pdf/15460986.pdf (accessed on 17th June 2025).

8. Anjum, A., Bloodsworth, P., Branson, A., Hauer, F., et al. (2007). The requirements for ontologies in medical data integration: A case study. http://arxiv.org/abs/0707.0763 (accessed on 17th June 2025).

9. Azuaga, A. B., Canete, J. D., Frade-Sosa, B., Gomez-Puerta, J. A., Morla, R., et al. (2022). Imaging findings in patients with immune checkpoint inhibitor-induced arthritis. https://diposit.ub.edu/dspace/bitstream/2445/201456/1/Imaging%20Findings%20in%20Patients%20with%20Immune%20Checkpoint%20Inhibitor-Induced%20Arthritis_Diagnostics.pdf (accessed on 17th June 2025).

10. Backhaus, M., Balint, P. V., Bruyn, G. A. W., Craig-Muller, N., et al. (2010). Self-directed learning of basic musculoskeletal ultrasound among rheumatologists in the United States. https://core.ac.uk/download/302079653.pdf (accessed on 17th June 2025).

11. Backhaus, M., Balint, P., Bruns, A., Bruyn, G. A., et al. (2016). Preliminary definitions for the

sonographic features of synovitis in children. https://core.ac.uk/download/54538633.pdf (accessed on 17th June 2025).

12. Backhaus, M., Burmester, G. R., Glimm, A. M., Haugen, D. R., et al. (2019). Fluorescence optical imaging for treatment monitoring in patients with early and active rheumatoid arthritis in a 1-year follow-up period. *Frontiers in Medicine*. https://core.ac.uk/download/286567847.pdf (accessed on 17th June 2025).

13. Badano, L., Bourji, K. I., Cozzi, F., Miatton, M., et al. (2015). Evaluation of right ventricular function performed by 3D-echocardiography in scleroderma patients. *European Heart Journal–Cardiovascular Imaging*. https://core.ac.uk/download/80154728.pdf (accessed on 17th June 2025).

14. Baraliakos, X., Betteridge, N., Braun, J., Burgos-Vargas, R., et al. (2013). Treating spondylarthritis, including ankylosing spondylitis and psoriatic arthritis, to target: Recommendations of an international task force. *Annals of the Rheumatic Diseases*. https://core.ac.uk/download/55764870.pdf (accessed on 17th June 2025).

15. Baraliakos, X., Dehoorne, J., Elewaut, D., Herregods, N., et al. (2015). Diagnostic value of pelvic enthesitis on MRI of the sacroiliac joints in enthesitis-related arthritis. *Annals of the Rheumatic Diseases*. https://core.ac.uk/download/55743217.pdf (accessed on 17th June 2025).

16. Barbulescu, A. L., Chisalau, B. A., Ciurea, P. L., Criveanu, M., et al. (2019). The effect of glucosamine, chondroitin and *Harpagophytum procumbens* on femoral hyaline cartilage thickness in patients with knee osteoarthritis–An MRI versus ultrasonography study. *Journal of Clinical Imaging Science*. https://core.ac.uk/download/216811083.pdf (accessed on 17th June 2025).

17. Basu, N., Goni, M., Murray, A. D., Waiter, G., et al. (2018). Neural indicators of fatigue in chronic diseases: A systematic review of MRI studies. *Neuroscience & Biobehavioral Reviews*. https://core.ac.uk/download/159067075.pdf (accessed on 17th June 2025).

18. Becce, F., Booij, R., Gallego Manzano, L., Mourad, A., et al. (2024). Chances and challenges of photon-counting CT in musculoskeletal imaging. *European Radiology*. https://core.ac.uk/download/610639100.pdf (accessed on 17th June 2025).

19. Benavent, D., & Sequí Sabater, J. M. (2025). Artificial intelligence in rheumatology research: What is it good for? *Clinical Rheumatology*. https://core.ac.uk/download/643237088.pdf (accessed on 17th June 2025).

20. Beschi, I. S., et al. (2023). Applications of deep learning and machine learning in healthcare domain–A literature review. *Health Informatics Journal*. https://core.ac.uk/download/596247273.pdf (accessed on 17th June 2025).

21. Biswas, S., Manohar, S., Steenbergen, W., van Es, P., et al. (2015). A method for delineation of bone surfaces in photoacoustic computed tomography of the finger. *Photoacoustic*. https://core.ac.uk/download/572182348.pdf (accessed on 17th June 2025).

22. Hendry, G. J., Watt, G. F., Brandon, M., Friel, L., Turner, D. E., Lorgelly, P. K., Gardner-Medwin, J., Sturrock, R. D., & Woodburn, J. (2013). The effectiveness of a multidisciplinary foot care program for children and adolescents with juvenile idiopathic arthritis: an exploratory trial. *Journal of rehabilitation medicine, 45*(5), 467–476. https://doi.org/10.2340/16501977-1130 (accessed on 17th June 2025).

23. Braun, J., Deppe, D., Diekhoff, T., Poddubnyy, D., et al. (2024). Diagnostic accuracy in axial spondylarthritis: A systematic evaluation of the role of clinical information in the interpretation of sacroiliac joint imaging. *Annals of the Rheumatic Diseases*. https://core.ac.uk/download/644526559.pdf (accessed on 17th June 2025).

24. Brogan, P., Burns, J. C., Cornish, J., Diwakar, V., et al. (2020). Lifetime cardiovascular management of patients with previous Kawasaki disease. *Archives of Disease in Childhood*. https://core.ac.uk/download/323066717.pdf (accessed on 17th June 2025).

25. Brown, K. K., Chung, L., Cottin, V., Distler, J. H. W., et al. (2022). Diagnosis and monitoring of systemic sclerosis-associated interstitial lung disease using high-resolution computed tomography. *Therapeutic Advances in Respiratory Disease*. https://www.zora.uzh.ch/id/eprint/222176/1/23971983211064463.pdf (accessed on 17th June 2025).

26. Bruni, C., Chen, S., Du, G., Furst, D. E., et al. (2024). A versatile role for lung ultrasound in systemic autoimmune rheumatic diseases related pulmonary involvement: A narrative review. *Frontiers in Medicine*. https://core.ac.uk/download/636776943.pdf (accessed on 17th June 2025).

27. Buisman, L. R., Hazes, J. M. W., Luime, J. J., Oppe, M., et al. (2016). A five-year model to assess the early cost-effectiveness of new diagnostic tests in the early diagnosis of rheumatoid arthritis. *Annals of the Rheumatic Diseases*. https://core.ac.uk/download/43291966.pdf (accessed on 17th June 2025).

28. Bykov, A., Doronin, A., Dunaev, A. V., Meglinski, I., et al. (2017). Combined use of laser Doppler flowmetry and skin thermometry for functional diagnostics of intradermal finger vessels. *Biomedical Optics Express*. https://core.ac.uk/download/222826363.pdf (accessed on 17th June 2025).

29. Cachia, M. J., & Vella, S. (2008). Charcot neuroarthropathy: Pathogenesis, diagnosis and medical management. *Malta Medical Journal*. https://core.ac.uk/download/46602192.pdf (accessed on 17th June 2025).

30. Chandramohan, M., Groves, C., Healy, P. J., Helliwell, P. S., et al. (2008). MRI changes in psoriatic dactylitis: Extent of pathology, relationship to tenderness and correlation with clinical indices. *Annals of the Rheumatic Diseases*. https://core.ac.uk/download/51789.pdf (accessed on 17th June 2025).

31. Chen, K., Terkeltaub, R., & Wu, Y. (2016). Systematic review and quality analysis of emerging diagnostic measures for calcium pyrophosphate crystal deposition disease. *Rheumatology International*. https://core.ac.uk/download/323065310.pdf (accessed on 17th June 2025).

32. Collin, M. (2023). Orofacial aspects of juvenile idiopathic arthritis in children. *European Archives of Pediatric Dentistry*. https://core.ac.uk/download/570950848.pdf (accessed on 17th June 2025).

33. Pizzorni, C., Sulli, A., Smith, V., Lladó, A., Paolino, S., Cutolo, M., & Ruaro, B. (2016). Capillaroscopy 2016: new perspectives in systemic sclerosis. Capillaroscopy 2016: new perspectives in systemic sclerosis. *Acta reumatologica portuguesa*, *41*(1), 8–14.(accessed on 17th June 2025).

34. Dancy, L. (2023). Defining the incidence of cardiac involvement in myositis using mapping based cardiovascular magnetic resonance imaging. *Cardiology in the Young*. https://core.ac.uk/download/595484228.pdf (accessed on 17th June 2025).

35. De Decker, S., Gielen, I., Lam, R., Packer, R. A., et al. (2015). Thoracic and lumbar vertebral bone mineral density changes in a natural occurring dog model of diffuse idiopathic skeletal hyperostosis. *Veterinary Radiology & Ultrasound*. https://core.ac.uk/download/55807446.pdf (accessed on 17th June 2025).

36. DE VINCENTIISet al. (2017). Sialendoscopic management of autoimmune sialadenitis: A review of literature. https://core.ac.uk/download/98339930.pdf (accessed on 17th June 2025).

37. El Asri, B., Mikram, M., Ounasser, N., Rhanoui, H., et al. (2024). A brief on artificial intelligence in medicine. https://core.ac.uk/download/642672219.pdf (accessed on 17th June 2025).

38. El Maghraoui, A., Unnanuntana, A., Schoenfeld, A. J., Mermerci Baskan, B., Riggs, B. L., Marshall, D., Resnick, D., et al. (2015). Thoracic and lumbar vertebral bone mineral density changes in a natural occurring dog model of diffuse idiopathic skeletal hyperostosis. https://core.ac.uk/download/36778322.pdf (accessed on 17th June 2025).

39. Elewaut, D., & Matucci-Cerinic, M. (2009). Treatment of ankylosing spondylitis and extra-articular manifestations in everyday rheumatology practice. https://core.ac.uk/download/55761196.pdf (accessed on 17th June 2025).

40. Espírito Santo, R. C. do, Fernandes, K. Z., Filippin, L. I., Lora, P. S., et al. (2018). Prevalence of rheumatoid cachexia in rheumatoid arthritis: A systematic review and meta-analysis. https://core.ac.uk/download/293631208.pdf (accessed on 17th June 2025).

41. Finucci, A., Iagnocco, A., Rutigliano, I. M., Scirocco, R., et al. (2015). Musculoskeletal ultrasonography in gout. https://core.ac.uk/download/74318651.pdf (accessed on 17th June 2025).

42. Gross, A. J., Kidambi, T. D., Lee, J. K., Ostroff, J. W., et al. (2017). Endoscopy is of low yield in the identification of gastrointestinal neoplasia in patients with dermatomyositis: A cross-sectional study. https://core.ac.uk/download/323074387.pdf (accessed on 17th June 2025).

43. Hügle, T. (2024). Advancing rheumatology care through machine learning. https://core.ac.uk/download/611826872.pdf (accessed on 17th June 2025).

44. Naredo, E., & Iagnocco, A. (2016). One year in review: ultrasound in arthritis. *Clinical and experimental rheumatology*, *34*(1), 1–10. Janta, I., Morán, J., Naredo, E., Nieto, J. C., Uson, J., Möller, I., Bong, D., Bruyn, G. A., D Agostino, M. A., Filippucci, E., Hammer, H. B., Iagnocco, A., Terslev, L., González, J. M., Mérida, J. R., & Carreño, L. (2016). How does a cadaver model work for testing ultrasound diagnostic capability for rheumatic-like tendon damage?. *Rheumatology international*, *36*(6), 863–869. https://doi.org/10.1007/s00296-016-3460-0 (accessed on 17th June 2025).

45. Kisten, Y. (2023). Ultrasound and fluorescence optical imaging biomarkers for early diagnosis and prediction of rheumatoid arthritis. https://core.ac.uk/download/552756762.pdf (accessed on 17th June 2025).

46. Ligtvoet, A., Bouter, L. M., Buxton, M., Fitch, K., Hanney, S., Grant, J., et al. (2008). Assessing the impact of health technology assessment in the Netherlands. https://core.ac.uk/download/337051.pdf (accessed on 17th June 2025).

47. Maffione, A. M., Anagnostou, C., Civitelli, L., Collorone, G., et al. (2015). Role of brain perfusion SPECT with 99mTc HMPAO in the assessment of response to drug therapy in patients with autoimmune vasculitis: A prospective study. https://core.ac.uk/download/54523723.pdf (accessed on 17th June 2025).

48. Manca, A., Mavidrou, A., Premkumar, A., Karmazyn, B., Wallace, C. A., Sherry, D. D., Turner, D. E., et al. (2009). Protocol for the Foot in Juvenile Idiopathic Arthritis trial (FiJIA): A randomized controlled trial of an integrated foot care programmed for foot problems in JIA. https://core.ac.uk/download/1396388.pdf (accessed on 17th June 2025).

49. Matcher, S. J. (2009). A review of some recent developments in polarization-sensitive optical imaging techniques for the study of articular cartilage. https://core.ac.uk/download/50699.pdf (accessed on 17th June 2025).

50. Palosaari, K. (2008). Quantitative and semiquantitative imaging techniques in detecting joint inflammation in patients with rheumatoid arthritis: Phase-shift water-fat MRI method for fat suppression at 0.23 T, contrast-enhanced dynamic and static MRI, and quantitative ^{99m}Tc-nano colloid scintigraphy. https://core.ac.uk/download/628859726.pdf (accessed on 17th June 2025).

51. Paltta, J. (2024). Diagnostic challenges in rheumatology–Improving validity of registry-based studies. https://core.ac.uk/download/619889197.pdf (accessed on 17th June 2025).

52. Patience, A., Speed, C. A., Bowen, C. J., Miller, D. L., Hendry, G. J., Siddle, H. J., et al. (2018). Survey of ultrasound practice amongst podiatrists in the UK. https://core.ac.uk/download/293885607.pdf (accessed on 17th June 2025).

53. Pfranjpe, G., et al. (2023). Digital health technologies in vision care: Transforming diagnostics and management. https://core.ac.uk/download/596247488.pdf (accessed on 17th June 2025).

54. Ruaro, B., Salton, F., Gandin, I., Confalonieri, M., D'Oria, M., Hughes, M., Confalonieri, P., et al. (2022). Correlation between microvascular damage and internal organ involvement in scleroderma: Focus on lung damage and endothelial dysfunction. *Diagnostics*. https://core.ac.uk/download/566469592.pdf (accessed on 17th June 2025).

55. Taimen, K. (2021). The many faces of vasculitis: Diagnostic challenges and economic burden. https://core.ac.uk/download/481513323.pdf (accessed on 17th June 2025).

56. van Alfen, N., Veltsista, D., & Vicino, A. (2024). Muscle ultrasound in myopathies. https://core.ac.uk/download/620697671.pdf (accessed on 17th June 2025).

MUSCULOSKELETAL BIOPSY AND HISTOPATHOLOGY

10

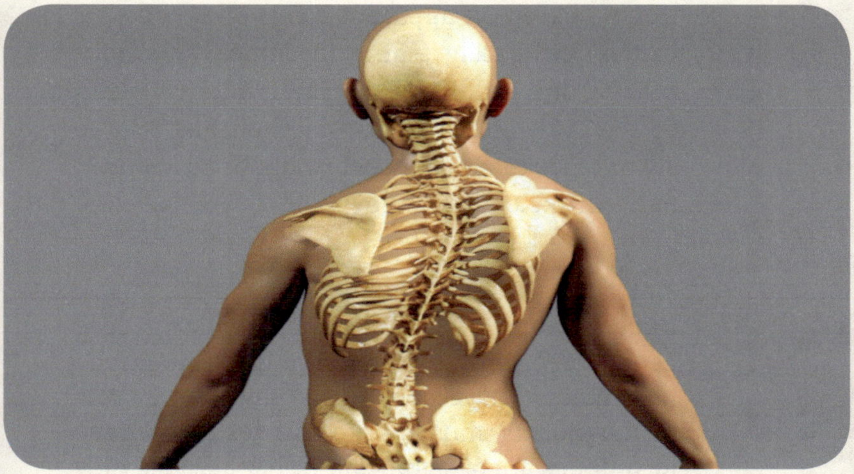

LEARNING OBJECTIVES

After studying this chapter, you will be able to:

1. Identify types of musculoskeletal biopsies;
2. Understand histopathological techniques;
3. Explain common musculoskeletal disorders diagnosed with biopsy;
4. Address complications and risks of biopsy.

Introduction

The musculoskeletal system, including bones, joints, muscles, and connective tissues, is in charge of mobility and health. Being a dense network, it is susceptible to many diseases and conditions, and therefore needs accurate diagnostic methods to differentiate between the several pathologies. Musculoskeletal histopathology and biopsy are obviously key instruments in diagnosis, as they allow direct visualization of tissue samples. This is an important leap towards learning about diseases , such as tumors and inflammatory processes through cellular and molecular processes. The inclusion of advanced imaging techniques, like elastography, has further increased diagnostic accuracy, particularly in the evaluation of soft tissue pathology (Ansari et al., 2023). With advances in specialization, research and updated guidelines also keep pace with changing practices, assisting healthcare professionals in managing the needs of patients effectively and avoiding risks associated with musculoskeletal disorders (Senneville et al., 2023) (Figure 10.1).

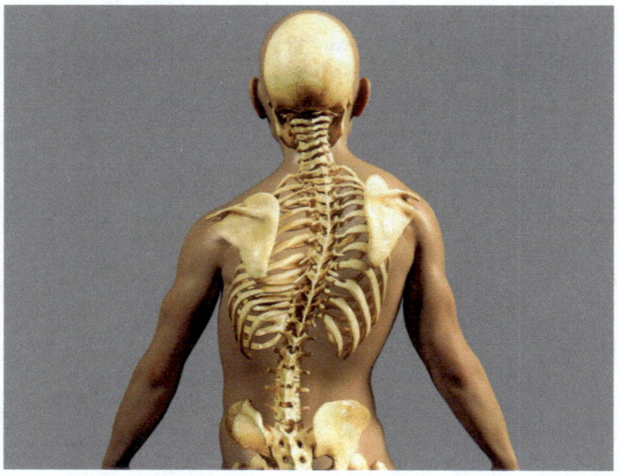

Figure 10.1. The musculoskeletal system, comprised of bones, joints, muscles, and connective tissues, plays a crucial role in maintaining mobility and overall health.

Source: https://shahalam.avisena.com.my/wp-content/uploads/2023/09/Scoliosis.jpg.

10.1. Types of Musculoskeletal Biopsies

Learning Outcome

1. Understand needle biopsy techniques;
2. Describe the open surgical biopsy technique;
3. Discuss the core needle biopsy technique;
4. Learn the image-guided biopsy technique;
5. Focus on the excisional biopsy technique;
6. Describe the incisional biopsy technique;
7. Know strengths and limitations of each type;
8. Explain indications for varied types of biopsies;
9. Focus on patient preparation for biopsies.

It is worth knowing the various types of musculoskeletal biopsies to make the diagnosis and proper planning of treatment. One of the most common ones is percutaneous needle biopsies, which can be classified into fine needle aspiration and core needle biopsies. Fine needle aspiration is less invasive, using a thin needle to suck out a small sample of tissue, best for cases where speed and less pain are needed. While core needle biopsies acquire larger tissue samples, which allow for enhanced histopathological assessment and retention of architecture (Cleary et al., 2017). This is particularly important when assessing bone and soft tissue tumors, where thorough examination is necessary.

Advanced imaging techniques, such as diffusion-weighted MRI, enhance biopsy accuracy by distinguishing between malignant and benign lesions based on apparent diffusion coefficient values, ultimately aiding in clinical decision-making and enabling early interventions (Azad et al., 2024). Each biopsy method has unique advantages to meet specific diagnostic needs in musculoskeletal pathology.

10.1.1. Needle Biopsy Techniques

Needle biopsy techniques, particularly core needle biopsy (CNB) and computed tomography (CT)-guided, have come to be invaluable tools in diagnosing musculoskeletal lesions. These techniques are of significant utility because they are highly precise and minimally invasive.

For instance, CNB has shown 74.4% diagnostic performance against post-excision histopathology, rising to 84.9% on the use of immunohistochemistry, quoting its success in distinguishing benign and malignant lesions with sensitivities of up to 98% (Giarso et al., 2016). Similarly, CT-guided percutaneous biopsies have a sensitivity of 95.4% and specificity of 85.7%, also an efficient agent in the identification of primary bone tumors (Dominic et al., 2017). This equilibrium of accuracy and safety positions needle biopsy techniques as a pillar in musculoskeletal biopsy and histopathology, allowing for precise diagnosis and subsequent treatment of many conditions affecting the musculoskeletal system (Figure 10.2).

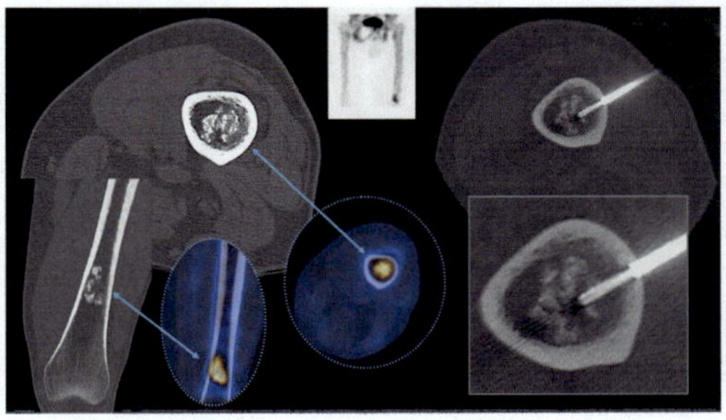

Figure 10.2. Needle biopsy techniques, particularly core needle biopsy (CNB) and computed tomography (CT)-guided procedures, have become essential tools in the diagnosis of musculoskeletal lesions.

Source: https://pub.mdpi-res.com/diagnostics/diagnostics-13-02350/article_deploy/html/images/diagnostics-13-02350-g001.png?1689155208.

10.1.2. Open Surgical Biopsy

Open biopsy surgery is a valuable procedure in the diagnosis of musculoskeletal lesions, particularly when the findings of less invasive techniques, such as core needle biopsy, are ambiguous. This procedure involved resecting a sample of the lesion for histopathological examination, which provides more precise information regarding tumor grade and type. Open surgical biopsy is especially helpful in cases where malignancy is suspected since it allows complete assessment and staging of the disease and eventually guides treatment protocols. According to studies, while core needle biopsy can reach satisfactory accuracy levels, the specificity and sensitivity of open biopsies are higher, especially in complex cases (Giarso et al., 2016). Additionally, advances in imaging technologies have assisted surgeons in safely and successfully performing these biopsies (Dominic et al., 2017). Accordingly, open surgical biopsy remains a valuable tool within the complex management of diagnosing and treating musculoskeletal tumors.

10.1.3. Core Needle Biopsy (CNB)

CNB is an essential diagnostic technique for musculoskeletal lesions because it offers a time-saving alternative to the traditional open techniques of biopsies. Interestingly, it is observed through research that CNB achieves comparable diagnostic accuracy to open biopsies, solidifying its place in clinical practice (Giarso et al., 2016). As a minimally invasive procedure, it is particularly valuable since it yields sufficient tissue for histopathological analysis while evading patient discomfort and reducing recovery time to a minimum. In addition to its application in malignant and benign lesions, CNB has proved more accurate when combined with immunohistochemical techniques, further refining diagnostic outcomes (Giarso et al., 2016). The incorporation of CT guidance further enhanced the efficacy of CNB, with a sensitivity of up to 95.4% for the diagnosis of primary bone tumors, accompanied by a low incidence of complications. Thus, CNB is set up as a valuable and reliable diagnostic tool in musculoskeletal pathology (Figure 10.3).

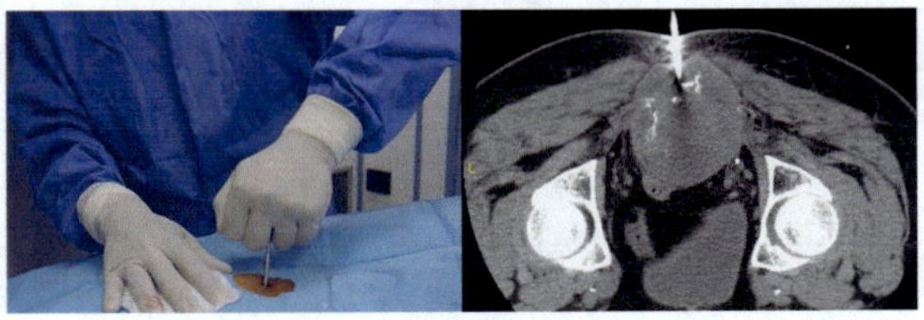

Figure 10.3. Core needle biopsy (CNB) has emerged as a pivotal technique in the diagnosis of musculoskeletal lesions, offering an efficient alternative to traditional open biopsy methods.

Source: https://pub.mdpi-res.com/curroncol/curroncol-31-00067/article_deploy/html/images/curroncol-31-00067-g001.png?1707114438.

10.1.4. Image-guided Biopsy

Image-guided biopsy has become a key facilitator in the diagnosis of musculoskeletal lesions due primarily to the ability to enhance the accuracy and dependability of tissue sampling. Imaging procedures , such as CT-guided biopsy enable precise localization of the lesion, which significantly improves diagnostic outcome. For instance, a study discovers that the CT-guided biopsy sensitivity in the diagnosis of primary bone tumors is as high as 95.4%, with a specificity of 85.7%, thus justifying its application as a diagnostic tool in orthopedic oncology (Dominic et al., 2017). Along with this, CNB has been shown to be as accurate as the traditional open biopsy method, and diagnostic accuracy is as high as 74.4%, which is increased to 84.9% using immunohistochemistry techniques (Giarso et al., 2016). Not only does this technological advancement reflect the superiority of image-guided procedures, but it also points to their superior position in the realm of histopathology and ultimately contributes to better patient care.

10.1.5. Excisional Biopsy

Excisional biopsy is an important procedure in the case of musculoskeletal biopsy and histopathology, as it allows for intensive examination of lesions while providing treatment simultaneously. Excisional biopsy is the removal of the whole mass, both in the diagnostic and therapeutic roles, enabling histopathological examination to exclude or confirm malignancies. The accuracy of excisional biopsies is improved over CNBs, where the rate of concordance for diagnosis is high according to research; for instance, the CNB study reported an accuracy of 74.4%, which can be up to 97.1% for benign tumors when coupled with adequate histopathological methods (Giarso et al., 2016). Moreover, excisional biopsies are especially significant in the instance of tumors like schwannomas, where histopathological examination is critical to make diagnoses without harming nerves during surgery (Behera et al., 2024). Such an element of diagnostic precision coupled with effective surgical intervention indicates the merit of excisional biopsy in musculoskeletal care (Figure 10.4).

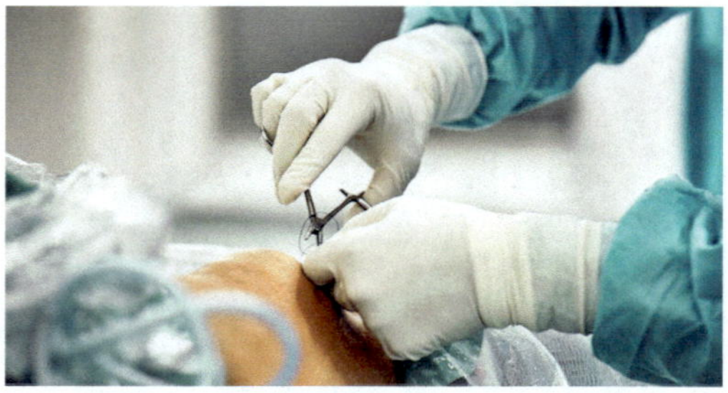

Figure 10.4. Excisional biopsy is a pivotal procedure in the realm of musculoskeletal biopsy and histopathology, as it enables comprehensive assessment of lesions while simultaneously providing treatment.

Source: https://media.post.rvohealth.io/wp-content/uploads/2022/08/surgeon-stitching-after-facebook-1200x628.jpg.

10.1.6. Incisional Biopsy

As techniques for musculoskeletal biopsy continue to advance, incisional biopsy is still an important procedure within the diagnostic pathway for musculoskeletal tumors. The technique is one in which surgical resection of a tumor segment is done, providing a vital histopathological specimen for analysis. The validity of incisional biopsies is exemplified by a study demonstrating that they are capable of specifically distinguishing benign from malignant lesions, thus impacting appropriate treatment protocols. For instance, CT-guided biopsy is shown to be 95.4% sensitive and 85.7% specific in the diagnosis of primary bone tumors, correlating with the precision of this method in clinical settings (Dominic et al., 2017). Besides, while cytology is used as a fast diagnostic technique on a regular basis, research has established that it may not be as sensitive in outlining specific histotypes, such as osteosarcoma, meaning that incisional biopsies should typically have priority when ordering for final diagnosis (Oikonomidis et al., 2021). Overall, incisional biopsy plays a critical role in the histological examination of musculoskeletal lesions (Figure 10.5).

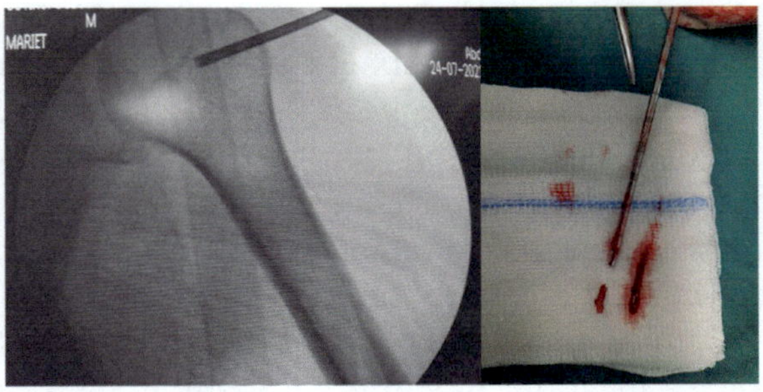

Figure 10.5. As musculoskeletal biopsy techniques evolve, the incisional biopsy remains a pivotal procedure in the diagnostic pathway for musculoskeletal tumors.

Source: https://www.mdpi.com/curroncol/curroncol-31-00067/article_deploy/html/images/curroncol-31-00067-g003.png.

10.1.7. Advantages and Disadvantages of Each Type

Various biopsy techniques for musculoskeletal lesions have varying merits and demerits, with implications for their clinical application. CNB is praised for its accuracy, with many times providing results similar to open biopsy without the need for an intricate surgical procedure. In research, the sensitivity of CNB diagnosis was 74.4%, and it was enhanced to 84.9% with the addition of immunohistochemistry, which showed its reliability in identifying benign and malignant lesions (Giarso et al., 2016).

On the other hand, CT-guided percutaneous core biopsy has good sensitivity (95.4%) and specificity (85.7%) in diagnosing primary bone tumors due to its non-invasive procedure and lower complication rates, which stood at merely 4.3% (Dominic et al., 2017). However, both of these approaches can be sample size and complication-limited, and patient selection and careful attention to the clinical context in which they are employed are thus crucial.

10.1.8. Indications for Different Biopsy Types

Choice of the most suitable type of biopsy is critical in differentiating between musculoskeletal diseases and each of a number of techniques has its applications under specific clinical circumstances. For instance, FNA is often used on palpable masses or lesions that are either malignant-suspected or benign due to the fact that it is minimally invasive and provides instant results.

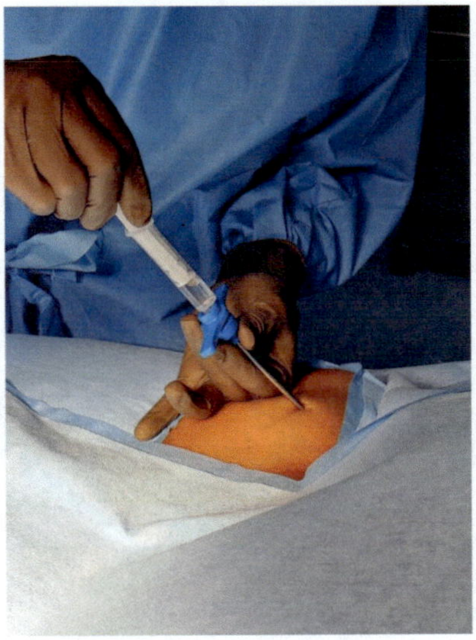

Figure 10.6. Determining the appropriate type of biopsy is crucial in achieving accurate diagnoses for musculoskeletal conditions, and various techniques are indicated based on specific clinical circumstances.

Source: https://media.springernature.com/lw685/springer-static/image/art%3A10.1007%2Fs13193-023-01788-8/MediaObjects/13193_2023_1788_Fig10_HTML.png.

Core needle biopsies, however, provide larger tissue samples and are thus vital in evaluating tumors where treatment depends on subtypes. In addition, where malignancy is suspected or intraoperative diagnosis is requested, frozen section biopsies facilitate immediate pathological examination, significantly impacting surgical decision and management (Kavitha, 2014). Additionally, imaging-guided biopsies, such as CT-guided tissue-core biopsies, may be requested in lesions occurring in areas of complex anatomy, so as to obtain accurate sampling and minimize complications (Felici et al., 2021). Thus, the choice of biopsy type must be appropriate for clinical situations, balancing the need for timely diagnosis against tissue quality for thorough histopathological examination (Figure 10.6).

10.1.9. Patient Preparation for Biopsy Procedures

Effective patient preparation for biopsy procedures is required in order to enhance benefits and minimize complications. Before a musculoskeletal biopsy, patients must be counseled comprehensively regarding the test in order to reduce anxiety and inform them of anticipated feelings or discomfort during biopsies. Preparation can include obtaining informed consent, where patients sign and acknowledge understanding of the risks versus the benefits of the test. Additionally, pre-procedure imaging is employed to ensure a precise location for biopsy, thereby enhancing the diagnostic efficacy of the procedures. FNAB is emphasized due to its simplicity and cost-effectiveness. Research has proven that FNAB possesses a highly impressive diagnostic yield of 86% in various musculoskeletal tumors (Dewo et al., 2016). Moreover, the process is very effective for soft tissue neoplasms and has a concordance rate of 94% (Dewo et al., 2016). Hence, preparation in a careful manner maximizes both patient comfort as well as the success of the biopsy as a whole.

Test Your Knowledge

1. When would a fine-needle aspiration (FNA) be adequate for musculoskeletal evaluation?
2. What are the indications for the performance of a muscle biopsy in suspected inflammatory myopathies?

10.2. Histopathological Techniques

Learning Outcome

1. Master tissue processing techniques;
2. Learn histopathology staining techniques;
3. Explain microscopic testing procedures;
4. Highlight immunohistochemistry uses;
5. Outline molecular techniques in histopathology;
6. Know the pathologists' role in diagnosis;
7. Interpret histopathological findings;
8. Identify frequent artifacts in tissue samples;
9. Understand histopathological technological developments.

Histopathological techniques have an integral role to play in the accurate diagnosis of musculoskeletal lesions, particularly those presenting as primary or metastatic tumors. Of all these techniques, CNB has emerged in importance due to its diagnostic accuracy, which is on par with open biopsy methods. For instance, studies have indicated that CNB can achieve a 74.4% accuracy rate compared to post-excision histopathological findings, and with a very high sensitivity of 98% if subsequently assayed by clinicopathological conferences (CPC) (Giarso et al., 2016). In addition, CT-guided biopsies have been shown to be 95.4% sensitive for the diagnosis of primary bone tumors and thus of proven value in the clinic (Dominic et al., 2017). These results emphasize the importance of the application of such histopathological techniques, not just to confirm the presence of malignancies but also to direct treatment modalities that deterministically affect patient outcome in musculoskeletal pathology.

10.2.1. Tissue Processing Methods

Processing tissue samples is a critical aspect of histopathological examination of musculoskeletal biopsies, with direct consequences for the validity of the diagnosis and subsequent treatment options. Initial fixation of the retrieved tissue to preserve cellular architecture and protein integrity is the first step, with formalin being the most common fixative used. Fixation is followed by embedding tissue samples into paraffin wax to facilitate the precise sectioning of thin tissue sections for microscopic analysis. Advanced techniques, such as ultrasound-guided biopsies, enhance tissue yield with great success rates in retrieving synovial tissue, as reported through an 81.6% success rate in histological examination after the procedure (Najm et al., 2016). The ability to analyze such samples at a transcriptomic level provides further insight into pathogenesis and therapeutic action, particularly in conditions like rheumatoid arthritis, where tissue response is critical to the creation of targeted therapy (Cope et al., 2016). Thus, tissue processing methods can be vital in diagnostic yields in musculoskeletal pathology (Figure 10.7).

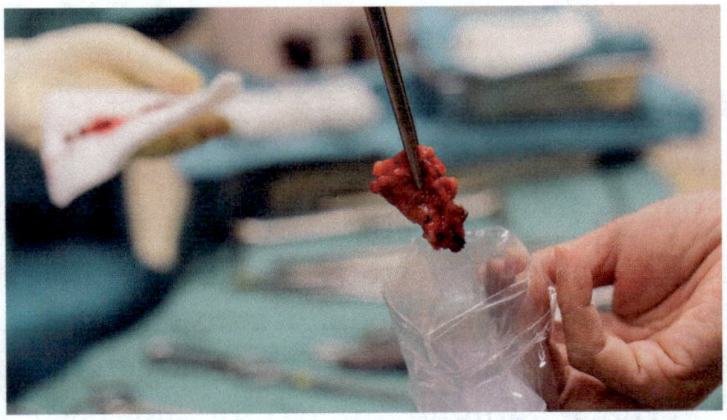

Figure 10.7. The processing of tissue samples is a critical step in the histopathological examination of musculoskeletal biopsies, directly impacting the accuracy of diagnosis and subsequent treatment decisions.

Source: https://ampath.com/category/1698666701.jpg.

10.2.2. Staining Techniques used in Histopathology

Histopathology relies heavily on various staining techniques that enhance the visualization of tissue structure and pathological changes, particularly in musculoskeletal biopsies. Among the most frequently used is hematoxylin and eosin (H&E) staining, which discriminates between nuclear and cytoplasmic structures with a straightforward protocol for benign and malignant lesion discrimination. Immunohistochemical staining once again refines the above diagnostic process by employing antibodies towards specific protein expressions of a range of pathologies. For instance, high-mobility group protein B1 (HMGB1) induction in tendinopathy has been said to regulate inflammatory mediators and critical matrix modifications, with significant importance of specific staining techniques in exploring disease processes (Akbar et al., 2017). Moreover, the specificity of CNB is significantly improved by the application of immunohistochemistry, from 74.4%–84.9%, thereby supporting the utility of such procedures in establishing consistent diagnoses in musculoskeletal pathology (Giarso et al., 2016).

10.2.3. Microscopic Examination Procedures

Microscopic examination procedures are the cornerstone of the study of musculoskeletal biopsies, enabling pathologists to differentiate between the inherent tissue characteristics of various pathologies. Before microscopic analysis, the appropriate tissue specimens must first be obtained, commonly through minimally invasive procedures , such as ultrasound-guided biopsies, which have had a whopping success rate of 81.6% in obtaining synovial tissue from undifferentiated arthritis patients (Aurélie Najm et al., 2016). After being obtained, the histological analysis involves a gentle process of fixation, embedding, sectioning, and staining to allow cellular structures and matrix components to be seen. This extent of minute observation is critical in diagnosing conditions , such as chondroblastomas, which, although usually benign, can present with aggressive forms necessitating urgent treatment (Alva et al., 2004). These microscopic techniques hence, not only optimize diagnostic precision but also direct therapy, thereby enhancing patient outcomes in musculoskeletal disease (Figure 10.8).

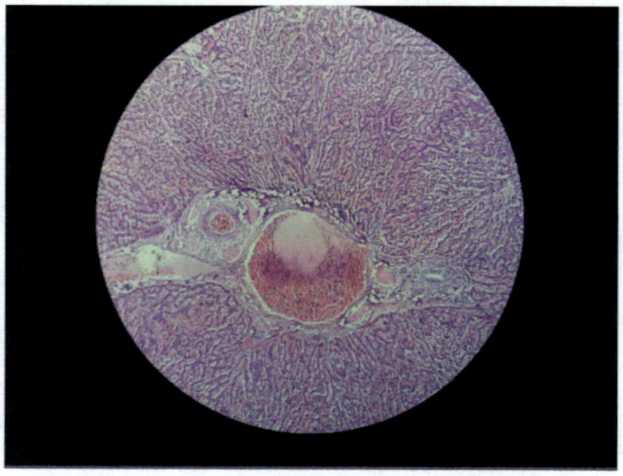

Figure 10.8. Microscopic examination procedures serve as a cornerstone in the analysis of musculoskeletal biopsies, enabling pathologists to discern the underlying tissue characteristics associated with various pathologies.

Source: https://qph.cf2.quoracdn.net/main-qimg-cb1515680e9fd0c8339a3de842233c24-lq.

10.2.4. Immunohistochemistry (IHC) Applications

IHC is a valuable method in the area of musculoskeletal biopsy and histopathology, which enhances the diagnostic performance for various bone and soft tissue pathologies. By binding specifically to target antigens in tissue sections using special antibodies, IHC allows visualization of protein expression patterns and differentiation between benign and malignant lesions. It is particularly valuable for tumor characterization because it allows lineage-specific markers to be identified and personalized therapeutic strategies to be developed. Further, integration of digital pathology in IHC protocols is set to ease the analysis, but challenges to clinical adoption and validation persist (Williams, 2020). Of note, innovation in ultrasonic surgical devices for bone biopsy allows for sample acquisition without compromising tissue architecture, thereby further adding to the value of IHC during subsequent histologic examination (Cleary et al., 2017). Hence, IHC is an important interface of pathology and technology in musculoskeletal medicine.

10.2.5. Molecular Techniques in Histopathology

The introduction of molecular methods in histopathology has tremendously enhanced the diagnostic power in musculoskeletal biopsies. These techniques, including immunohistochemistry and reverse transcriptase PCR (RT-PCR), enable pathologists not only to recognize the morphological characteristics of tissues but also to decode intricate molecular pathways involved in diseases.

For instance, HMGB1 has also been found to be a significant mediator of inflammation in tendon pathologies, whose expression is greater in tendinopathic tissues compared with controls, which may provide insight into the application of specific therapeutic interventions (Akbar et al., 2017). Along with that, CNB, a routine assessment method of musculoskeletal lesions, has been enhanced in its accuracy of diagnosis by adding immunohistochemical analysis, from a baseline of 74.4%–84.9% post-immunohistochemistry (Giarso et al., 2016). Hence, application of molecular tools not only enhances diagnostic precision but also creates opportunities for personalized treatment modalities in musculoskeletal disorders (Figure 10.9).

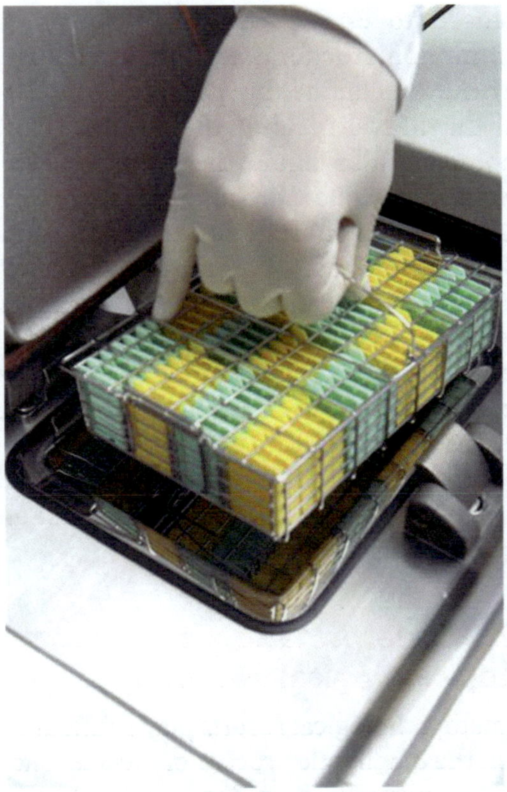

Figure 10.9. The integration of molecular techniques in histopathology has profoundly enhanced the diagnostic capabilities in musculoskeletal biopsies.

Source: https://www.leicabiosystems.com/sites/default/files/styles/720_tablet_portrait_fallback/public/media_image-file/2021-04/csm_inserting_basket__5_02_974c4a0100.jpg?itok=KOkxfyW1.

10.2.6. Role of Pathologists in Diagnosis

Pathologists are significant in the diagnosis of musculoskeletal conditions as they provide invaluable experience in the interpretation of biopsy specimens retrieved from various lesions. Specifically, techniques , such as CNB have become accepted practices for musculoskeletal tumor diagnosis with high accuracy rates. For instance, a study uncovered that CNB had a diagnostic accuracy rate of 74.4%, which increased to 84.9% with the incorporation of immunohistochemistry, highlighting the contributions made by pathologists toward ideal diagnostic results (Giarso et al., 2016). Pathologists also allow the determination of inflammatory conditions by methods , such as ultrasound-guided synovial biopsies with an 81.6% success rate in obtaining tissue. Such biopsies not only enhance disease pathology knowledge but also contribute significantly towards patient management through making definitive diagnoses in a majority of patients (Aurélie Najm et al., 2016). Pathologists are therefore a critical team member in the diagnostic process within musculoskeletal biopsy and histopathology.

10.2.7. Interpretation of Histopathological Findings

The histopathological results play a fundamental role in the diagnostic process of musculoskeletal diseases, particularly in determining benign or malignant lesions. Histopathology is literally a microscopic examination of tissue sections from biopsies wherein cellular structure and abnormal cell groups or inflammation markers can be detected. In chronic enteropathy among canine patients, for example, significant histopathological changes , such as increased eosinophils and ultrastructural damage to enterocytes have a pivotal role in making a diagnosis and maximizing appropriate dietary treatment (Alam et al., 2013). Similarly, musculoskeletal neoplasms can be reliably defined with more sophisticated imaging modalities , such as diffusion-weighted MRI, which maximize the precision of histopathological diagnoses by correlating imaging results with pathological results (Azad et al., 2024). The integration of histopathological interpretation and imaging studies is therefore essential to offer a comprehensive insight into musculoskeletal pathologies and guide effective treatment planning (Figure 10.10).

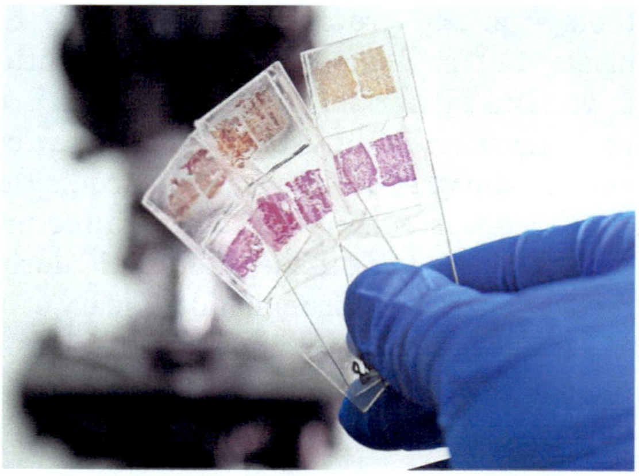

Figure 10.10. Histopathology provides a microscopic examination of tissue samples obtained from biopsies, allowing for the identification of cellular architecture and the presence of abnormal cell types or inflammatory markers.

Source: https://www.apexhospitals.com/_next/image?url=https%3A%2F%2Fbed.apexhospitals.com%2Fuploads%2Fhisto_b78d7b5894.jpg&w=1200&q=75.

10.2.8. Common Artifacts in Tissue Samples

In the area of musculoskeletal biopsy and histopathology, the accuracy of the diagnostic results is usually impaired by the common artifacts that arise while preparing tissue sampling. The artifacts, such as freezing artifacts, variation in fixation, and abnormalities in sectioning, tend to overshadow significant histological details that are important in diagnosis. As an illustration, in frozen section procedures, ice crystal formation may interfere with cellular architecture, leading to misinterpretation of tissue pathology (Kavitha, 2014).

In addition, fixation failure may result in inadequate nuclear staining or cytoplasmic artifact retention, complicating the differentiation between benign and malignant lesions (Felici et al., 2021). Awareness of these potential drawbacks is significant for surgeons and pathologists alike, as the development of artifacts can have a significant bearing on clinical decision-making, ultimately resulting in the quality of patient outcomes. It is therefore paramount to pay close attention to preprocessing so as to minimize such artifacts as well as enhance the integrity of musculoskeletal biopsy results.

10.2.9. Advances in Histopathological Technology

Advanced histopathological technology of recent times has dramatically altered the landscape of musculoskeletal biopsy and tissue diagnosis. Imaging techniques, such as reflectance confocal microscopy and optical coherence tomography enhance high-resolution, non-invasive tissue inspection, with increased diagnostic efficiency and accuracy.

Using these technologies, pathologists can optically view cellular morphology with previously unattainable resolution, allowing for earlier malignancy detection and treatment planning. Laser-based imaging tools have also emerged, offering real-time data on tumor vasculature and optimizing surgical planning—important factors in treating musculoskeletal tumors. While the techniques advance, their integration into routine practice has the promise of decreased patient distress and a shorter time gap from diagnosis to cure, catering to contemporary healthcare goals of speed and precision.

Additionally, institutions like the Instituto de Ciências Biomédicas de Abel Salazar are a pioneer in this work, highlighting the ongoing necessity of enhanced methodologies for histopathology (Amorim et al., 2014). Equipment designed for dermatologic use also provides valuable information, showing how imaging support devices can effectively guide surgical planning and follow-up treatment in musculoskeletal oncology (Figure 10.11).

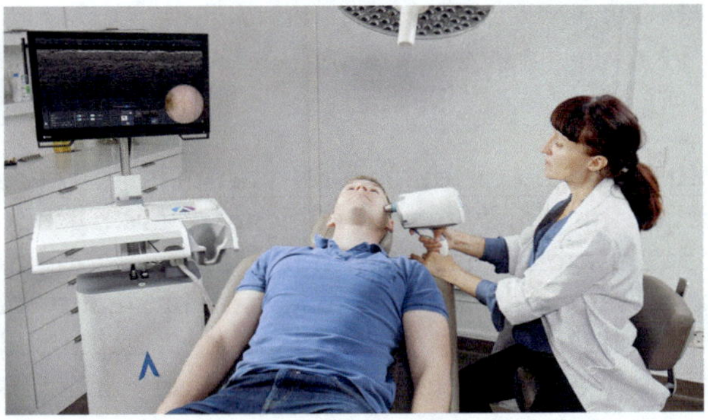

Figure 10.11. Enhanced imaging techniques , such as reflectance confocal microscopy and optical coherence tomography, allow for high-resolution, non-invasive examinations of tissue, significantly improving diagnostic accuracy and efficiency.

Source: https://www.mdpi.com/life/life-13-02268/article_deploy/html/images/life-13-02268-g001.png.

Test Your Knowledge

1. How do pathologists utilize immunohistochemistry in the diagnosis of inflammatory myopathies?
2. What histological features are typical of dermatomyositis versus polymyositis?

10.3. Common Musculoskeletal Disorders Diagnosed by Biopsy

Learning Outcome

1. Learn osteosarcoma;
2. Highlight Ewing's sarcoma;
3. Describe rheumatoid arthritis;
4. Summarize osteomyelitis, and soft tissue tumors;
5. Define degenerative joint diseases;
6. Identify inflammatory myopathies;
7. Define gout and crystal arthropathies;
8. Highlight metastatic bone disease.

Musculoskeletal disorders, particularly those requiring biopsy for final diagnosis, are a group of conditions that potentially have the ability to significantly compromise patient quality of life. The most common disorders diagnosed through a biopsy include inflammatory arthritis and systemic lupus erythematosus (SLE). The histopathological examination of the synovial tissue or other areas of damage allows for classification of the disease, with some patterns being obvious, e.g., prevalence of diffuse proliferative lupus nephritis in SLE patients, and can direct treatment (Karki et al., 2017).

Moreover, musculoskeletal manifestations of cancer and its immunotherapy also validate the role of biopsy. Immune-related toxicities, particularly of musculoskeletal origin, have been rising in number in patients undergoing these therapies and hence need rigorous histopathological evaluation to diagnose underlying situations (Puzanov et al., 2017). In general, these findings validate the pivotal position of biopsies in establishing accurate diagnoses and managing different musculoskeletal illnesses.

10.3.1. Osteosarcoma

Osteosarcoma, an underlying bone cancer that affects mostly young people and adolescents, poses significant diagnosis and treatment problems. The tumor develops in the metaphysis of long bones, making early detection challenging and necessitating precise histopathological tests. In this context, fine needle aspiration biopsy (FNAB) emerges as a significant diagnostic technique, which is easy with minimal procedure risk as opposed to core needle biopsy. Studies assessing its efficacy indicate a concordance rate of 60% in the diagnosis of tumors of bones, such as osteosarcoma, highlighting its significance in obtaining accurate diagnoses (Dewo et al., 2016). It is crucial that this diagnostic precision occurs, as timely intervention can remarkably transform patient outcomes. Therefore, enhancing the accuracy of FNAB in osteosarcoma through recurrent adjustment of methods and standards is essential in planning treatment and enhancing patient outcomes (Dewo et al., 2016) (Figure 10.12).

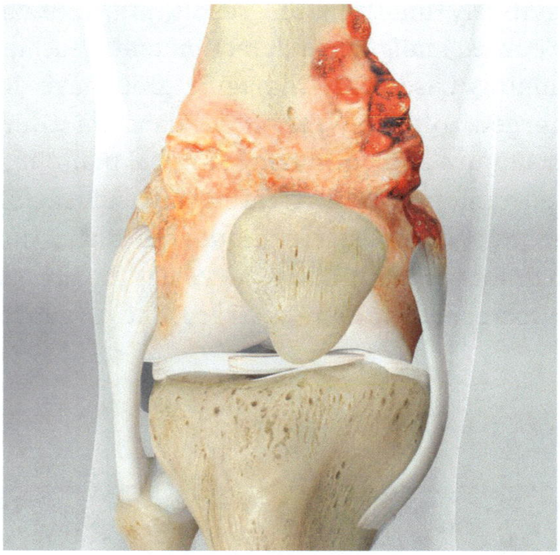

Figure 10.12. Osteosarcoma.

Source: https://d2yjegym0lbr1w.cloudfront.net/thumbs/osteosarcoma_1280.jpg?v=20191103.

10.3.2. Ewing's Sarcoma

Ewing's sarcoma, a malignant small round cell tumor of adolescents and young adults, necessitates accurate histopathological diagnosis to plan proper treatment. This tumor is most often seen in the limbs, spine, and pelvis bones and presents unique challenges in differentiation from other sarcomas. According to studies, biopsy procedures are important in obtaining representative tissue samples; the clinic-based biopsies' sensitivity has been reported to be comparable to theatre-based ones at 95.5% and 97.7% respectively (Ahmed et al., 2015). Furthermore, biopsy procedures undertaken at the clinic have been found to be safe and cost-reducing, with a clinical success rate of 94% compared to operating room biopsies, substantially reducing the costs of the procedure (Ahmed et al., 2015). This further attests to the worth of selecting appropriate biopsy modalities in the management of Ewing's sarcoma to promote patient outcome through timeliness and accuracy.

10.3.3. Rheumatoid Arthritis (RA)

RA is a severe problem in the field of musculoskeletal disorders, characterized by persistent inflammation and joint destruction. It is an autoimmune condition, commonly presenting itself through persistent synovitis with resulting grievous pain, joint deformity, and loss of function. Sophisticated understanding of the disease pathogenesis in recent years underlines the importance of examination of the synovial tissue. Synovial biopsy is now a major tool not only in the diagnosis of RA but also in evaluating the efficacy of treatment procedures. Ultrasound guidance has rendered these biopsies safer and more effective, and studies have indicated that they are as successful as 81.6% in recovering tissue and have an appreciable rate of certain diagnoses in certain cases (Najm et al., 2016). This indicates the potential of synovial tissue analysis to elucidate inflammatory mechanisms, directing future treatment to achieve disease remission, now at the center of modern RA management (Cope et al., 2016) (Figure 10.13).

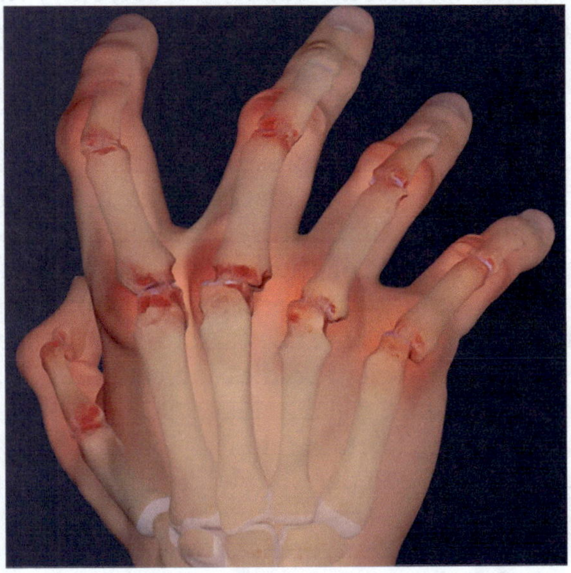

Figure 10.13. Rheumatoid arthritis (RA).

Source: https://integrativedoctorclinic.com/wp-content/uploads/2023/01/Rheumatoid-arthritis.jpg.

10.3.4. Osteomyelitis

Osteomyelitis, a bone inflammation caused by infection, is very difficult to diagnose and treat in musculoskeletal pathology. The success of image-guided core needle biopsy (ICNB) has also been particularly notable, as it was concluded that in 68.4% of the cases examined, osteomyelitis was diagnosed histopathologically, demonstrating the role of the biopsy in the diagnosis of the condition (Baker et al., 2024). Furthermore, the study determined that microbiological cultures were found to be positive in nearly 30% of cases, implying the difficulties in treating osteomyelitis efficiently. These observations are in agreement with the significance of adequate histopathological examination, as diagnostic mistakes can largely determine treatment plans for patients, as evidenced by the 9-40% rate of bone tumor misdiagnosis of cases under consideration (Carter et al., 2001). Thus, active multidisciplinary efforts remain valuable to enhance diagnostic quality in osteomyelitis cases.

10.3.5. Soft Tissue Tumors

Soft tissue tumors represent a heterogeneous category of neoplasms that can arise in various anatomical locations, with each location having unique challenges in their diagnosis. Diagnosis of such tumors can be critically dependent on biopsies that allow histopathological examination. Recent studies indicate that CNB has also been a reliable diagnostic procedure for musculoskeletal lesions, yielding 74.4% accuracy in comparison with post-excision histopathology, rising to 84.9% after the application of immunohistochemistry (Giarso et al., 2016).

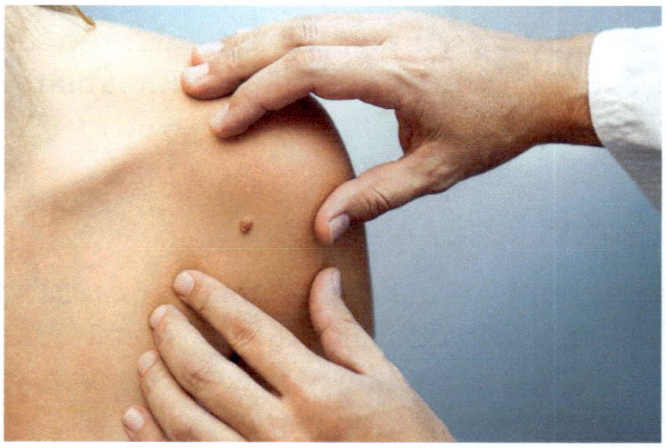

Figure 10.14. Soft tissue tumors represent a diverse group of neoplasms that can arise in various anatomical locations, posing unique diagnostic challenges.

Source: https://sa1s3optim.patientpop.com/assets/images/provider/photos/2576311.jpg.

On top of that, the role of advanced imaging modalities , such as CT-guided biopsies, has increasingly been realized and has been proven to be highly sensitive at 95.4% and specific at 85.7% in the diagnosis of primary bone tumors (Dominic et al., 2017). These measures demonstrate the importance of accuracy in the diagnosis of soft tissue tumors because precise histological evaluation is crucial in determining treatment plans and overall patient outcomes in musculoskeletal oncology (Figure 10.14).

10.3.6. Degenerative Joint Diseases

Degenerative joint diseases, characterized by progressive loss of joint components, represent a significant challenge in musculoskeletal health, particularly as they produce pain and loss of function. Histopathological diagnosis plays a crucial role in elucidation of the mechanisms underlying such disorders. For instance, the HMGB1 expression has been described in research as an important factor in tendinopathy, and its overexpression is linked to inflammatory pathways as well as matrix remodeling (Akbar et al., 2017). All these findings indicate the complex interplay between inflammatory mediators in degenerative diseases. In addition, Modic change studies in the spine illustrate the importance of histopathological examination for the elucidation of bone marrow lesions associated with disc degeneration and low back pain, demonstrating increased numbers of CD90-positive cells associated with inflammatory and fibrotic changes (Betz et al., 2022). These observations emphasize the utility of biopsies and histopathology in elucidating degenerative joint diseases.

10.3.7. Inflammatory Myopathies (IIM)

IIMs are a heterogeneous collection of autoimmune skeletal muscle disorders with muscle inflammation and accompanied by levels of weakness. Clinical findings, serologic markers, and histological findings are mainly employed in the diagnosis, which are important in differentiating IIM from other myopathies. Histopathologic examination has revealed typical patterns, including fibrosis and vascular changes, which may be important markers of the disease processes underlying (Agliano et al., 2016). Besides, as information on IIM continues to increase, treatment methods become increasingly sophisticated, with mechanisms increasingly specific to patients' individual autoantibody profiles as decided by biopsy assessment (Cooper et al., 2016). The problem in this case is the heterogeneity of such diseases since symptoms can overlap with non-inflammatory myopathies, hence the challenge in diagnosis and management. Effective management is not only measured by inflammation control but also by vigilance for associated complications, underscoring the specific value of musculoskeletal biopsy for that (Figure 10.15).

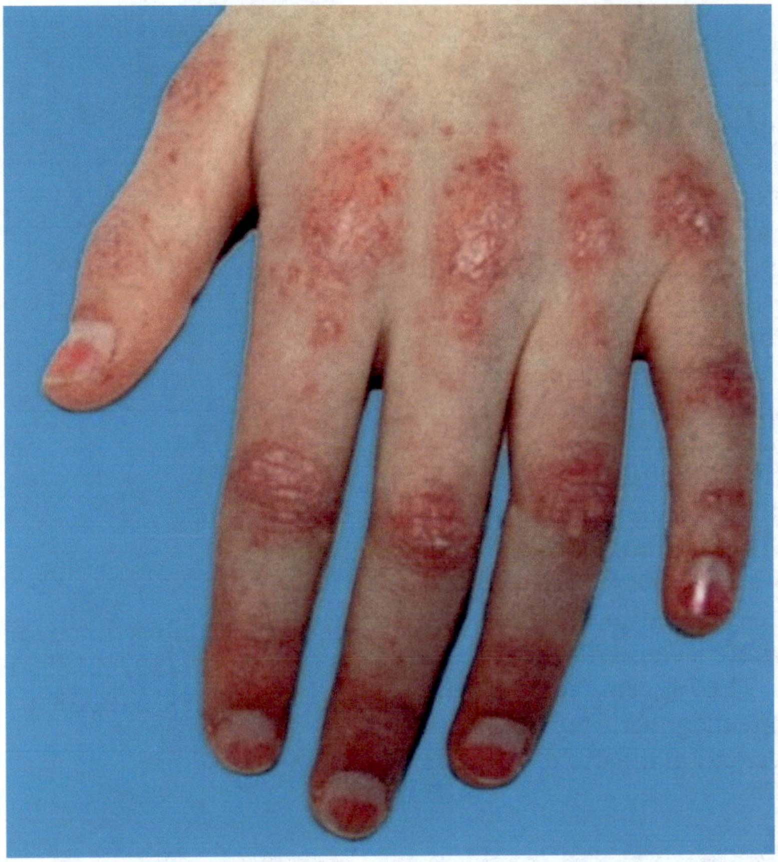

Figure 10.15. Inflammatory myopathies (IIM) represent a complex group of autoimmune skeletal muscle disorders characterized by muscle inflammation and varying degrees of weakness.

Source: https://elimrheumaticcentre.com/wp-content/uploads/2023/04/gottron1.jpg.

10.3.8. Gout and Crystal Arthropathies

Gout and crystal arthropathies are characterized by the deposition of monosodium urate crystals in the joints, leading to intense inflammation and pain. Because these conditions often present in the form of acute attacks of swelling and pain, synovial biopsy and histopathologic study have a key role in making the diagnosis and designing treatment. The utility of ultrasound-guided synovial biopsy has evolved into a primary method of obtaining tissue specimens among undifferentiated arthritic patients, with a high success rate of tissue procurement and meaningful histological results (Najm et al., 2016). Synovial tissue examination can also elucidate disease pathogenesis mechanisms and aid in the identification of typical histological patterns for specific arthropathies (Caporali et al., 2021). This combined approach is essential not only for the accurate diagnosis of gout and crystal arthropathies but also for the individualized therapeutic management to resist their debilitating effect.

10.3.9. Metastatic Bone Disease

Metastatic bone disease is a formidable clinical condition due to the complexity of its pathology and the patient care implications. This refers to cancer spread from an original site to the bone, leading to pain, fractures, and dysfunction. It is important to properly diagnose it since it will influence the treatment plan and prognostic evaluation. CNB is found to be a reliable method of making the diagnosis of musculoskeletal lesions, including metastatic disease, with a success rate of 74.4% against post-excision histopathology, with a further improvement when combined with immunohistochemical techniques (Giarso et al., 2016). Also, FNAC has been reported to be used in the diagnosis of bone tumors, where sensitivity was 90% and specificity was 91.67%, emphasizing the potential as a first-line diagnostic tool (Rathi et al., 2018). These advances in the use of biopsies are essential to the successful management of metastatic bone disease, allowing for both accurate diagnoses and early intervention (Figure 10.16).

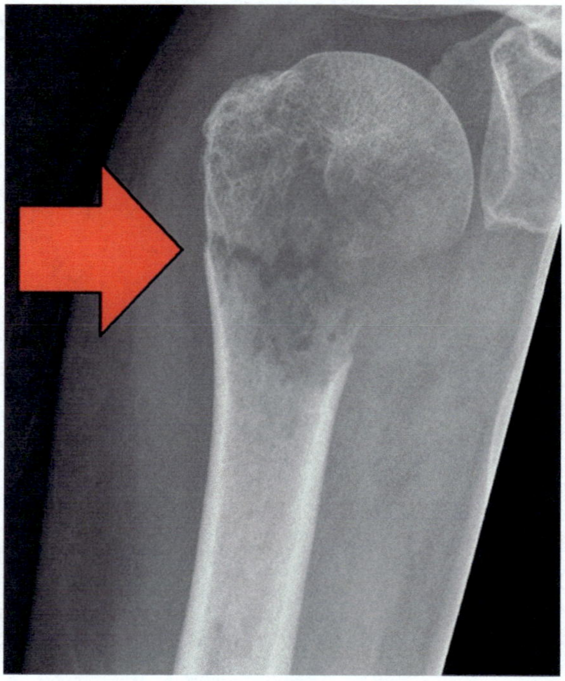

Figure 10.16. Metastatic bone disease.

Source: https://orthopaedia.com/wp-content/uploads/2023/10/a278b017-807e-4a0e-9273-908eafeb7715-1649987901703.png.

Test Your Knowledge

1. What are the characteristics of gout and pseudogout biopsies?
2. What are the histopathologic aspects of osteomyelitis?

10.4. Complications and Risks Associated with Biopsy

Learning Outcome

1. Focus on risk of infection;
2. Discuss bleeding complication;
3. Understand risk for nerve damage;
4. Describe management of post-biopsy pain;
5. Know psychological impact on patients;
6. Discuss misdiagnosis due to sampling error;
7. Focus on need for repeat biopsies;
8. Explain long-term effects of biopsy;
9. Identify methods for minimizing complications.

The biopsy process itself, although required for final diagnosis in musculoskeletal oncology, carries a large number of complications and risks that have to be carefully weighed. Open biopsies, although extremely accurate, have the risk of dissemination of tumor, particularly for aggressive malignancies , such as osteosarcoma. As pointed out in Roa (2006), the biopsy location is of prime concern, considering that the involved tract may be contaminated with the tumor, resulting in subsequent operations being more complex. Moreover, the risk of complications , such as infection, hemorrhage, and nerve injury presents an added threat to the procedure. However, FNAC, as noted in Rathi et al. (2018), can reduce some of the risks of surgery and provide immediate results, but cannot replace histopathological evaluation completely. Physicians need to be aware of such risks to make logical choices regarding the modality of biopsy to achieve minimum patient complications and maximum diagnostic yield.

10.4.1. Infection Risks

Risk of infection is a significant concern with musculoskeletal biopsy procedures because such procedures violate the skin barrier, which can be a gateway to pathogens in the body. Infection not only complicates the operative site but also affects patient outcomes in a negative way, particularly in osteosarcoma where tumor cells can contaminate the biopsy tract. A research reviewing biopsy tracts noted that in about 80.8% of the cases, there was no infiltration of the tumor, and it is likely that with proper technique, infection risk-related complications can be avoided, hence improving safety in limb-sparing operations (Roa, 2006). Additionally, a combined diagnostic modality based on ultrasonography and elastography has been demonstrated to improve the accuracy of tissue assessments, potentially decreasing the need for invasive biopsies, which carry inherent infection risk. This synergy of diagnostic precision with fewer invasive procedures is necessary for maintaining patient safety as well as effective treatment plans (Bagri et al., 2020) (Figure 10.17).

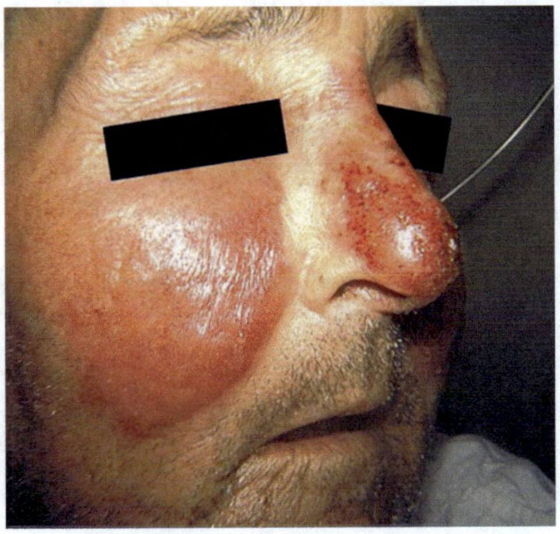

Figure 10.17. The risk of infection is a significant concern in musculoskeletal biopsy procedures, as these interventions breach the skin barrier, potentially allowing pathogens to enter the body.

Source: https://www.id.theclinics.com/cms/10.1016/j.idc.2020.10.011/asset/278be946-17d7-40ff-8b2d-22b311b19b70/main.assets/gr3_lrg.jpg.

10.4.2. Bleeding Complications

The possibility of hemorrhagic complications is a consideration in musculoskeletal biopsies, particularly with the risks inherent from interposing with vascular tissues in close proximity to bone tumors. Although the complication rate of CT-guided biopsies has been reported to be quite low at 4.3%, the impact of even minimal bleeding can significantly alter patient outcome, especially if the lesion was large or near important anatomy (Dominic et al., 2017). Moreover, veterinary medicine research confirms that while procedures like FNAB and tissue-core biopsy (TCB) yield high rates of diagnosis, minor hemorrhage complications occur in approximately 30.6% of instances (Felici et al., 2021). This is important in highlighting careful pre-procedure assessment and the necessity of strictly monitoring post-operative times in order to successfully manage and avoid bleeding complications. Awareness of these factors is essential in order to enhance patient safety in the diagnostic process.

10.4.3. Nerve Damage Potential

Risk of musculoskeletal biopsy and histopathology is one of the significant risks of damaging nerves, resulting in painful complications and impaired function. The risk of inadvertently damaging nearby nerves during the procedure makes precise anatomical knowledge and imaging skills imperative. For instance, schwannomas, the tumors that grow from nerve sheath cells but are benign, can lead to increased pain and sensory alterations due to their proximity to peripheral nerves. The tumors are responsible for a few upper limb tumors, but they show the need for accurate appraisal in a biopsy situation because they can be mistaken for ganglion cysts (Roa, 2006). In addition, improvement in ultrasound imaging technology has enhanced visualization of nerve structures during procedures, and that can reduce the incidence of nerve complications. Thus, achieving an equilibrium between diagnostic efficiency and minimal nerve damage is paramount to achieve the best patient results for musculoskeletal biopsies (Figure 10.18).

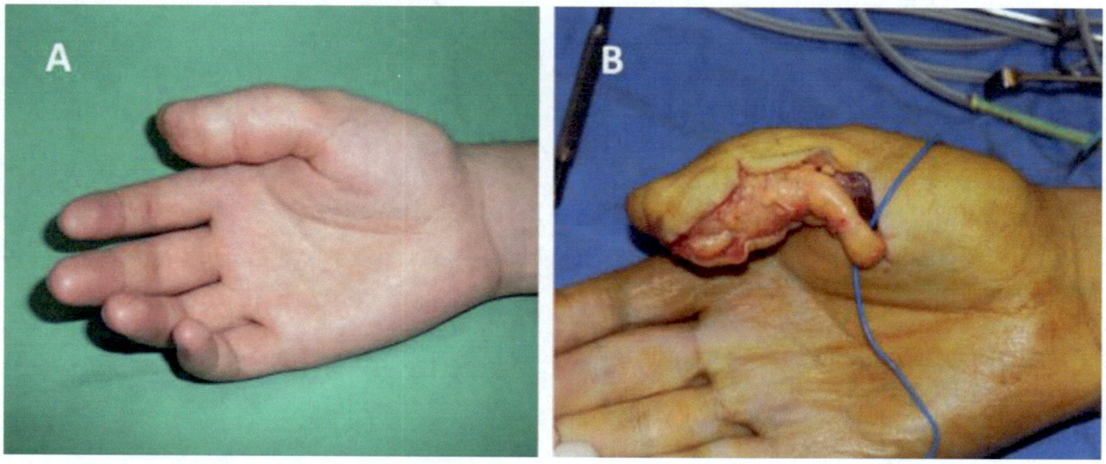

Figure 10.18. Schwannomas of the upper limb.

Source: https://www.mdpi.com/diagnostics/diagnostics-12-01319/article_deploy/html/images/diagnostics-12-01319-g001.png.

10.4.4. Pain Management Post-biopsy

Post-musculoskeletal biopsy, effective pain management is needed to prevent patient discomfort and facilitate healing. The procedure generally induces varying degrees of pain, primarily dependent upon the location of the biopsy and technique employed. Relief of pain initially is typically the administration of analgesics, i.e., nonsteroidal anti-inflammatory agents (NSAIDs) or opioids, titrated to the individual's pain threshold and expected post-procedure pain. In addition, multidisciplinary care with the incorporation of physical therapy and patient counseling in managing expectations and activity restrictions can be applied to maximize pain management methods. Early detection and intervention are necessary, especially because some patients may develop immune-related adverse events (irAEs) complicating recovery, particularly those being treated for malignancies. Detailed guidelines, as highlighted by the Society for Immunotherapy of Cancer for the management of toxicity, emphasize the importance of a multi-disciplinary approach to effectively address these concerns (Puzanov et al., 2017; Hospital et al., 2023).

10.4.5. Psychological Impact on Patients

The psychological impact of musculoskeletal biopsies on the patients can be tremendous, such as fear, uncertainty, and even depression. Getting a biopsy typically triggers anxiety about potential diagnoses, especially in diseases with complex presentations beyond simple musculoskeletal symptoms (Both et al., 2017). The patients always question the implications of their biopsy results on their trajectory of health, thus higher levels of stress. Moreover, the results concerning Modic changes in bone marrow can increase concern as they include chronic disability and pain (Betz et al., 2022). Psychological impacts are not to be underestimated; they can affect the general quality of life and compliance with treatment. Therefore, healthcare workers need to address such emotional components, offering patients coping skills and proper information, empowering them in the ambiguity inherent in diagnostic procedures and chronic disease (Figure 10.19).

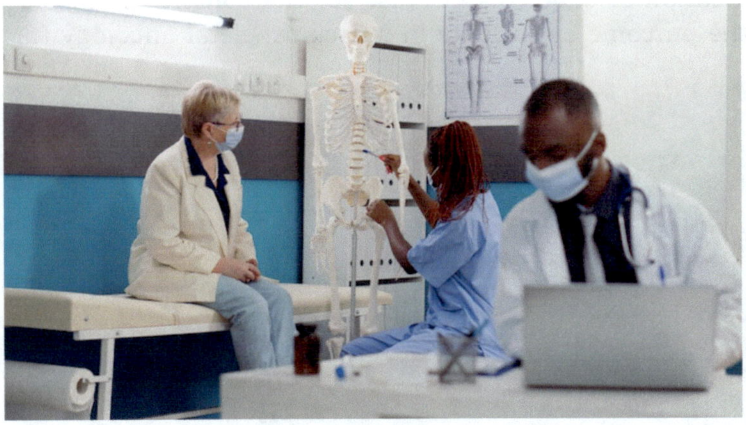

Figure 10.19. The psychological impact of musculoskeletal biopsies on patients can be profound, encompassing anxiety, uncertainty, and even depression.

Source: https://img.freepik.com/free-photo/old-woman-nurse-with-face-masks-analyzing-human-skeleton-bones-osteopathy-consultation-medical-worker-explaining-orthopedic-diagnosis-anatomy-spinal-cord-checkup-visit_482257-48507.jpg?semt=ais_hybrid&w=740.

10.4.6. Misdiagnosis Due to Sampling Error

Misdiagnosis in musculoskeletal conditions is most often due to sampling error during biopsies, which has the potential to significantly influence patient outcomes. With histopathological assessment based on a small sample size, the chances of missing crucial tumor characteristics increase, leading to underdiagnosis or misclassification. For instance, in differentiating lipomas and well-differentiated liposarcomas, it was found in one study that MRI diagnoses agreed with end pathology only 69% of the time because it described the diagnostic difficulty presented by overlapping imaging findings (Eward et al., 2013). This is an even more serious mistake where sampling fails to accurately represent tumor heterogeneity, since a biopsy that is too small may miss malignant tissue behind, which might have distinctive histological findings. Hence, increased recognition of sampling practices and stringent assessments are imperative to enhance diagnostic performance and minimize the risk of misdiagnosis in musculoskeletal biopsies (Sternheim et al., 2013). By embracing better practices, clinicians will be able to cope more effectively with the challenges posed by sampling errors in histopathology.

10.4.7. Need for Repeat Biopsies

The need for repeat biopsies in the context of musculoskeletal tumors emphasizes the intricacies of correct diagnosis. Though percutaneous core needle biopsy (PCNB) has been shown to have a high diagnostic rate of 93.4% and a staggering accuracy rate of 97.9% (Kumar et al., 2024), there are certain cases where initial attempts provide inconclusive results. These are the cases where repeat biopsies are useful in order to arrive at final diagnoses, as they are more likely to provide the needed clarity provided by preliminary samples. Similarly, FNAB likewise was proven to have adequate sensitivity and specificity with a total accuracy of 83% (Sumpono et al., 2024). However, its tendency to be misleading in the case of lesions showing similar morphologic features warrants greater consideration for ambiguous cases. The significance of the repeat biopsies is thus important not only for the verification of diagnosis but also for the construction of future treatment plans, ultimately affecting the outcome of patients in musculoskeletal oncology (Figure 10.20).

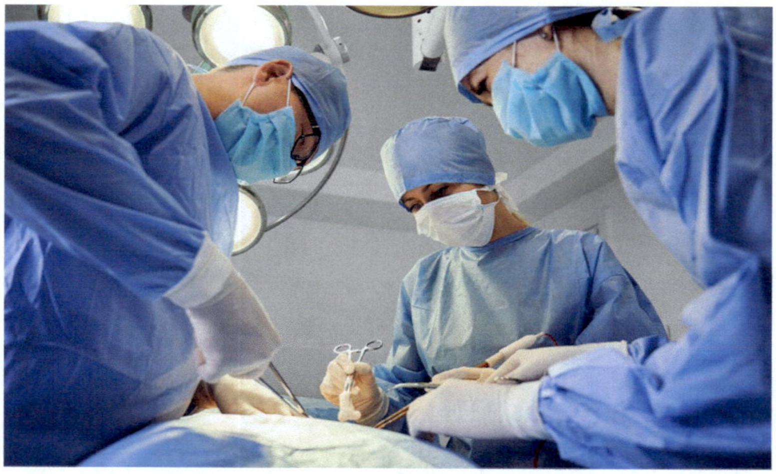

Figure 10.20. Need for repeat biopsies.

Source: https://www.emjreviews.com/wp-content/uploads/2024/10/WN2-16.jpg.

10.4.8. Long-term Effects of Biopsy

The long-term effects of musculoskeletal biopsy procedures extend beyond short-term diagnostic benefit to affect both the physiological and functional results in patients. Therapeutic interventions , such as limb-sparing surgery in soft tissue sarcomas, demonstrate how biopsy results can inform treatment modalities that seek to preserve function without jeopardizing oncological security. For instance, studies show that patients receiving classifications of nerve involvement at the time of biopsy can do well, with a first-line limb salvage rate of 100% in certain groups, attesting to the central role of biopsy in surgical planning (Tamimi, 2020). Conversely, use of adjunct treatments, such as platelet-rich plasma (PRP) plus surgery, calls to attention potential complications; while PRP is used to promote recovery, evidence shows that it actually has the opposite effect and suppresses tissue vascularity and apoptotic cell numbers without improving clinical gains (Carr et al., 2015). The role of biopsy in the management of musculoskeletal disorders is thus complex, and its use calls for careful consideration in treatment.

10.4.9. Strategies to Minimize Complications

Complications in musculoskeletal biopsy and histopathology should be avoided to provide the optimal patient outcome. Proper pre-operative assessment is a must and facilitates an assessment of possible risks in an individual patient, particularly if there exist associated comorbidities. The employment of advanced imaging techniques, i.e., MRI and ultrasound, makes it possible to precisely localize the lesion, and thus reduces the possibility of damaging nearby tissues while obtaining the biopsy. Also, application of limb-sparing surgical modalities, especially in the case of neurovascular, has been observed to yield satisfactory oncological outcomes with enhancement in functional recovery (Tamimi, 2020). Further, maintaining a multidisciplinary practice, including inter-profession collaboration among orthopedic surgeons, radiologists, and pathologists, ensures appropriate communication regarding patient care, thereby avoiding post-operative complications (Aga Khan University Hospital et al., 2023). Finally, all these measures come together to improve patient safety and reduce adverse outcome rates in musculoskeletal biopsy procedures (Figure 10.21).

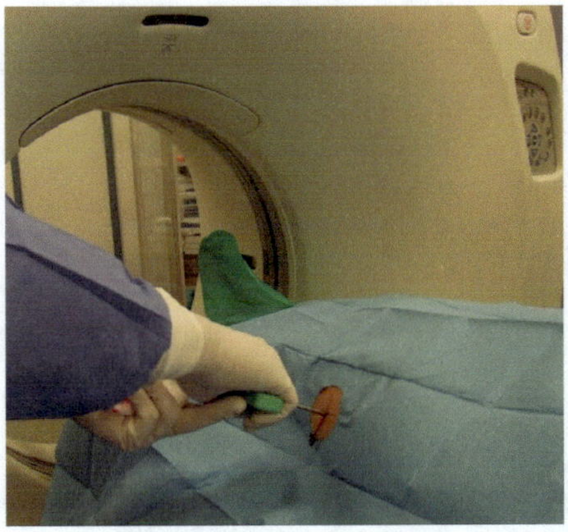

Figure 10.21. Minimizing complications during musculoskeletal biopsy and histopathology is paramount for ensuring optimal patient outcomes.

Source: https://onlinelibrary.wiley.com/cms/asset/24065dbd-e21d-4cc7-8924-55a82eaca42d/tswj538152-fig-0002d-m.jpg.

Test Your Knowledge

1. What are the risks of nerve damage in soft tissue biopsy?
2. How can a suboptimal biopsy technique lead to non-diagnostic or misleading diagnoses?

Summary

The advancement in musculoskeletal biopsy techniques, particularly CNB and CT-guided biopsy, has significantly enhanced diagnostic accuracy for musculoskeletal tumors and thus patient care. As documented by recent studies, CNB has an accuracy of 74.4%, rising to 84.9% when supplemented with immunohistochemistry, and a superb sensitivity of 98% for benign and malignant lesions (Giarso et al., 2016). Further, CT-guided biopsies are highly effective in their yield, with a sensitivity of 95.4% and specificity of 85.7% as reported, making it a good predictor of primary bone tumors (Dominic et al., 2017). It implies that, with proper diagnostic methods, clinicians are able to better differentiate between tumor types, thereby leading to focused treatment. Continued evaluation and development of musculoskeletal biopsy techniques are necessary to enhance the accuracy and efficacy of tumor diagnoses in clinical practice.

KEY TERMS FROM THIS CHAPTER

- Musculoskeletal system
- Joints
- Connective tissues
- Elastography
- Fine needle aspiration
- Musculoskeletal lesions
- Image-guided biopsy
- Histopathology
- Incisional biopsy
- Bones
- Muscles
- Tumors
- Specialization
- Core needle biopsy (CNB)
- Open biopsy surgery
- Excisional biopsy
- Benign tumors

Critical Thinking Questions

1. **Which of the following is a common indication for rheumatology muscle biopsy?**
   a. Gout diagnosis
   b. Systemic lupus erythematosus
   c. Polymyositis or dermatomyositis
   d. Rheumatoid arthritis
2. **Which histological finding is characteristic of dermatomyositis?**
   a. Endomysial inflammation with $CD8^+$ T cells
   b. Non-caseating granulomas
   c. Perifascicular atrophy
   d. Ragged red fibers
3. **A bone biopsy showing "mosaic" lamellar bone pattern is diagnostic of:**
   a. Osteoporosis
   b. Osteomalacia
   c. Paget's disease of bone
   d. Osteoarthritis
4. **Synovial biopsy in rheumatoid arthritis typically reveals:**
   a. Normal synovial lining
   b. Suppurative inflammation
   c. Hyperplastic synovium with lymphoid aggregates
   d. Caseating granulomas
5. **Which biopsy technique is most appropriate for evaluating suspected vasculitis affecting muscle?**
   a. Fine-needle aspiration
   b. Incisional muscle biopsy
   c. Core needle biopsy of bone
   d. Bone marrow biopsy

Short Answer Questions

1. What are the different types of musculoskeletal biopsies (e.g., needle, core, open, incisional)?
2. Under what circumstances is a core needle biopsy preferable to an open biopsy?
3. What kinds of staining methods are used to evaluate muscle pathology (e.g., H&E, trichrome, NADH)?
4. What are the key features met in a rheumatoid arthritis patient's synovial biopsy?
5. What are the classical histological features of inclusion body myositis (IBM)?
6. How is giant cell arteritis diagnosed via biopsy?
7. What are the most common complications of musculoskeletal biopsy procedures?
8. How does bleeding risk vary between muscle and bone biopsies?

Answers to Critical Thinking Questions

1. (c); 2. (c); 3. (c); 4. (c); 5. (b)

References

1. Puzanov, I., Diab, A., Abdallah, K., Bingham, C. O., 3rd, Brogdon, C., Dadu, R., Hamad, L., Kim, S., Lacouture, M. E., LeBoeuf, N. R., Lenihan, D., Onofrei, C., Shannon, V., Sharma, R., Silk, A. W., Skondra, D., Suarez-Almazor, M. E., Wang, Y., Wiley, K., Kaufman, H. L., ... Society for Immunotherapy of Cancer Toxicity Management Working Group (2017). Managing toxicities associated with immune checkpoint inhibitors: consensus recommendations from the Society for Immunotherapy of Cancer (SITC) Toxicity Management Working Group. *Journal for immunotherapy of cancer*, *5*(1), 95. https://doi.org/10.1186/s40425-017-0300-z(accessed on 17th June 2025).
2. Aga Khan University Hospital, Karachi. (2023). *LABRAD: Vol 48, Issue 1–July 2023*. https://core.ac.uk/download/578442137.pdf (accessed on 17th June 2025).
3. Agliano,' M., Chirico, C., Corallo, C., Cutolo, M., et al. (2016). Histopathological findings in systemic sclerosis-related myopathy: Fibrosis and microangiopathy. https://core.ac.uk/download/84485025.pdf (accessed on 17th June 2025).
4. Ahmed, W., Kadir, M. M., Mohib, Y., Rashid, R., et al. (2015). Clinic-based biopsy with a small curette: Is it a reliable and safe option in extremity tumors? https://core.ac.uk/download/84855134.pdf (accessed on 17th June 2025).
5. Ahmed, W., Mohib, Y., Rashid, R. H., Umer, M., et al. (2015). Clinic-based biopsy vs. theatre biopsy of bone and soft tissue extremity tumors: Comparable diagnostic modalities. https://core.ac.uk/download/84854887.pdf (accessed on 17th June 2025).
6. Akbar, M., Crowe, L. A. N., Garcia-Melchor, E., Gilchrist, D. S., et al. (2017). Targeting danger molecules in tendinopathy: The HMGB1/TLR4 axis. https://core.ac.uk/download/84340439.pdf (accessed on 17th June 2025).
7. Al Azad, M. S., Chowdhury, P., Karki, B. P., Rahman, S., et al. (2024). Accuracy of diffusion-weighted magnetic resonance imaging in diagnosing malignant musculoskeletal tumors. https://core.ac.uk/download/613693867.pdf (accessed on 17th June 2025).
8. Alam, S., Allenspach, K., Batt, R., Biempica, E., et al. (2013). A comprehensive pathological survey of duodenal biopsies from dogs with diet-responsive chronic enteropathy. https://core.ac.uk/download/36777044.pdf (accessed on 17th June 2025).
9. Alva, N. K., Harish, K., & Janaki, M. G. (2004). "Primary" aggressive chondroblastoma of the humerus: A case report. https://core.ac.uk/download/pdf/3459230.pdf (accessed on 17th June 2025).
10. Amorim, I., Caseiro, A. R., Da Silva Bartolo, P. J., Gartner, A., et al. (2014). Cell therapy with human MSCs isolated from the umbilical cord Wharton jelly associated to a PVA membrane in the treatment of chronic skin wounds. https://core.ac.uk/download/pdf/24067325.pdf (accessed on 17th June 2025).
11. Ansari, M. Y., Qaraqe, M., Righetti, R., Serpedin, E., & Qaraqe, K. (2023). Unveiling the future of breast cancer assessment: A critical review on generative adversarial networks in elastography ultrasound. *Frontiers in Oncology, 13*. https://doi.org/10.3389/fonc.2023.1282536 (accessed on 17th June 2025).
12. Bagri, N., Baloji, A., Chandra, R., K., et al. (2020). Diagnostic accuracy of an integrated approach

using conventional ultrasonography, and Doppler and strain elastography in the evaluation of superficial soft tissue lesions. https://core.ac.uk/download/344355268.pdf (accessed on 17th June 2025).

13. Baker, J. C., Dettorre, G. M., Gandra, S., George, J., et al. (2024). Diagnostic efficacy and clinical impact of image-guided core needle biopsy of suspected vertebral osteomyelitis. https://core.ac.uk/download/643771785.pdf (accessed on 17th June 2025).

14. Behera, S. S., Kumar, N. N., Ray, C. S., Sahoo, S., et al. (2024). Management of extracranial schwannomas in head and neck region–An observational study. https://core.ac.uk/download/613707956.pdf (accessed on 17th June 2025).

15. Betz, M., Brunner, F., Distler, O., Dudli, S., et al. (2022). CD90-positive stromal cells associate with inflammatory and fibrotic changes in Modic changes. https://www.zora.uzh.ch/id/eprint/224699/1/1_s2.0_S2665913122000553_main.pdf (accessed on 17th June 2025).

16. Bodla, A. K., Peddamadyam, S., Krishna, V., Kancherla, N. R., Nayak, K. N., Cherukuri, N., & Uppin, S. (2024). An image-guided percutaneous core needle biopsy for accurate assessment of musculoskeletal tumors: A targeted diagnosis. *Cureus, 16*. https://www.semanticscholar.org/paper/330d846d484875ae2db859fd0cf5ab7df9745320 (accessed on 17th June 2025).

17. Both, T. (T.), van Daele, P. L. A., Dalm, V. A. S. H., Hagen, M., et al. (2017). Reviewing primary Sjögren's syndrome: Beyond the dryness–aFrom pathophysiology to diagnosis and treatment. https://core.ac.uk/download/154414050.pdf (accessed on 17th June 2025).

18. Caporali, R., Coletto, L., Compagnoni, R., Ingegnoli, F., et al. (2021). The crucial questions on synovial biopsy: When, why, who, what, where, and how? https://core.ac.uk/download/603235514.pdf (accessed on 17th June 2025).

19. Carr, A., Murphy, R., Dakin, S., Rombach, I., et al. (2015). Platelet-rich plasma injection with arthroscopic acromioplasty for chronic rotator cuff tendinopathy: A randomized controlled trial. https://core.ac.uk/download/35283358.pdf (accessed on 17th June 2025).

20. Carter, S. R., Grimer, R. J., Sneath, R. S., Spooner, D., et al. (2001). Diagnosing musculoskeletal tumors. https://core.ac.uk/download/pdf/8062968.pdf (accessed on 17th June 2025).

21. Cleary, R., Li, L., Lucas, M., Mathieson, L., et al. (2017). Ultrasonic needles for bone biopsy. https://core.ac.uk/download/74230568.pdf (accessed on 17th June 2025).

22. Cooper, R., Lilleker, J., & Murphy, S. (2016). Selected aspects of the current management of myositis. https://core.ac.uk/download/74197598.pdf (accessed on 17th June 2025).

23. Cope, A., Filkova, M., Galloway, J., Mant, T., et al. (2016). Is there a role of synovial biopsy in drug development? https://core.ac.uk/download/77066279.pdf (accessed on 17th June 2025).

24. Dewo, P. (P.), Lanodiyu, Z. (Z.), Magetsari, R. (R.), Marseno, D., et al. (2016). Accuration of fine needle aspiration biopsy in musculoskeletal tumour. https://media.neliti.com/media/publications/300741-accuration-of-fine-needle-aspiration-bio-a1b11c75.pdf (accessed on 17th June 2025).

25. Dominic, K. P., Dijoe, D., & Toms, J. (2017). A retrospective analysis of computed tomography guided biopsy in the diagnosis of primary bone tumors. *International Journal of Research in Orthopaedics, 3*(3), 569–572. https://doi.org/10.18203/issn.2455-4510.IntJResOrthop20171903(accessed on 17th June 2025).

26. Eward, W. C., Ferguson, P. C., Griffin, A. M., O'Donnell, P. W., et al. (2013). Can experienced

observers differentiate between lipoma and well-differentiated liposarcoma using only MRI? https://core.ac.uk/download/232564543.pdf (accessed on 17th June 2025).

27. Felici, A., Ghiraldelli, A., Dettori, A., Miglio, A., Del Signore, F., Simeoni, F., Falerno, I., et al. (2021). Clinical value of CT-guided fine needle aspiration and tissue-core biopsy of thoracic masses in the dog and cat. https://core.ac.uk/download/534179724.pdf (accessed on 17th June 2025).

28. Giarso, P., Kamal, A. F., & Siregar, N. C. (2016). Accuracy of Core Needle Biopsy for Musculoskeletal Lesion in Cipto Mangunkusumo Hospital Jakarta. *eJournal Kedokteran Indonesia, 4*(1). https://doi.org/10.23886/ejki.4.5901.8-14(accessed on 17th June 2025).

29. Gurumurthy, B., Pramod, B. M., Sujanatheja, J. S., et al. (2023). Diagnostic dilemma: Schwannoma or ganglion cyst. https://core.ac.uk/download/595817252.pdf (accessed on 17th June 2025).

30. Karki, S., Kayastha, G. K., Pandey, B., Poudyal, N., et al. (2017). Histopathological findings of renal biopsy in systemic lupus erythematosus. https://core.ac.uk/download/228863289.pdf (accessed on 17th June 2025).

31. Kavitha, K. (2014). Validation of frozen section in intraoperative decision making in malignancies. https://core.ac.uk/download/288215552.pdf (accessed on 17th June 2025).

32. Najm, A., Beaulé, B. L. G., Orr, C., Della Beffa, C., Veale, D. J., Forestier, R., et al. (2016). Success rate and utility of ultrasound-guided synovial biopsies in clinical practice. https://core.ac.uk/download/59921584.pdf (accessed on 17th June 2025).

33. Oikonomidis, I., & Tsouloufi, T. (2021). Diagnostic accuracy of cytology for canine osteosarcoma compared to histopathology. https://core.ac.uk/download/429844935.pdf (accessed on 17th June 2025).

34. Rathi, M., Sharma, S. P., Singh, P., Tyagi, R., et al. (2018). Incidence of bone tumors and tumor-like lesions at a tertiary center–A study of 64 cases. https://core.ac.uk/download/539909936.pdf (accessed on 17th June 2025).

35. Roa, M. (2006). The incidence of malignant infiltration in human osteosarcoma biopsy tract. https://core.ac.uk/download/333873488.pdf (accessed on 17th June 2025).

36. Senneville, É., Albalawi, Z., van Asten, S. A. V., Abbas, Z. G., Allison, G., Aragón-Sánchez, J., Embil, J. M., et al. (2023). IWGDF/IDSA guidelines on the diagnosis and treatment of diabetes-related foot infections (IWGDF/IDSA 2023). *Clinical Infectious Diseases.* https://doi.org/10.1093/cid/ciad527 (accessed on 17th June 2025).

37. Sternheim, A., Griffin, A. M., Wunder, J. S., White, L. M., O'Donnell, P. W., Ferguson, P. C., & Eward, W. C. (2013). Can experienced observers differentiate between lipoma and well-differentiated liposarcoma using only MRI? https://core.ac.uk/download/193691648.pdf (accessed on 17th June 2025).

38. Sumpono, A. S., Yunus, J., Krisnugraha, Y., & Dwianingsih, E. (2024). The accuracy of fine needle aspiration biopsy (FNAB) in diagnosing musculoskeletal lesion. *Indonesian Journal of Biomedicine and Clinical Sciences.* https://www.semanticscholar.org/paper/3fbd53295f5c111d9fc62503bc49724495e3613b (accessed on 17th June 2025).

39. Tamimi, N. N. (2020). Results of limb-sparing surgery of soft tissue sarcoma of the lower extremity with sciatic nerve involvement. https://core.ac.uk/download/287790231.pdf (accessed on 17th June 2025).

CLINICAL PHARMACOLOGY IN RHEUMATIC DISEASES

11

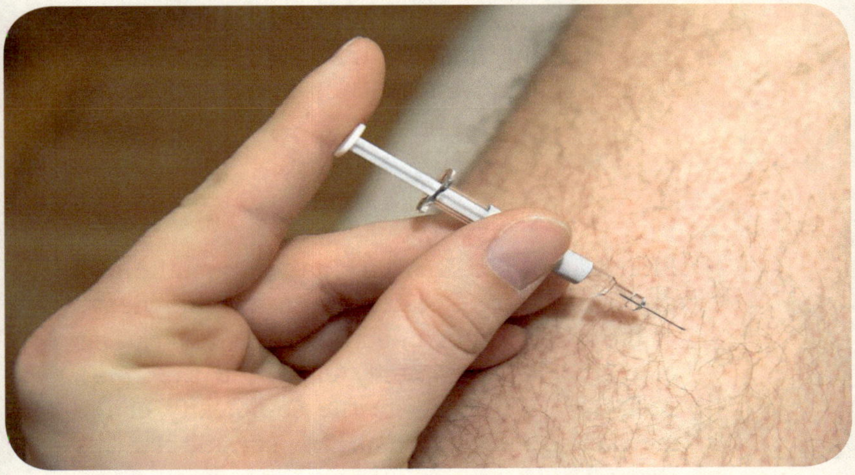

LEARNING OBJECTIVES

After studying this chapter, you will be able to:

1. Understand mechanisms of action of pharmacological agents;
2. Explain pharmacotherapy in individual rheumatic diseases;
3. Discuss safety profiles and adverse effects;
4. Know future directions in clinical pharmacology.

Introduction

Clinical pharmacology plays a pivotal role in the treatment of rheumatic diseases, which encompass a vast array of inflammatory disorders of joints and connective tissues. The sophisticated interaction between pharmacotherapy and patient-specific factors necessitates a comprehensive understanding of drug action, dosing, and interactions. Indeed, contemporary evidence has highlighted the importance of prescription behavior in this context; therefore, while gastroprotective drugs are crucial in preventing NSAID-induced gastrointestinal lesions, their prescribed doses under real practice are often lower than recommended by guidelines, indicating a discrepancy in clinical practice (Bilušić et al., 2006). Secondly, the pursuit of novel therapeutic options shows the ongoing need for effective pharmacological therapies. This is particularly the case where investigators seek to optimize treatment results through the identification of drugs that can be optimized for specific patient groups, further improving all-around outcomes for patients suffering from such challenging conditions (Alturkmani et al., 2016).

11.1. Mechanisms of Action of Pharmacological Agents

Learning Outcome

1. Appreciate an overview of drug mechanisms in rheumatic diseases;
2. Define non-steroidal anti-inflammatory drugs (NSAIDs);
3. Highlight disease-modifying antirheumatic drugs (DMARDs);
4. Define biologic agents and their targets;
5. Educate on corticosteroids and their pharmacodynamics;
6. Acknowledge analgesic role in pain relief;
7. Understand new therapy mechanisms of action;
8. Define pharmacogenomics in rheumatic disease treatment;
9. Define drug interaction and implications.

The mechanisms of action of pharmacologic agents used in the treatment of rheumatic diseases are diverse, yet centrally related to the inflammatory pathways that underlie these diseases. Tumor necrosis factor inhibitors (TNFi), for instance, are pivotal in modulating immune responses by selectively binding to and neutralizing TNF-alpha, one of the major cytokines of inflammation, which reduces disease activity and risk of radiographic progression in psoriatic arthritis (Mantravadi et al., 2017). Besides, the clinical significance of the pharmacokinetics of TNFi can be helpful in personalizing treatment to the individual patient, taking into consideration the heterogeneity of drug response due to immunogenicity (Mantravadi et al., 2017). Similarly, spa treatment and mud-bath treatment are found to exert therapeutic effects on knee osteoarthritis that enhance the quality of life by reducing pain and functional impairment by non-surgical means. The combined findings of these observations highlight the multidimensionality of treatment strategies for rheumatic diseases (Figure 11.1).

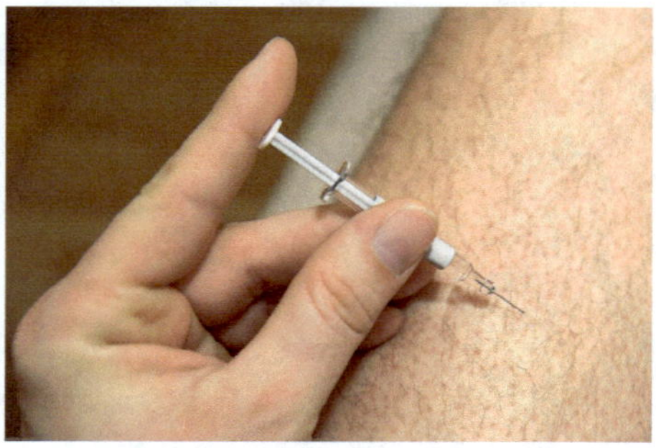

Figure 11.1. Tumor necrosis factor.

Source: https://cdn-prod.medicalnewstoday.com/content/images/articles/324/324841/person-being-given-injection-into-thigh.jpg.

11.1.1. Overview of Drug Mechanisms in Rheumatic Diseases

Pharmacological treatment of rheumatic diseases is largely founded on the knowledge of the mechanisms of action of various classes of medicines. Commonly employed therapies, such as TNFi, illustrate the complexity of the mechanisms in conditions like psoriatic arthritis (PsA). TNFi have also been shown to significantly influence the outcomes of therapy by suppressing inflammatory pathways to reduce symptomatic burden and inhibit radiographic progression in involved joints (Mantravadi et al., 2017).

Disease-modifying antirheumatic drugs (DMARDs) and non-steroidal anti-inflammatory drugs (NSAIDs) also play a role in preventing inflammation and pain in numerous rheumatic diseases, such as osteoarthritis (OA). The efficacy of these medications is typically patient by patient and with the occurrence of comorbidities, which continue to pose ongoing challenges to pharmacotherapy. For these reasons, continued research into the pharmacokinetics and potential immunogenicity of these medications continues to be important to optimize treatment modalities and improve patient quality of life (Ceccarelli et al., 2018).

11.1.2. Non-steroidal Anti-inflammatory Drugs (NSAIDs)

Their application has been a standard in the management of rheumatic disorders, particularly those characterized by chronic inflammation and pain, such as OA. Given that about 65% of OA patients in the United States are treated with NSAIDs, their efficacy to improve pain and physical function is well established (Conway et al., 2021). But the benefits of NSAIDs are often countered by the risk of severe adverse effects, including gastrointestinal complications, renal failure, and cardiovascular incidents. For instance, there is evidence that while knowledge of potential gastrointestinal side effects due to NSAIDs is high with medical professionals, the practice of guidelines for gastroprotection is poor. In studies, few risk NSAID users were administered gastroprotectives in the recommended dosage, indicating a lack of optimal patient care (Bilušić et al., 2006). Therefore, the balance process between maximum pain relief and safety remains a fundamental issue in rheumatological clinical pharmacology (Figure 11.2).

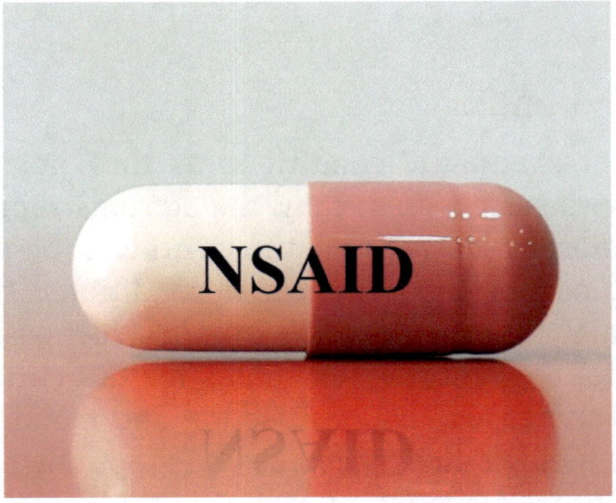

Figure 11.2. Utilization of non-steroidal anti-inflammatory drugs (NSAIDs).

Source: https://complete-physio.co.uk/wp-content/uploads/2020/07/nsaids-art-1-1024x826-1.jpg.

11.1.3. Disease-modifying Antirheumatic Drugs (DMARDs)

DMARDs play an integral role in the management of rheumatic disease, with a particular role in altering the course of disease and preventing chronic joint destruction. The medication, such as methotrexate, sulfasalazine, and biologic agents like tumor necrosis factor inhibitors, is designed to downregulate the underlying inflammation that characterizes rheumatoid arthritis and psoriatic arthritis. Recent studies propose that treatment with DMARDs can significantly improve patient outcomes; for instance, TNF inhibitors are very effective in the management of psoriatic arthritis but also show a need for alternatives in non-responders (Mantravadi et al., 2017). Additionally, the safety and potential impact of some vaccines, e.g., COVID-19 vaccination, on the flare of arthritis have been investigated with no significant associations detected between vaccinated patients (Chan et al., 2021). Therefore, the strategic use of DMARDs, as attested by the continued research work, reasserts their place in the clinical pharmacology of rheumatic disorders.

11.1.4. Biologic Agents and their Targets

The introduction of biologic agents has revolutionized the therapy of rheumatic disorders, with the advent of targeted drugs aimed at specific pathologic processes. Of all these agents, TNFi have been most pivotal, particularly in conditions , such as PsA, where they have significantly enhanced therapeutic outcomes and reduced radiographic progression (Mantravadi et al., 2017). Not every patient responds to TNFi, though, which leaves room for an immediate need for alternative modes and agents. For instance, new biologics with interleukin (IL)-23 and IL-17 pathway targets have shown promise in modulating the manifestation of the disease. Of most interest are drugs like ustekinumab, which cure arthralgia and psoriatic arthritis effectively but with inconsistent efficacy in various presentations. Therefore, the pharmacokinetics and immunogenicity of such biologics have to be understood to the fullest in order to optimize treatment regimens and ultimately personalize patient outcomes in rheumatic conditions (Figure 11.3).

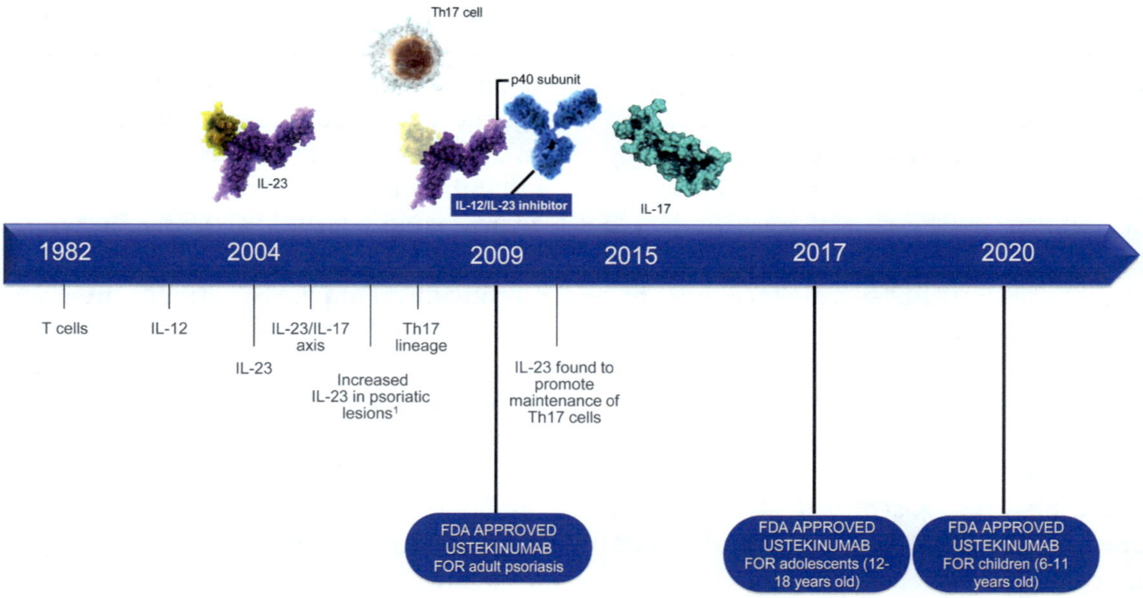

Figure 11.3. Treatments like USTEKINUMAB effectively target arthralgia and psoriatic arthritis, albeit with variable efficacy across different presentations.

Source: https://publinestorage.blob.core.windows.net/d2072d86-130f-4107-81da-331b43aeec96/jerp-22-44-g001.jpg.

11.1.5. Corticosteroids and their Pharmacodynamics

Corticosteroids are also crucial in the management of rheumatic conditions as they possess potent anti-inflammatory and immunosuppressive activities. Mechanistically, the steroids repress the transcription of inflammatory response genes, thereby decreasing the synthesis of pro-inflammatory cytokines. This pharmacodynamic effect is particularly beneficial in conditions , such as rheumatoid arthritis, which is due to persistent inflammation that leads to joint destruction and incapacitation. While corticosteroids provide rapid relief and improve outcomes for the patient, chronic use poses significant challenges in the form of increased risk of infection and metabolic side effects. Furthermore, following the introduction of biologic therapies like TNFi, options have been revolutionized but still leave patients with suboptimal response to corticosteroids or TNFi (Mantravadi et al., 2017). Therefore, corticosteroid pharmacodynamics must be grasped to achieve the best therapy and management of unmet rheumatic disease patients' needs (Nimbalkar, 2016).

11.1.6. Role of Analgesics in Pain Management

The analgesic function in pain therapy of rheumatic disease patients has an important role, particularly in situations like OA, which greatly deteriorates the quality of life. Analgesics, particularly the NSAIDs, represent typical treatment options to alleviate pain and increase physical functionality in patients. In fact, approximately 65% of OA patients in the United States take NSAIDs as part of their pain management regimen, a testament to their pivotal role in clinical practice. Although the analgesics are not risk-free, as they have the potential to have serious side effects like gastrointestinal and cardiovascular events (Ceccarelli et al., 2018). Interestingly, studies have indicated that the use of non-invasive therapy, such as mud-pack therapy and balneotherapy, can reduce the dependency on NSAIDs but effectively manage pain and consequently result in patient improvement and quality of life (Ceccarelli et al., 2018). Therefore, a multifaceted approach of analgesic utilization is needed in the treatment of rheumatic conditions (Figure 11.4).

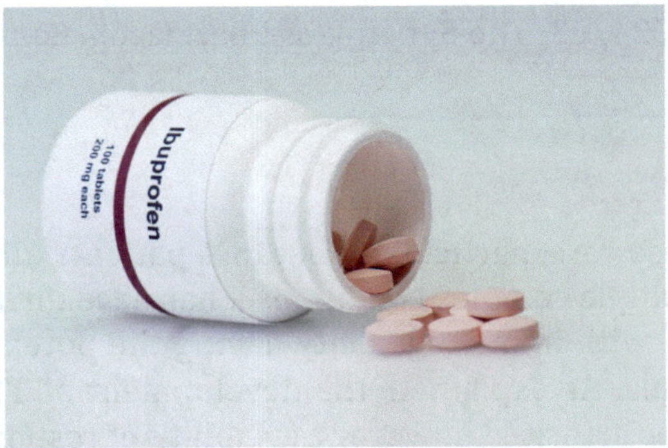

Figure 11.4. Analgesics, particularly non-steroidal anti-inflammatory drugs (NSAIDs), are frequently prescribed to alleviate pain and improve physical functionality among patients.

Source: https://i0.wp.com/sems-journal.ch/wp-content/uploads/2017/01/shutterstock_173323913.jpg?resize=770%2C515&ssl=1.

11.1.7. Mechanisms of Action of Newer Therapies

The state-of-the-art science of rheumatic disease treatment is focused on a better understanding of the mechanisms of the disease so that more targeted interventions can be developed. Notably, TNFi have revolutionized the management of diseases like PsA by greatly averting inflammation and joint destruction through clearly understood mechanisms of action. The biologics exert their effects by blocking TNF-alpha, a cytokine that signals for inflammatory pathways, which has led to monumental improvements in patient outcomes, particularly those resistant to standard therapies (Mantravadi et al., 2017). Parallel to this, studies on endothelin-1 (ET-1) antagonists represent another new line of therapeutic approach, especially for conditions like pulmonary arterial hypertension secondary to rheumatic diseases. The potent vasoconstrictor activity of ET-1 initiates vascular remodeling and thus forms a key target of drug therapy (Chester et al., 2014). This is a welcome direction towards personalized therapy in the clinical pharmacology of rheumatic diseases.

11.1.8. Pharmacogenomics in Rheumatic Disease Treatment

Pharmacogenomics plays a pivotal role in the treatment of rheumatic illnesses by allowing for individualized medication based on individual genetic profiles. Pharmacogenomics plays the most significant role in the treatment of juvenile idiopathic arthritis (JIA), where standard therapy, such as methotrexate, is less effective in patients. Research has indicated that 35-45% of patients are resistant to methotrexate due to differences in genes controlling drug metabolism and response pathways (Alessandro eVentura et al., 2015).

Advances in genomic technology, including genome-wide studies, have begun to uncover new biological mechanisms involved in drug response, and further validation may permit more directed treatment strategies in JIA. In addition, ongoing research into pharmacogenomic markers of other rheumatic illnesses, like gout, emphasizes the need for the development of treatment strategies with reference to genetic susceptibility. Finally, the integration of pharmacogenomics in the clinic has the potential to significantly improve outcomes in rheumatic disease care (Figure 11.5).

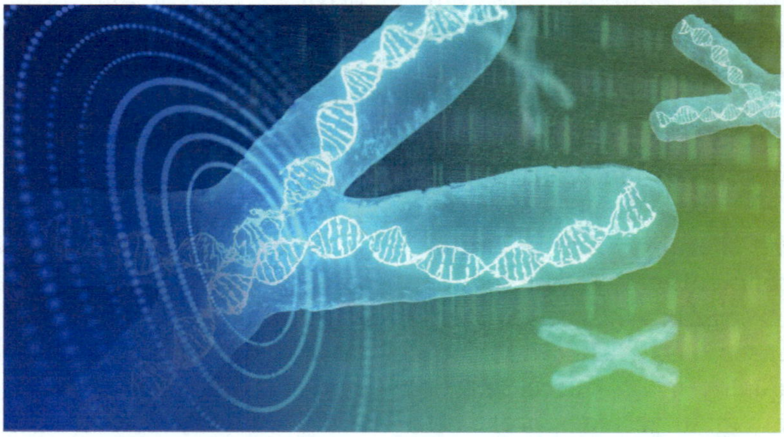

Figure 11.5. Pharmacogenomics plays a pivotal role in the treatment of rheumatic diseases by enabling personalized medicine tailored to individual genetic profiles.

Source: https://incitehealth.com/wp-content/uploads/2024/03/The-Synergy-of-Pharmacogenomics.jpg.

11.1.9. Drug Interactions and their Implications

Drug interactions are a critical factor in rheumatic disease care, particularly because patients might have to use multiple drugs to effectively manage their multiple complex conditions. Pharmacokinetics of drugs , such as TNFi is influenced by several factors, with immunogenicity having the potential to compromise therapeutic efficacy in certain individuals. As explained, the development of TNFi has transformed outcomes for diseases , such as psoriatic arthritis; however, variability of response among individuals makes cautious consideration of potential interactions with other therapeutic interventions a necessity (Mantravadi et al., 2017). Furthermore, the prevalence of polypharmacy among elderly patients contributes to the likelihood of inadmissible prescribing, thus the merit of systematic screening in clinical practice to identify and avert harmful interactions (Boussery et al., 2015). Finally, understanding such interactions is crucial in optimizing treatment regimens and improving patient outcomes in the framework of clinical pharmacology of rheumatic disorders.

Test Your Knowledge

1. What is the mechanism by which rituximab reduces ANCA-associated vasculitis disease activity?
2. How do JAK inhibitors (e.g., tofacitinib, baricitinib) influence intracellular signaling in autoimmune arthritis?

11.2. Pharmacotherapy in Specific Rheumatic Diseases

Learning Outcome

1. Understand treatment guidelines for rheumatoid arthritis;
2. Describe osteoarthritis management approaches;
3. Describe systemic lupus erythematosus management approaches to drugs;
4. Emphasize psoriatic arthritis and its treatment;
5. Describe gout management and urate-lowering therapy;
6. Emphasize scleroderma and pharmacological management;
7. Describe ankylosing spondylitis treatment horizon;
8. Understand the pharmacotherapy of juvenile idiopathic arthritis;
9. Outline new therapies in rheumatic disorders.

Rheumatic disease pharmacotherapy requires an individualized approach considering multiple factors of the patient, including age and comorbidities. As the incidence of diseases , such as rheumatoid arthritis and osteoarthritis is on the rise, particularly in the elderly, issues regarding pharmacologic therapy are all the more prominent.

Notably, the intricacy of therapy with analgesic and anti-inflammatory therapy in geriatric patients emphasizes the necessity of individualized care plans for these patients that consider altered pharmacokinetics and pharmacodynamics (Bajorek et al., 2014). Furthermore, current evidence is indicative of the promise of herbal medications as adjunct therapies, which have the ability to bestow analgesic and anti-inflammatory action with reduced toxicity, thus complementing standard pharmacotherapy (Kriukova et al., 2018). Such integrated methods not only add strength to the efficacy of treatment but also ensure patient safety, ultimately yielding superior overall outcomes in the treatment of rheumatic diseases, especially in the context of complex aging populations.

11.2.1. Rheumatoid Arthritis (RA) Treatment Protocols

Treatment regimens for RA aim to decrease inflammation, alleviate symptoms, and prevent long-term damage to joints. Current treatment with DMARDs and corticosteroids is the pharmacological foundation, but these drugs have limitations in the form of side effects, as well as variable efficacy between patient groups (Lee et al., 2021). More recent evidence has identified that circadian rhythms have an important influence on the modulation of RA symptoms and that the timing of medication can improve outcomes.

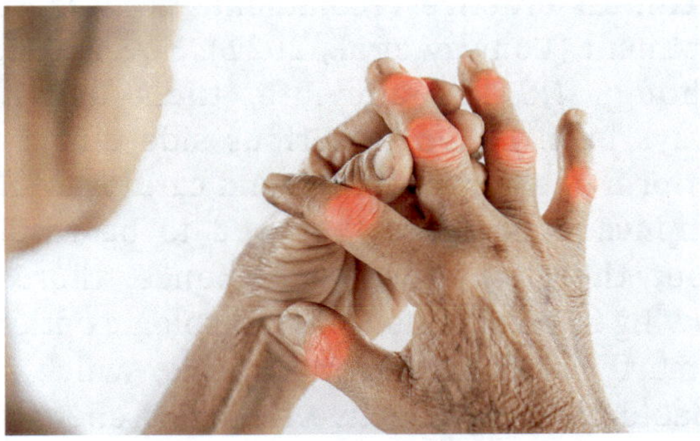

Figure 11.6. The treatment protocols for rheumatoid arthritis (RA) aim to mitigate inflammation, alleviate symptoms, and prevent long-term joint damage.

Source: https://midamortho.com/wp-content/uploads/2023/12/midamortho1.png.

For example, pro-inflammatory cytokines exhibit a diurnal variation with increased levels in morning hours, which impact the severity of RA symptoms during that time (Lee et al., 2021). In recent years, adjunct therapies like Montelukast, a leukotriene receptor antagonist, have been of interest for the potential to slow disease progression, offering a new target to augment existing treatment regimens (Nimbalkar, 2016). As research advances, optimization of treatment regimens with new medications in conjunction with existing therapies will maximize patient quality of life (Figure 11.6).

11.2.2. Osteoarthritis Management (OA) Strategies

Optimal management strategies for OA are crucial to minimizing pain and maximizing physical functioning in patients, particularly as the disease more prominently involves the burgeoning population of older adults. According to current studies, it is revealed that most OA patients take NSAIDs as part of their therapy. In the USA, about 65% of OA patients receive NSAIDs to manage their pain, which indicates the high reliance on these medications in clinical practice recommendations for OA treatment (Conway et al., 2021). Nevertheless, although NSAIDs alleviate, their use has always been linked to serious side effects in the form of gastrointestinal and cardiovascular complications, hence the need to be careful about their long-term use. Hence, there is growing interest in non-pharmacologic options, primarily bioactive nutraceuticals, which are capable of being effective for pain relief with fewer side effects, hence ensuring patient safety as well as the general outcome of the treatment (Conway et al., 2021).

11.2.3. Systemic Lupus Erythematosus (SLE) Pharmacological Approaches

The therapy of SLE is a particular challenge for clinical pharmacology owing to its complexity and heterogeneity. Its therapy is frequently grounded in immunosuppressive treatment to suppress the autoimmune disease process. Historical therapeutics , such as corticosteroids and antimalarials, play crucial roles in the management of acute flares and symptom suppression; however, the development of biologics, such as monoclonal antibodies targeting discrete cytokines and immune mechanisms, has revolutionized treatment models.

The study of chemokines , such as fractalkine/CX3CL1 is a very promising avenue for therapeutic targeting, offering new insights into SLE inflammation (Ahmed et al., 2012). Moreover, careful preconception assessment is important in women with undifferentiated connective tissue disease (UCTD) because they may have unpredictable courses of disease and it can be challenging to control with medication in pregnancy (Clemenza et al., 2022).

In general, an individualized approach to pharmacotherapy is required for optimizing the result in SLE patients (Figure 11.7).

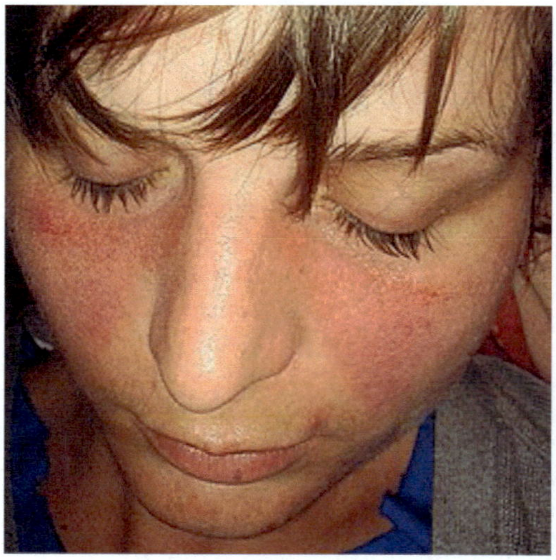

Figure 11.7. The management of systemic lupus erythematosus (SLE) presents a unique challenge in clinical pharmacology due to its complex and heterogeneous nature.

Source: https://upload.wikimedia.org/wikipedia/commons/thumb/5/52/Lupusfoto.jpg/250px-Lupusfoto.jpg.

11.2.4. Psoriatic Arthritis (PsA) and its Treatment Options

PsA is an indolent inflammatory disease, both in terms of joint inflammation and skin symptoms, which causes severe physical disability and reduced quality of life. Since the advent of the biologic agents, most importantly the TNFi, treatment for PsA has been radically changed, with significant improvement in therapy for the majority of patients. Evidence demonstrates that TNFi not only enhances symptoms but also delays radiographic progression of joint damage, which is essential to long-term patient management (Mantravadi et al., 2017). Of the various TNFi alternatives, adalimumab has documented the highest drug survival and efficacy, outperforming etanercept and infliximab in maintenance of therapeutic response (Berardesca et al., 2018). However, there is still an unmet need for those patients who do not adequately respond to these medications. As a result, ongoing assessment of biosimilars and other treatments must be undertaken to plug these gaps in PsA treatment (Figure 11.8).

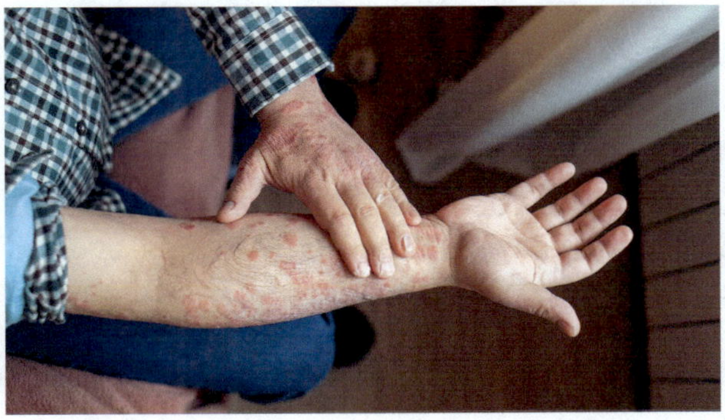

Figure 11.8. Psoriatic arthritis (PsA) is a chronic inflammatory disorder characterized by both joint pain and skin lesions, which can lead to significant physical impairment and reduced quality of life.

Source: https://post.healthline.com/wp-content/uploads/2022/11/senior-male-psoriasis-1296-728-header.jpg.

11.2.5. Gout Management and Urate-lowering Therapies

Effective management of gout is primarily dependent on the employment of urate-lowering therapies, which play an important role in symptom relief and flare prevention for gout's inflammatory disease. Options for managing the disease include allopurinol and febuxostat, both of which effectively lower serum urate levels, thus reducing the frequency of acute gout attacks and chronic joint damage. There have been recent research that has indicated treatment regimen inconsistencies, some of which have demonstrated suboptimal medication adherence and inconsistent gout definitions in electronic health record (EHR)-based literature (Baxter et al., 2019). New treatments as well as new treatment approaches are ongoing, highlighting the necessity of updating clinical guidelines based on emerging research evidence. Therefore, clinicians must be vigilant for patient response to treatment in an attempt to deliver tailored care plans to optimize outcomes in gout treatment within the overall framework of rheumatic disorders.

11.2.6. Scleroderma and Available Pharmacological Interventions

Scleroderma, or systemic sclerosis, is an autoimmune disorder where excessive collagen is deposited to result in fibrosis of tissues and derangement of the vessels. The management of this complex condition often involves pharmacotherapies to manage symptoms and prevent disease progression. The evidence of present systematic reviews of literature has shown the efficacy of various treatments, particularly in managing Raynauds phenomenon and digital ulcers, which are frequent in patients with scleroderma. Calcium channel blockers, phosphodiesterase-5 inhibitors, and intravenous prostacyclin analogues have been found to be moderately effective in minimizing the frequency and intensity of Raynauds attacks, whereas treatments , such as bosentan have proved to be effective in preventing new digital ulcers (Cordeiro et al., 2024). Furthermore, the linkage of endothelin-1 with pulmonary arterial hypertension in scleroderma patients highlights the use of endothelin receptor antagonists and the promising path in the treatment of vascular manifestations of the disease (Chester et al., 2014). These drug treatments play a vital role in improving the well-being of people affected by the disease (Figure 11.9).

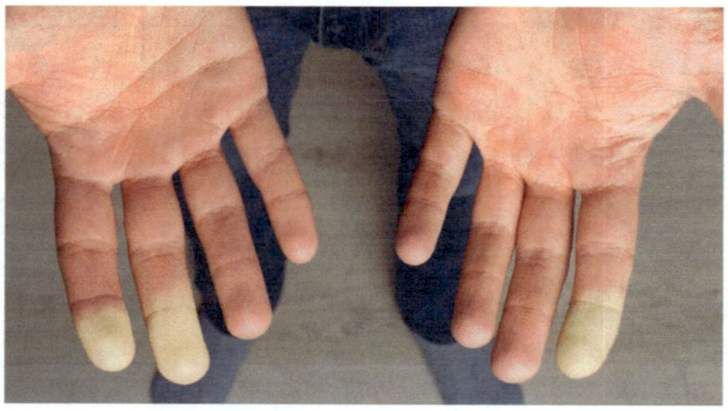

Figure 11.9. Scleroderma, or systemic sclerosis, is an autoimmune disorder characterized by excessive collagen deposition leading to tissue fibrosis and vascular abnormalities.

Source: https://www.heal-medical.com/media/images/service/Scleroderma.jpg.

11.2.7. Ankylosing Spondylitis (AS) Treatment Landscape

Treatment of AS has changed dramatically, mostly because biologic agents that target tumor necrosis factor (TNF) have been introduced. These drugs have shown great effectiveness in reducing the disabling signs and symptoms of AS, such as inflammation and pain in the sacroiliac joints, with a uniform capacity to prevent radiographic disease progression. As has been mentioned, TNF blockers , such as infliximab and adalimumab not only control the joint signs of AS but also its extra-articular manifestations, i.e., uveitis and inflammatory bowel disease, and therefore are a central selection in the therapeutical arsenal of patients with AS (Elewaut et al., 2009). But it is important to explain the heterogeneity of patient response to these drugs, where some patients fail to achieve sufficient relief and thus constitute an unmet need for alternative treatments (Mantravadi et al., 2017). This kind of complexity mandates the use of a multidimensional approach to treatment in choosing treatment to optimally manage AS (Figure 11.10).

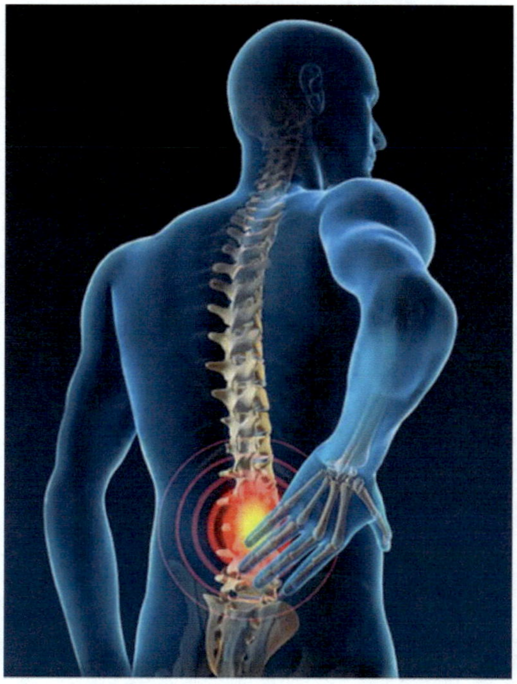

Figure 11.10. The treatment landscape for ankylosing spondylitis (AS) has evolved significantly, primarily due to the introduction of biologic therapies that target tumor necrosis factor (TNF).

Source: https://bestmadenaturalproducts.com/cdn/shop/files/Captura_de_ecra_2022-11-07_as_12.20.52_480x480.webp.

11.2.8. Juvenile Idiopathic Arthritis (JIA) Pharmacotherapy

JIA is an excellent pediatric rheumatology dilemma, for which in-depth knowledge of pharmacotherapy is needed to minimize disease impact. Cornerstone therapy is constituted by NSAIDs, which are pain- and inflammation-reducing, but may be inadequate in certain patients. Because of this, DMARDs, such as methotrexate, are frequently utilized to modify disease course and improve long-term outcomes. As the pathology of JIA has improved, biologic agents targeted at distinct immune targets have entered as a significant component of the pharmacotherapy arsenal and have been found to be efficacious in the management of refractory disease. These advances underscore the need for individually tailored treatment regimens based on both safety and efficacy, particularly with the risk of devastating side effects associated with long-term steroid therapy and other systemic agents (Jiang et al., 2012). Ultimately, a composite pharmacotherapy strategy is needed to induce quality of life improvement in affected children while addressing the complexities of this multimodal condition.

11.2.9. Emerging Therapies in Rheumatic Diseases

The treatment landscape for rheumatic diseases is rapidly evolving, with new opportunities to improve outcomes for patients. New therapies, particularly those acting on anti-inflammatory mechanisms, represent a dramatic advance in the management of conditions like PsA. have transformed therapeutic regimens, with remarkable efficacy in controlling disease manifestations and halting structural damage in PsA. Yet there exists a subset of patients who are not sufficiently responsive to TNFi, highlighting the need for new alternatives and therapies (Mantravadi et al., 2017). Moreover, ongoing research into the immunogenicity of these agents also informs their use, allowing for patient-specific treatment modalities that take into account individualized responses. Additional emphasis on vascular inflammation and its role in rheumatic disease also offers means of possible therapeutic interventions to minimize complications due to the diseases (Abbas et al., 2017). This evolving environment also impinges on the potential of improved pharmacological interventions within clinical practice (Figure 11.11).

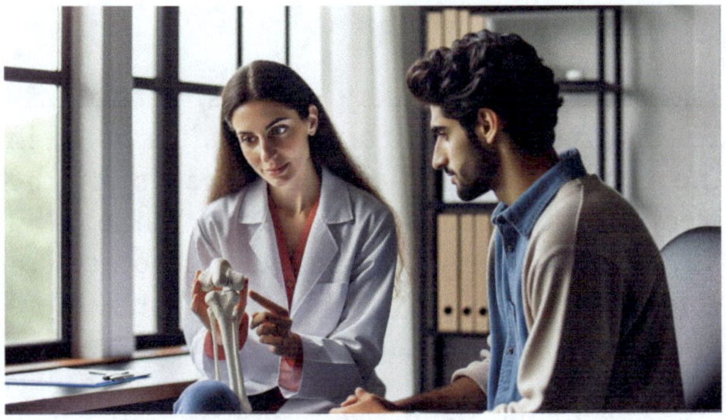

Figure 11.11. The landscape of therapeutic options for rheumatic diseases is rapidly evolving, providing new avenues for improving patient outcomes.

Source: https://regenerative.nz/wp-content/uploads/2024/03/Untitled.png.

Test Your Knowledge

1. What are the goals of treatment and drug management of ankylosing spondylitis?
2. What medications are used for acute versus chronic gout treatment?

11.3. Adverse Effects and Safety Profiles

Learning Outcome

1. Understand common adverse effects of NSAIDs;
2. Describe long-term effects of DMARDs;
3. Discuss safety concerns with biologic therapy;
4. Highlight corticosteroid-related complications;
5. Monitoring for adverse drug effects;
6. Identify risk factors for drug toxicity;
7. Highlight patient education regarding drug safety;
8. Learn how to counteract adverse effects;
9. Understand drug safety regulatory factors.

The biologic drug safety profiles, particularly TNFi, present important considerations in the context of their clinical benefits for the treatment of rheumatic diseases. While TNFi have remarkably improved outcomes of conditions , such as psoriatic arthritis, there remain issues with their side effects.

The drugs have been reported to cause increased susceptibility to infections and potential malignancies, which necessitate close monitoring of patients and screening protocols. Secondly, immunogenicity matters in the efficacy and safety of TNFi since antibodies to certain drugs can form in patients, hence diminishing the effectiveness of therapy (Mantravadi et al., 2017).

Biosimilars have created a door for increased availability but have raised alarms regarding their safety profiles compared to reference biologics. Awareness of the regulatory setting and pharmacovigilance of biosimilars is important, since it will influence their application in clinical practice and ultimately affect patient management of rheumatologic disease.

11.3.1. Common Adverse Effects of Nonsteroidal Anti-Inflammatory Drugs (NSAIDs)

The NSAIDs are also widely utilized in the management of pain in rheumatic disease; however, they possess a multitude of typical side effects that can complicate treatment. Gastrointestinal adverse effects, such as dyspepsia and peptic ulceration, are among the most frequent adverse effects and tend to produce considerable morbidity in long-term patients on these drugs. The drugs also have a tendency to elevate blood pressure and, in certain groups of patients, result in renal impairment, for which they have to be monitored carefully when prescribed. Such concerns are more relevant in elderly patients, who will have pre-existing risks for such side effects.

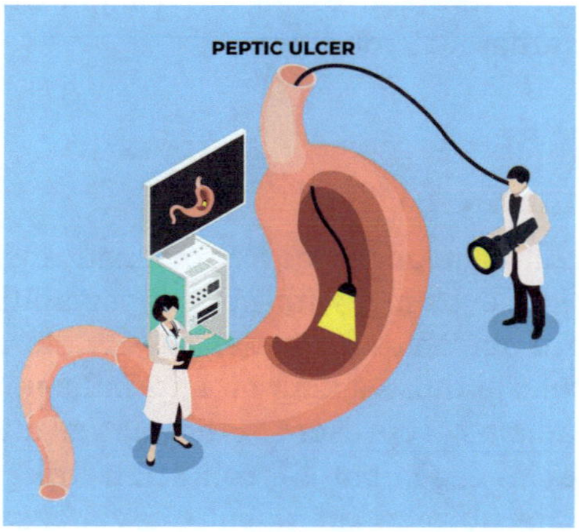

Figure 11.12. Gastrointestinal disturbances, such as dyspepsia and peptic ulceration, are among the most prevalent side effects, often leading to considerable morbidity in patients using these agents long-term.

Source: https://ca-times.brightspotcdn.com/dims4/default/2942fc9/2147483647/strip/true/crop/2428x1366+1+0/resize/1200x675!/quality/75/?url=https%3A%2F%2Fcalifornia-times-brightspot.s3.amazonaws.com%2F21%2F96%2F24839b72403db29487e619a1ed4b%2Fpeptic-ulcer-lead.jpeg.

Furthermore, while NSAIDs are revealed to be efficacious in the relief of symptoms in rheumatoid arthritis and osteoarthritis, a significant proportion of patients may rely on co-therapy with gastroprotectives to minimize such complications, demonstrating how careful one has to be when optimizing clinical outcomes (Gupta et al., 2018). This serves to emphasize the importance of understanding the pharmacological profiles of NSAIDs in the context of overall management of rheumatic diseases (Mantravadi et al., 2017) (Figure 11.12).

11.3.2. Long-term Effects of Disease-Modifying Anti-Rheumatic Drugs (DMARDs)

The long-term effects of DMARDs play a vital role in the treatment of rheumatic diseases, including rheumatoid arthritis (RA). These drugs not only alleviate symptoms but also have a profound impact on the course of the disease and on the maintenance of the joints. Clinical data confirm that early intervention with DMARDs is associated with better outcomes, avoiding joint damage and improved patient quality of life in the long term. For instance, cost-effectiveness analysis has proved that methotrexate (MTX) is marginally better in outcome in direct cost, but on the whole effect on disease activity improvement is equivalent among various DMARDs like hydroxychloroquine and MTX with hydroxychloroquine (C S et al., 2018). Moreover, studies show that certain DMARDs , such as adalimumab, retain higher drug survival rates than others , such as infliximab and etanercept, which is an indicator of their success in long-term disease treatment regimens for conditions , such as psoriatic arthritis and psoriasis (Berardesca et al., 2018).

11.3.3. Safety Concerns with Biologic Therapies

Biologic therapies have revolutionized the treatment of rheumatic disease by offering targeted mechanisms, symptomatic relief, and increased quality of life for patients. However, the emergence of these treatments has also raised some serious safety concerns. The possibility of adverse side effects, such as malignancies and infections, requires careful observation and risk evaluation in treated patients. Studies have indicated high patient satisfaction with intravenous (IV) biologic treatment, with the majority expressing positive perceptions once treatment is begun, but it is essential to understand the impact of these medications on outcomes in the long term (Black et al., 2017). Biologics are very costly, and this has prompted efforts to introduce biosimilars as a lower-cost alternative, but also one that needs to be evaluated for its safety profile and long-term efficacy. Thus, a personalized strategy to patient education and shared decision-making is needed to efficiently address these complex safety challenges (Figure 11.13).

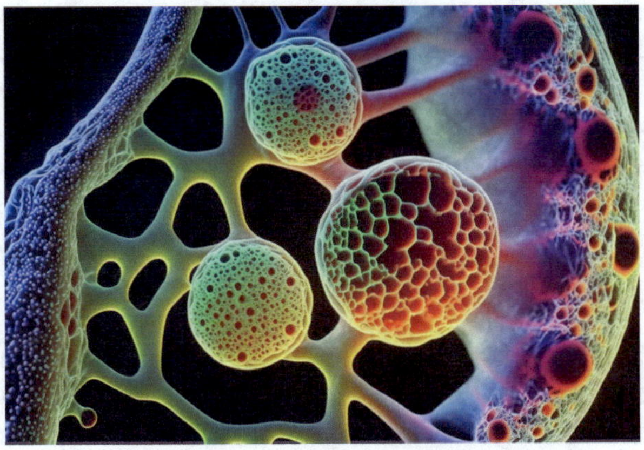

Figure 11.13. Biologic therapies have revolutionized the treatment of rheumatic diseases, offering targeted mechanisms that alleviate symptoms and improve patients' quality of life.

Source: https://cdn.prod.website-files.com/5d9667bad4a41e222995e15b/63dc3a32be7bef61606d0e19_RA%20copy.webp.

11.3.4. Corticosteroid-related Complications

Complications of corticosteroids are a significant problem in rheumatic disease management because these medications, although effective at reducing inflammation and controlling the disease, may introduce many complications. Among them are metabolic complications, for instance, hyperglycemia and osteoporosis, which in turn can worsen the overall condition of the patient and complicate treatment. Current studies indicate that education regarding the safe prescription of adjunctive medicines, such as gastroprotection agents, is lacking in prescribers, particularly in high-risk patients for gastrointestinal intolerance to simultaneous NSAIDs and corticosteroids (Bilušić et al., 2006). Besides, oral manifestations of autoimmune diseases can also influence patients' quality of life significantly, which emphasizes the importance of early intervention and integral care in avoiding corticosteroid-induced side effects (Bossù et al., 2018). Hence, correct education and a multidisciplinary team are inevitable in preventing these side effects as well as achieving optimal therapeutic outcomes in rheumatology.

11.3.5. Monitoring for Adverse Drug Reactions (ADRs)

In clinical pharmacology, particularly when the patient has rheumatoid diseases, ADR monitoring is extremely vital in upholding both the patient's safety and the clinical effectiveness of treatment. The fact that drugs , such as NSAIDs, DMARDs, and biologics are multiple suggests the need for vigilant monitoring to suppress risks due to ADRs. For instance, in a trial of cardiovascular drugs, many patients developed ADRs, dominated by myalgia as a reaction to statins and cough as a reaction to angiotensin-converting enzyme inhibitors, indicating the requirement for cautious monitoring practices (Mantravadi et al., 2017). Similarly, the use of rituximab among rheumatic disease patients has been linked to serious side effects, for example, increased susceptibility to infection and potential reactivation of tuberculosis, which necessitates careful monitoring and reporting through pharmacovigilance platforms (Malhotra et al., 2018). This proactive measure not only adds to optimizing therapeutic strategies but also highlights the importance of patient-focused care in rheumatology (Figure 11.14).

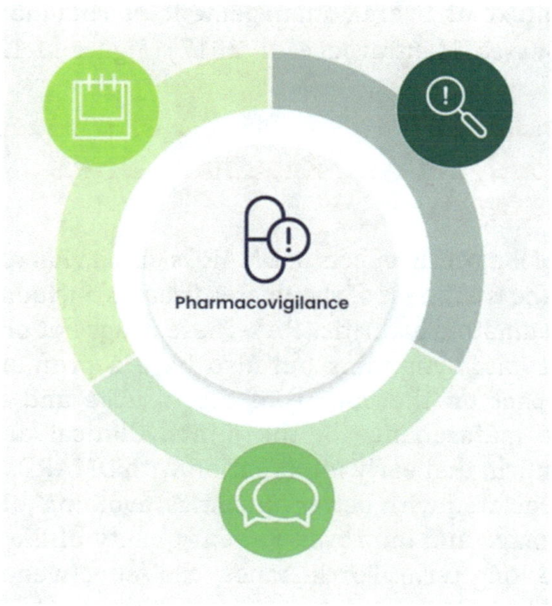

Figure 11.14. In the realm of clinical pharmacology, particularly within the treatment of rheumatic diseases, the monitoring for adverse drug reactions (ADRs) is paramount in ensuring patient safety and treatment efficacy.

Source: https://www.pharmaceuticalpress.com/wp-content/uploads/2024/08/what-is-pharmacovigilance.png.

11.3.6. Risk Factors for Drug Toxicity

There is a need to understand the risk factors of drug toxicity among rheumatic disease patients to maximize therapeutic outcomes and minimize adverse effects. Several variables, including age, comorbidities, and concomitant medication administration, are responsible for rendering the patient susceptible to drug toxicity. For instance, the elderly patient may possess altered pharmacokinetics, hence increasing the risk for adverse drug effects. In clinical practice, the presence of concomitant risk factors has the tendency to increase the need for precise monitoring and individually tailored pharmacological therapy. A study revealed that patients who received NSAID treatment and other risk factors were prescribed more gastroprotective agents; however, most were given them in amounts less than the recommended doses, potentially putting them at higher risk for gastrointestinal complications (Bilušić et al., 2006). Besides, the effect of some biomarkers and conditions on treatment outcomes guarantees that clinicians must remain vigilant to modify therapies for the purposes of minimizing the risks of drug toxicity (Chester et al., 2014).

11.3.7. Patient Education on Medication Safety

Effective patient education regarding medication safety is a critical component of managing rheumatic disorders, particularly where the complexity of regimens is likely to cause polypharmacy. It is critical that healthcare practitioners support patients in making informed choices so that they understand the implications of their drugs, such as side effects and interactions. It is proven that before IV treatment, a very large percentage of patients are informed about therapy options, and this enhances their perception of the effectiveness of treatment and of care by a very significant amount (Black et al., 2017). Furthermore, because the ageing population is more susceptible to potentially inappropriate prescribing (PIP), community pharmacists play an imperative role in the identification and resolution of such issues through overt screening tools like the GheOP3S (Boussery et al., 2015). Through the establishment of patient education and the utilization of the pharmacist's skills, the therapeutic outcome and safety of the patient can be improved in rheumatology (Figure 11.15).

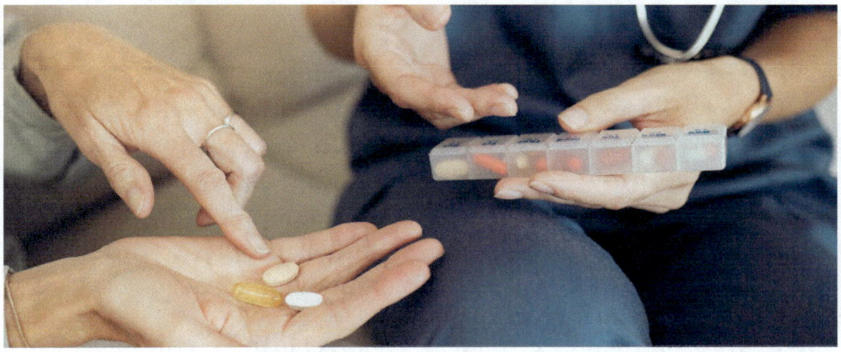

Figure 11.15. Effective patient education on medication safety is a critical component of managing rheumatic diseases, particularly where the complexity of treatment regimens often leads to polypharmacy.

Source: https://navinurses.com/wp-content/uploads/2024/03/Med-Management-Hero.jpg.

11.3.8. Strategies to Mitigate Adverse Effects

In their counteraction against the adverse effects that pharmacological treatment in rheumatic diseases presents, having effective strategies in place is of prime importance for enhancing patient outcomes. One of the popular methods is therapeutic drug monitoring (TDM), which facilitates individualized adjustment of biologic treatment through monitoring the drug in the patient's system. Although TDM has tremendous potential, its extensive application is limited by barriers , such as disagreement about clinical integration and cost-effectiveness, which limit reimbursement systems (Altepeter et al., 2025). Besides, some agents , such as hydroxychloroquine (HCQ), have been noted to have positive results in the treatment of conditions , such as recurrent miscarriage, but are also excessively dangerous for adverse effects, e.g., ocular toxicity. This calls for constant monitoring of potential adverse effects under treatment regimens (Zhang et al., 2024). Ultimately, coordinated action by healthcare providers, policymakers, and patients must be undertaken to optimize treatment regimens while minimizing risk in the field of rheumatic disorders.

11.3.9. Regulatory Considerations for Drug Safety

In the field of clinical pharmacology, especially where rheumatic disorders are concerned, regulatory issues relating to drug safety become predominant. The arrival of biologic drugs has transformed the era of therapy, but also calls for stringent regulation to guarantee efficacy and safety for the patient. With the advent of biosimilars, which have been designed to be highly similar to existing biologics, the regulatory framework must adapt to accommodate them to occupy space in clinical practice without diminishing rigorous safety standards. TDM for biologics is another example of a crucial regulatory concern; TDM is also an emerging tool for optimizing drug dosing and advancing patient outcomes. However, obstacles , such a lack of consensus on clinical guidelines and reimbursement issues prevent it from being used on a broad scale (Altepeter et al., 2025). These regulatory obstacles must be addressed to advance treatment options and ensure confidence in the safety and efficacy of therapies for rheumatologic conditions (Figure 11.16).

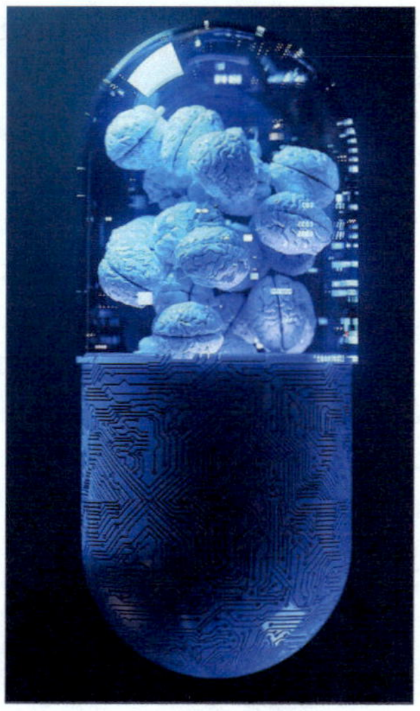

Figure 11.16. With the advent of biosimilars, which are designed to be highly similar to existing biologics, the regulatory framework must adapt to facilitate their integration into clinical practice while maintaining rigorous safety standards.

Source: https://cdn.sanity.io/images/03hnmfyj/production/651843bef421e05762fccb4c8ccef4ed351451f0-1600x900.jpg.

Test Your Knowledge

1. What are the hematologic and hepatic risks of leflunomide therapy?
2. Which rheumatologic medications require regular renal function monitoring?

11.4. Future Directions in Clinical Pharmacology

Learning Outcome

1. Learn advances in personalized medicine;
2. Understand the artificial intelligence function in drug creation;
3. Explain innovations in drug delivery systems;
4. Discuss gene therapy potential in rheumatic disease;
5. Learn therapeutic agent development in new areas;
6. Know patient-reported outcome significance;
7. Explain global health perspectives on the treatment of rheumatic disease;
8. Describe collaborative study efforts;
9. Identify challenges in future clinical pharmacology.

As the course of clinical pharmacology continues to evolve, future advancements are more personalized medicine, and particularly the treatment of rheumatic disease. With the advent of biologic therapy, such as TNFi, therapeutic management has been revolutionized, with improved efficacy in the case of PsA (Mantravadi et al., 2017). Challenges remain, particularly in the case of those who do not respond adequately to treatment. The future will be based on paying attention to learning about pharmacokinetics and immunogenicity as a means of customizing treatment strategies (Mantravadi et al., 2017). Besides, the potential for biosimilars to enhance accessibility and cost-effectiveness of biologic therapy underscores the imperative for ongoing research and education regarding pharmacologic agents (Mantravadi et al., 2017). At the same time, studying dietary factors, e.g., total fat intake in knee osteoarthritis, illuminates the complex interplay among pharmacotherapy and lifestyle and calls for a multidimensional approach to patient management.

11.4.1. Advances in Personalized Medicine

The concept of personalized medicine has come a long way, particularly in the management of rheumatic disorders, characterized by their heterogeneity and multifactorial pathophysiology. These advances have introduced a new generation of treatment modalities tailored to the individual patient's genetic constitution, environment, and lifestyle to optimize therapeutic gain. In RA, for instance, identification of specific innate immune signatures, i.e., upregulation of TLR3 and IL1RAP/IL1R3, has revealed the potential for selective therapies that might greatly improve patient treatment (Fillerová et al., 2019).

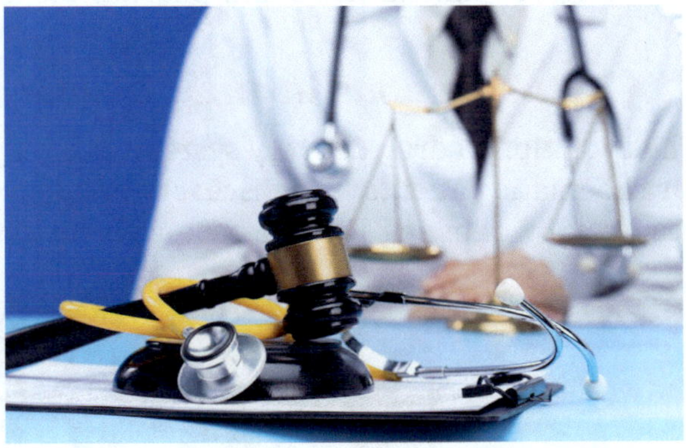

Figure 11.17. The integration of personalized medicine principles will be essential in refining clinical pharmacology practices in rheumatology, ultimately leading to more effective and individualized care strategies.

Source: https://media.licdn.com/dms/image/v2/D5612AQGmY0SNiq5UTg/article-cover_image-shrink_720_1280/article-cover_image-shrink_720_1280/0/1705453232531?e=2147483647&v=beta&t=2irsvbpfj4keUHaHydftSCzDzOdE2O7wXMeD9-wSURQ.

Again, as with current research into gout, personalized interventions not only improve efficacy but also limit side effects, thereby improving patient compliance and quality of life. As the discipline evolves, the use of personalized medicine principles will become essential in making clinical pharmacology practice in rheumatology more streamlined, thereby leading to more effective and tailored care approaches (Figure 11.17).

11.4.2. Role of Artificial Intelligence (AI) in Drug Development

The role of AI in drug discovery is rapidly transforming the landscape of clinical pharmacology, particularly for rheumatic diseases. By utilizing machine learning algorithms and predictive analysis, researchers can mechanize the drug discovery process, reducing time and cost to provide new treatments. AI facilitates more precise data analysis through minimization of errors in data collection, which is critical in sensing complex relationships in multidimensional diseases. Moreover, automated systems have shifted towards the inclusion of real-time user assistance and continuous quality monitoring, enhancing diagnostic precision and treatment efficacy, as noted in the development of intelligent healthcare technologies (Djumanov, 2011). In the treatment of inflammatory bowel disease, AI can decide the optimal therapy for extraintestinal manifestations, showing promise in individualizing treatment regimens. Lastly, recent developments in AI for drug development have the potential not only to offer better patient outcomes but also to usher in a new paradigm for the design of clinical trials and pharmacologic interventions.

11.4.3. Innovations in Drug Delivery Systems

The evolution of drug delivery systems has played a key role in optimizing therapeutic effectiveness for rheumatic patients. The discovery of nanoparticles and liposomes revolutionized drug targeting accuracy by allowing local release without systemic side effects.

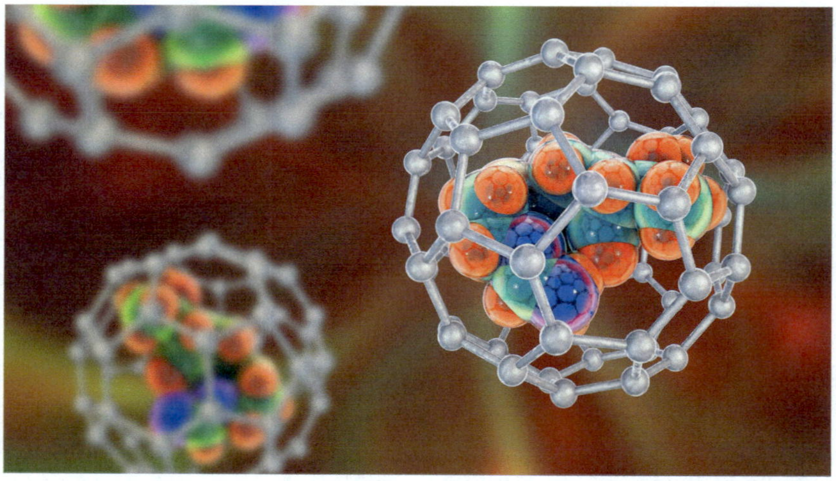

Figure 11.18. Innovations , such as nanoparticles and liposomes have revolutionized the precision of drug targeting, allowing for localized treatment while minimizing systemic side effects.

Source: https://cdn.prod.website-files.com/650867962272bf8f15c1034b/66d0e3d935f8122db13547aa_GettyImages-1423889653_CAS-Insights-Hero-Image.jpg.

These advanced systems allow for controlled release, promoting patient compliance and total efficacy, particularly for chronic diseases common in rheumatology. Moreover, biosimilar and targeted biologic development accommodates the need for cheaper alternatives without sacrificing patient access to needed drugs and without exerting excessive financial burdens on health systems. In particular, drug assessment models, as discussed above, bring out the convergence of stakeholders in maximizing the utilization of these innovative therapies, thereby maintaining healthcare systems. Such collaborative environments are essential to the recovery of trust and to the effective integration of new as well as existing medicines into therapeutic regimens for individuals suffering from these disabling disorders (Kitsiou et al., 2013; Godman et al., 2014) (Figure 11.18).11.4.4. Potential of Gene Therapy in Rheumatic Diseases

The therapeutic potential of gene therapy in rheumatic illnesses is quickly emerging in the forefront, providing opportunities for specifically targeted intervention not easily replicable with conventional pharmacological interventions. Through direct manipulation of the genetic elements involved in inflammatory processes, gene therapy can potentially provide a more durable solution to the management of conditions like RA. For instance, understanding the molecular mechanisms of RA, such as the roles of tumor necrosis factor-α (TNF-α) and lymphotoxin-α (LT-α) in joint inflammation, could lead to gene therapies aimed at regulating their expression (Neregård, 2013).

Moreover, highlighting inflammatory mechanisms and their molecular regulation with a specific emphasis on those transcription factors that are in charge, for instance, NF-κB, highlights the promise gene therapy holds to modulate inflammatory responses where they start (Kim et al., 2016). Ultimately, gene therapy's incorporation into routine clinical practice could revolutionize the treatment paradigm of rheumatic diseases, with the expectation of improved patient outcomes.

11.4.5. Development of Novel Therapeutic Agents

There is a need to find new medications as treatment options, with the limitations of the existing medications. Current strategies, particularly TNFi, have been found effective in controlling disease conditions like PsA; yet, a significant proportion of patients respond poorly or lose response with time (Mantravadi et al., 2017). This necessitates new treatments that will fill these gaps and limitations. Research on the molecular mechanism of inflammation, such as the role of proinflammatory mediators and transcription factors, has created opportunities for the identification of new anti-inflammatory medications. Specifically, research on drugs , such as cerulenin that suppress significant inflammatory processes , such as the Nuclear Factor Kappa-B, holds promise for creating therapeutic derivatives that are efficacious (Kim et al., 2016). By strategically creating agents that can modulate these pathways, investigators hope to improve the patient's outcomes in rheumatic diseases through individualized pharmacologic therapy (Figure 11.19).

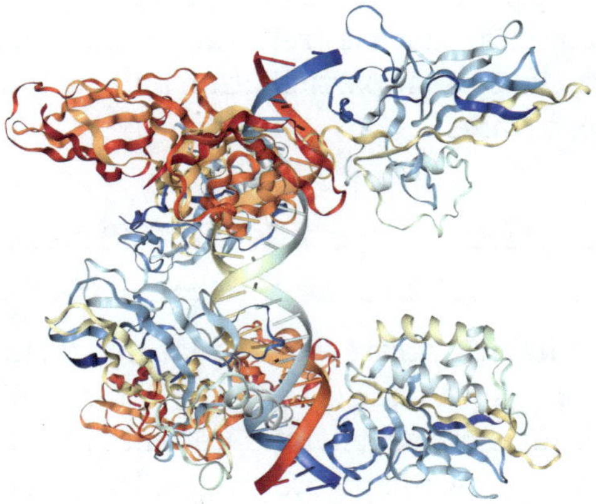

Figure 11.19. Nuclear factor kappa-B.

Source: https://cdn1.sinobiological.com/styles/default/images/protein-structure/RELA-protein-structure.jpg.

11.4.6. Importance of Patient-reported Outcomes (PROs)

PROs are a concept increasingly appreciated for being at the center of clinical pharmacology in rheumatic diseases. Involving patients in their own assessment allows practitioners to become attuned to the symptomatology experienced, but also to more closely tailor the treatment strategies. For instance, patients with undifferentiated connective tissue disease (UCTD) will tend to have complex symptomatology that can be subjective and so calling for their involvement in management measures (Anderson, 2018). Additionally, the use of PROs supports conventional clinical evaluations by including patients' assessments of the effectiveness and quality of therapy, allowing for a comprehensive overview of treatment outcomes. In addition to targeted therapies like JAK inhibitors, their effects on patients can be understood through PROs, which aid clinicians in making informed choices about treating patients based on their pharmacokinetic and pharmacodynamic characteristics (Shehata et al., 2024). Lastly, the integration of PROs in clinical practice increases the aggregate care of rheumatic disease, reiterating the need for aggressive patient participation and customized care programs.

11.4.7. Global Health Perspectives on Rheumatic Disease Treatment

Global health strategy in treating rheumatic disease emphasizes the need for tailored therapeutic interventions to ensure patient outcomes across disparate groups. The creation of TNFi has significantly improved the management of conditions , such as psoriatic arthritis, demonstrating how new pharmacotherapy is able to halt disease progression and alleviate symptoms in the majority of patients. However, a significant number of patients are nonresponsive or experience declining effectiveness with time, emphasizing the necessity for ongoing research and adjustment of treatment protocols (Mantravadi et al., 2017). Moreover, the recent global health crisis caused by the COVID-19 pandemic has revealed complex interplays between infectious and autoimmune diseases, and an even-handed balance between immunosuppression and infection management must be achieved (Diamanti et al., 2020). In response to this, healthcare systems worldwide encounter this challenge; there must be an inter-coordinated effort towards increasing knowledge about the pharmacokinetics and immunogenicity of the therapy to maximize therapy in rheumatic disease (Figure 11.20).

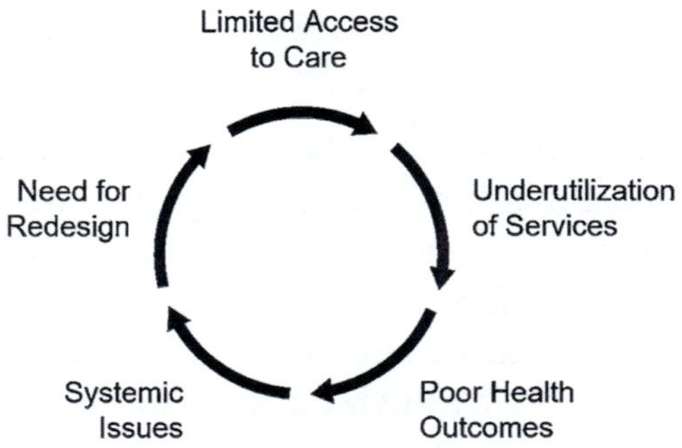

Figure 11.20. Global health perspectives on rheumatic disease treatment.

Source: Santosa A, Li JW, Tan TC. Digital Health for Equitable Rheumatic Care: Integrating Real-World Experiences to Guide Policy Pathways. Healthcare. 2025; 13(4):438. https://doi.org/10.3390/healthcare13040438

11.4.8. Collaborative Research Initiatives

Interdisciplinary research efforts are the core of solving the complex complications surrounding rheumatic diseases in clinical pharmacology. Interdisciplinary collaborations have the potential to integrate various stakeholders' knowledge in institutional environments, healthcare organizations, and pharmaceutical companies to facilitate in-depth studies that enhance the precision of therapeutic methods.

For instance, studies like those from Open Heart International in Fiji can provide useful insight into the long-term impact of mechanical valve replacement within rheumatic heart disease and highlight post-operative surveillance and self-care (Mangnall et al., 2017). Moreover, innovative models of partnership can maximize medicine use and expenditure, and novel rheumatic disease treatments will be effective and affordable (Godman et al., 2014). By the establishment of a collaborative community of shared resources and knowledge, these activities enhance the care of patients while maintaining healthcare sustainability in situations where there is a lack of resources.

11.4.9. Future Challenges in Clinical Pharmacology

There are gigantic challenges in store for clinical pharmacology as it continues evolving, particularly in rheumatological disease treatment. Among the key challenges is the attainment of effective therapies amidst contrasting economic realities, primarily in the setting of low-resource contexts. For instance, the epidemic of hypertension in sub-Saharan Africa demonstrates how financial constraints limit access to medicines to induce prevention and early treatment strategies in line with local circumstances (Twagirumukiza & Van Bortel, 2011). Furthermore, the trend of Undifferentiated Connective Tissue Disease (UCTD) shows the intricacy of pharmacological therapy for rheumatology. Patients are more likely to present with comorbid symptoms, complicating diagnosis and treatment and further exacerbating pressure on limited rheumatology resources (Anderson, 2018). They create the imperative for innovative solutions in clinical practice, including the development of evidence-based treatment algorithms and training of primary care professionals in disease-modifying antirheumatic drug use, in order to enhance timely and appropriate management of patients within diverse healthcare environments.

Test Your Knowledge

1. How are biosimilars revolutionizing the landscape of rheumatologic pharmacotherapy?
2. What are some of the emerging small molecules being studied for inflammatory arthritis?

Summary

Rheumatic diseases clinical pharmacology emphasizes the importance of personalized therapeutic strategies to optimize patient results. As shown, patients' beliefs about drugs are significant in adherence, with increased concerns related to increased rates of non-adherence in chronic disease patients, including rheumatoid arthritis (Bo et al., 2017). Belief modification through intervention can be valuable in practice. Furthermore, the current advancements in early clinical trial methods, such as modeling and simulation, indicate the evolving nature of drug development and the need for clinical pharmacologists to adapt accordingly (Caplain et al., 2019). By incorporating patient experience and using innovative trial designs, medical practitioners can improve medication compliance and treatment of rheumatic diseases in general, leading to better health outcomes. Thus, ongoing research and the development of new practices will be essential to addressing the issues of pharmacological management in this field.

The study of clinical pharmacology in rheumatic disorders raises several important points that inform our understanding of drug efficacy and patient outcomes. For instance, the close link between skin psoriasis and developing psoriatic arthritis highlights early detection as crucial, with late diagnosis being associated with adverse long-term outcomes. Screenings with particular questionnaires have also opened up undiagnosed prevalence, and the potential of lifestyle and genetic factors guiding risk assessment has been brought into the limelight (McHugh, 2015). Further, pragmatic trials , such as the REDES-TNF trial emphasize the need for evidence-based guidelines through analyzing the impact of dose reduction in tumor necrosis factor antagonists in spondyloarthritis treatment. The project aims at determining resounding evidence that may enhance the treatment strategies and finally better inform clinical practices, capturing the complexity of treating rheumatic disease (Avendaño et al., 2015).

KEY TERMS FROM THIS CHAPTER

- Dosing
- Gastrointestinal lesions
- Tumor necrosis factor inhibitors (TNFi)
- Psoriatic arthritis
- Drug response
- Spa treatment
- Quality of life
- Non-steroidal anti-inflammatory drugs
- Pharmacotherapy
- Prescription
- Discrepancy
- Radiographic progression
- Pharmacokinetics
- Immunogenicity
- Mud-bath treatment
- Disease-modifying antirheumatic drugs
- Medications

Critical Thinking Questions

1. **Which of the following is a disease-modifying antirheumatic drug (DMARD)?**
   a. Acetaminophen
   b. Methotrexate
   c. Ibuprofen
   d. Prednisone
2. **What is the mechanism of action of methotrexate in rheumatoid arthritis?**
   a. TNF-alpha inhibition
   b. Inhibition of cyclooxygenase enzymes
   c. Folic acid antagonism affecting DNA synthesis
   d. Calcium channel blockade
3. **Which biologic agent is a TNF-alpha inhibitor?**
   a. Tocilizumab
   b. Rituximab
   c. Etanercept
   d. Abatacept
4. **Hydroxychloroquine is typically used in:**
   a. Osteoarthritis
   b. Gout
   c. Systemic lupus erythematosus
   d. Ankylosing spondylitis
5. **Which of the following is a significant toxicity to watch for with chronic hydroxychloroquine treatment?**
   a. Nephrotoxicity
   b. Retinal toxicity
   c. Hepatotoxicity
   d. Bone marrow suppression

Short Answer Questions

1. How is methotrexate's immunomodulatory effect in rheumatoid arthritis?
2. What is the mechanism of action of TNF-alpha inhibitors infliximab and adalimumab?
3. What is the initial pharmacologic management of early rheumatoid arthritis?
4. What is the management of refractory systemic lupus erythematosus?
5. What are the major adverse effects of long-term corticosteroid use?
6. What are methotrexate's toxicities, and how do they monitor them?
7. What new biologic agents are being developed for refractory rheumatoid arthritis?
8. How could precision medicine strategies enhance drug choice in SLE?

Answers to Critical Thinking Questions

1. (b); 2. (c); 3. (c); 4. (c); 5. (b)

References

1. Abbas, A., Agca, R., Ait-Oufella, H., Albert, M. A., Alexander, J., Alexander, K., et al. (2017). Targeting inflammation to reduce cardiovascular disease risk: A realistic clinical prospect? https://core.ac.uk/download/80697766.pdf (accessed on 17th June 2025).

2. Godman, B., Malmström, R. E., Diogene, E., Gray, A., Jayathissa, S., Timoney, A., Acurcio, F., Alkan, A., Brzezinska, A., Bucsics, A., Campbell, S. M., Czeczot, J., de Bruyn, W., Eriksson, I., Yusof, F. A., Finlayson, A. E., Fürst, J., Garuoliene, K., Guerra Júnior, A., Gulbinovič, J., ... Gustafsson, L. L. (2015). Are new models needed to optimize the utilization of new medicines to sustain healthcare systems?. *Expert review of clinical pharmacology*, *8*(1), 77–94. https://doi.org/10.1586/17512433.2015.990380(accessed on 17th June 2025).

3. Ahmed, S., Jones, B., & Koch, A. E. (2012). Pathological role of fractalkine/CX3CL1 in rheumatic diseases: A unique chemokine with multiple functions. https://core.ac.uk/download/pdf/8720785.pdf (accessed on 17th June 2025).

4. Altepeter, T., Bray, K., Cheifetz, A. S., Chevalier, A., et al. (2025). Therapeutic drug monitoring of biologics: Current practice, challenges and opportunities–A workshop report. https://core.ac.uk/download/653314005.docx (accessed on 17th June 2025).

5. Alturkmani, H., Baltezor, M., Butte, A. J., Chen, B., et al. (2016). *In silico* and *in vitro* drug screening identifies new therapeutic approaches for Ewing sarcoma. https://core.ac.uk/download/323072722.pdf (accessed on 17th June 2025).

6. Amit, B., Baljit, K., Gautam, S. P., Z. L., et al. (2020). A never-ending story of rheumatoid arthritis. https://core.ac.uk/download/482241560.pdf (accessed on 17th June 2025).

7. Anderson, L. A. (2018). Treatment of undifferentiated connective tissue disease with csDMARD's through primary care providers in the absence of intervention via rheumatology. https://core.ac.uk/download/235066358.pdf (accessed on 17th June 2025).

8. Avendaño, C., Calvo, G., de Miguel, E., Gratacós Masmitjà, J., et al. (2015). Evaluation of dose reduction versus standard dosing for maintenance of remission in patients with spondylarthritis and clinical remission with anti-TNF (REDES-TNF): Study protocol for a randomized controlled trial. https://core.ac.uk/download/43551498.pdf (accessed on 17th June 2025).

9. Bajorek, B., & Singh, S. (2014). Defining 'elderly' in clinical practice guidelines for pharmacotherapy. https://opus.lib.uts.edu.au/bitstream/10453/35163/1/Defining%20%27elderly%27%20in%20clinical%20practice%20guidelines%20for%20pharmacotherapy.pdf (accessed on 17th June 2025).

10. Baxter, P., Conaghan, P. G., Crossfield, S. S. R., Johnson, B., et al. (2019). Variation in methods, results and reporting in electronic health record-based studies evaluating routine care in gout: A systematic review. https://core.ac.uk/download/228166851.pdf (accessed on 17th June 2025).

11. Berardesca, E., Bernardini, N., Bianchi, L., Chimenti, S., et al. (2018). Use of biological drugs in patients with psoriasis and psoriatic arthritis in Italy: Results from the PSONG survey. https://core.ac.uk/download/154948747.pdf (accessed on 17th June 2025).

12. Bilušić, M., Erdeljić, V., Francetić, I., Huić, M., et al. (2006). Use of gastroprotective agents in recommended doses in hospitalized patients receiving NSAIDs: A drug utilization study. https://core.ac.uk/download/11699264.pdf (accessed on 17th June 2025).

13. Black, S., DeHoratius, R. J., Gaylis, N. B., Kafka, J., et al. (2017). Patient-reported outcome assessment of inflammatory arthritis patient experience with intravenously administered biologic therapy. https://core.ac.uk/download/129192309.pdf (accessed on 17th June 2025).

14. Bo, N., Champman, S., Chater, A. M., Chen, X., et al. (2017). Beliefs about medicines and non-adherence in patients with stroke, diabetes mellitus and rheumatoid arthritis: A cross-sectional study in China. https://core.ac.uk/download/130975487.pdf (accessed on 17th June 2025).

15. Bossù, M., Di Carlo, G., Giovarruscio, F., Polimeni, A., et al. (2018). Autoimmune diseases and their manifestations on oral cavity: Diagnosis and clinical management. https://core.ac.uk/download/159635803.pdf (accessed on 17th June 2025).

16. Boussery, K., Mehuys, E., Petrovic, M., Somers, A., et al. (2015). Older patients' prescriptions screening in the community pharmacy: Development of the Ghent Older People's Prescriptions Community Pharmacy Screening (GheOP3S) tool. https://core.ac.uk/download/55843875.pdf (accessed on 17th June 2025).

17. Caplain, H., Douglas, D., Hardman, T., Rottey, S., et al. (2019). *European Federation for Exploratory Medicines Development Lyon Conference 2019: The Changing Landscape of Early Medicines Development: Be Prepared*. https://core.ac.uk/download/395605450.pdf (accessed on 17th June 2025).

18. Ceccarelli, F., Fontana, M., Fraioli, A., Mennuni, G., et al. (2018). Efficacy of spa-therapy, mud-pack therapy, balneotherapy and mud-bath therapy in the management of knee osteoarthritis: A systematic review. https://core.ac.uk/download/159267875.pdf (accessed on 17th June 2025).

19. Chan, E. W. Y., Chui, C. S. L., Lai, F. T. T., Lau, M., et al. (2021). Two-dose Covid-19 vaccination and possible arthritis flare among patients with rheumatoid arthritis in Hong Kong. https://core.ac.uk/download/480393079.pdf (accessed on 17th June 2025).

20. Chester, A. H., & Yacoub, M. H. (2014). The role of endothelin-1 in pulmonary arterial hypertension. https://core.ac.uk/download/77008841.pdf (accessed on 17th June 2025).

21. Clemenza, S., Mecacci, F., Ottanelli, S., Petraglia, F., et al. (2022). Undifferentiated connective tissue disease in pregnancy: A topic yet to be explored. https://core.ac.uk/download/610511386.pdf (accessed on 17th June 2025).

22. Conway, G. E., & Heffernan, S. M. (2021). Nutraceutical alternatives to pharmaceutical analgesics in osteoarthritis. https://core.ac.uk/download/392256349.pdf (accessed on 17th June 2025).

23. Cordeiro, A., Costa, E., Cunha-Santos, F., Dourado, A., et al. (2024). Systematic literature review to inform the Portuguese recommendations for the management of Raynaud's phenomenon and digital ulcers in systemic sclerosis and other connective tissue diseases. https://core.ac.uk/download/614518814.pdf (accessed on 17th June 2025).

24. Diamanti, A. P., Lagana, B., Pioli, C., Rosado, M. M., et al. (2020). Cytokine release syndrome in COVID-19 patients, a new scenario for an old concern: The fragile balance between infections and autoimmunity. https://core.ac.uk/download/323191917.pdf (accessed on 17th June 2025).

25. Djumanov, D. (2011). Intelligent technologies for real-time monitoring and decision support systems. https://core.ac.uk/download/30696016.pdf (accessed on 17th June 2025).

26. Elewaut, D., & Matucci-Cerinic, M. (2009). Treatment of ankylosing spondylitis and extra-articular manifestations in everyday rheumatology practice. https://core.ac.uk/download/55761196.pdf (accessed on 17th June 2025).

27. Ezhil Ramya, J., Kannan, M. S., Mansoora Shahiba, R., et al. (2019). Prescribing pattern and adverse drug reactions of cardiovascular drugs in out-patient department of a tertiary care hospital. https://core.ac.uk/download/539896133.pdf (accessed on 17th June 2025).

28. Fillerová, R., Horák, P., Kriegová, E., Kudělka, J., et al. (2019). Cross-disease innate gene signature: Emerging diversity and abundance in RA comparing to SLE and SSc. https://core.ac.uk/download/237018692.pdf (accessed on 17th June 2025).

29. Gupta, R., Malhotra, A., & Malhotra, P. (2018). Study of prescription pattern of drugs used in the treatment of osteoarthritis in a tertiary care teaching hospital: An observational study. https://core.ac.uk/download/551598747.pdf (accessed on 17th June 2025).

30. Jiang, A., Cebulla, C. M., Wang, J., Christoforidis, J. B., & Chang, S. (2012). Systemic treatment of vitreous inflammation. https://core.ac.uk/download/194611210.pdf (accessed on 17th June 2025).

31. Kim, M. J. (2016). SAR studies on the inhibitors for the treatment of inflammatory diseases. https://core.ac.uk/download/79712516.pdf (accessed on 17th June 2025).

32. Kitsiou, A., Caforio, A. L. P., Porta-Sanchez, A., Vahanian, A., Iung, B., Carrera, C., Szymanski, C., et al. (2013). *ESC Core Curriculum for The General Cardiologist (2013)*. https://core.ac.uk/download/55756305.pdf (accessed on 17th June 2025).

33. Mantravadi, S., Ogdie, A., & Kraft, W. K. (2017). Tumor necrosis factor inhibitors in psoriatic arthritis. *Expert review of clinical pharmacology*, *10*(8), 899–910. https://doi.org/10.1080/17512433.2017.1329009(accessed on 17th June 2025).

34. Krishnan, S., Balan, C. S., & Mohamedali, S. P. (2018). *A Cost-Effective Analysis of Various Disease Modifying Anti-Rheumatic Drugs for Patients with Rheumatoid Arthritis*. https://core.ac.uk/download/539895924.pdf (accessed on 17th June 2025).

35. Kriukova, A., & Vladymyrova, I. (2018). Determination of technological parameters and indicators of the quality of new herbal collection. https://core.ac.uk/download/322516348.pdf (accessed on 17th June 2025).

36. Lacy, A. (2017). Dietary fat and the prevalence of hand osteoarthritis: Data from the osteoarthritis initiative. https://core.ac.uk/download/142080935.pdf (accessed on 17th June 2025).

37. Lee, Y. (2021). Circadian rhythms and the treatment of rheumatoid arthritis. https://core.ac.uk/download/614775583.pdf (accessed on 17th June 2025).

38. Malhotra, S., Pandya, S., Parikh, N., Patel, A., et al. (2018). A case series of rituximab-induced tuberculosis. https://core.ac.uk/download/543134475.pdf (accessed on 17th June 2025).

39. Mangnall, T., & Jane, L. J. (2017). Outcomes of adolescents and younger adults who have mechanical valve replacement surgery for rheumatic heart disease in a low-middle-income country. https://core.ac.uk/download/212692600.pdf (accessed on 17th June 2025).

40. McHugh, N. J. (2015). Early psoriatic arthritis. https://core.ac.uk/download/542186223.pdf (accessed on 17th June 2025).

41. Neregård, P. (2013). Studies on the therapeutic modulation of inflammation in the synovial membrane of rheumatoid arthritis. https://core.ac.uk/download/70340474.pdf (accessed on 17th June 2025).

42. Nimbalkar, V. V. (2016). Montelukast and cetirizine may ameliorate progression of rheumatoid arthritis. https://core.ac.uk/download/327998772.pdf (accessed on 17th June 2025).

43. Shehata, H., Nasr, M., & Naser, M. (2024). Role of Janus kinase inhibitors (JAKis) in autoimmune disorders: Review. https://core.ac.uk/download/636457488.pdf (accessed on 17th June 2025).

44. Twagirumukiza, M., & Van Bortel, L. M. (2011). Management of hypertension at the community level in sub-Saharan Africa (SSA): towards a rational use of available resources. *Journal of human hypertension*, *25*(1), 47–56. https://doi.org/10.1038/jhh.2010.32 (accessed on 17th June 2025).

45. Ventura, A., Taddio, A., Favretto, D., Stocco, G., Decorti, G., et al. (2015). Genetic determinants for methotrexate response in juvenile idiopathic arthritis. https://core.ac.uk/download/53745632.pdf (accessed on 17th June 2025).

46. Zhang, A., Zheng, J., Zheng, X., Zhu, Y., et al. (2024). The therapeutic effect of hydroxychloroquine on patients with recurrent miscarriage and the risk assessment of its ocular retinal toxicity. https://core.ac.uk/download/616936560.pdf (accessed on 17th June 2025).

PSYCHOSOCIAL ASPECTS OF RHEUMATIC DISEASES

12

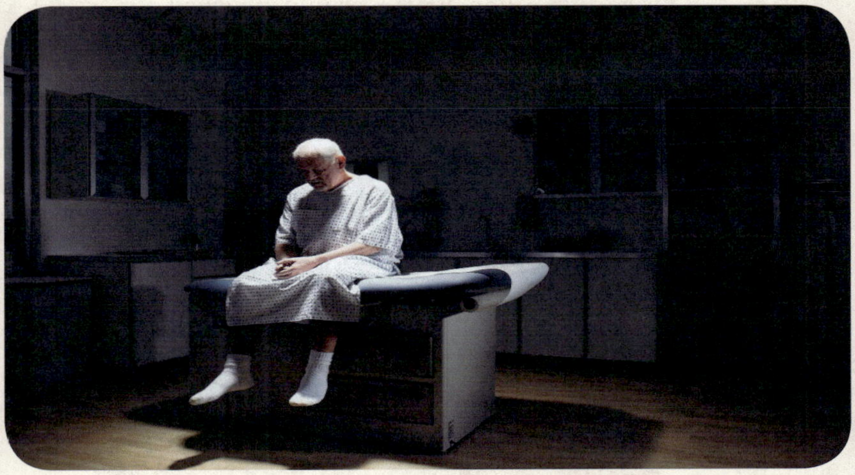

LEARNING OBJECTIVES

After studying this chapter, you will be able to:

1. Identify psychological impacts of rheumatic conditions;
2. Explain the social implications of developing rheumatic conditions;
3. Highlight the economic burden of rheumatic conditions;
4. Discuss treatments and support measures.

Introduction

Rheumatic conditions are a diverse collection of conditions that cause significant impacts on both physical function and psychosocial function. It is also important to understand the psychosocial determinants of these diseases because stressors are believed to be a major contributor to the acceleration of symptoms and the course of the disease. Studies have shown that stressful events lead to initiation and perpetuation of rheumatic diseases, with the psychosocial setting being of high relevance for disease regulation (Creemers et al., 2010). Also, a biopsychosocial model has become acknowledged as required for effective treatment services, emphasizing that biological demands are insufficient to address the complex realities of patients (Burton et al., 2008). The multidisciplinary model promotes the inclusion of psychosocial care alongside medical interventions in order to improve not only physical health status but also the overall quality of life of patients who have these chronic conditions. Hence, managing psychosocial factors becomes a critical component in the total management of rheumatic diseases.

12.1. Psychological Impact of Rheumatic Diseases

Learning Outcome

1. Identify key psychological symptoms endured;
2. Understand chronic pain and mental health;
3. Emphasize the occurrence of anxiety and depression;
4. Discuss patient coping mechanisms;
5. Acknowledge the role of psychological support in therapy;
6. Explain the role played by severity of disease on mental health;
7. Learn about rheumatoid disease stigma;
8. Discuss psychological factors in disease progression;
9. Understand the importance of mental health screenings.

The psychological impact of rheumatic diseases transcends the physical manifestation of such diseases, strongly affecting patients' mental health and well-being. Many of these patients with such diseases , such as rheumatoid arthritis have high levels of depression and anxiety, primarily due to the chronic pain and functional disability associated with their disease. These psychological issues may be compounded by the necessity for long-term treatment regimens, necessitating frequent adaptation of exercise, rest, and medication by patients to control disease activity. Successful patient education initiatives have been demonstrated to play an important role in reducing these challenges through improved self-management abilities and enhanced self-efficacy. For instance, group education programs can improve patients' knowledge about their illness and treatment to produce improved health outcomes. However, although the programs may improve physical health and self-management behaviors, improved psychosocial health status is less consistently achieved (Taal et al., 1993; Taal et al., 1997).

12.1.1. Common Psychological Symptoms Experienced

The psychological impact of rheumatic diseases is powerful and tends to manifest itself in common symptoms , such as anxiety and depression. All these conditions significantly affect the quality of life of patients and are further accompanied by the chronic pain and physical limitations that come with rheumatic conditions. Researchers have identified that approximately 20% of individuals who have chronic physical illness develop depression, which is also associated with poor treatment compliance and negative health outcomes (Chipping et al., 2016).

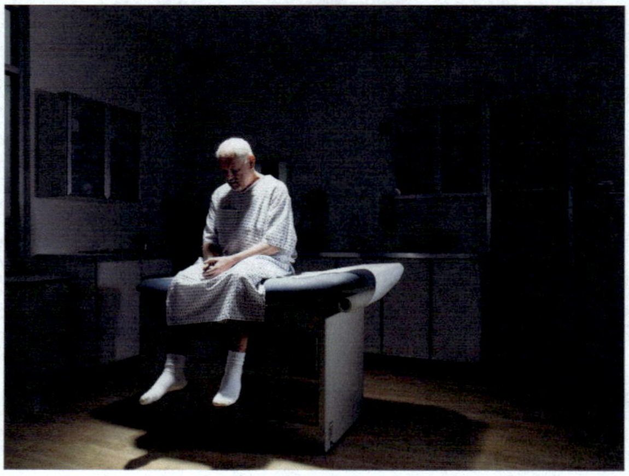

Figure 12.1. The psychological impact of rheumatic diseases is profound, often manifesting as common symptoms , such as anxiety and depression.

Source: https://www.rheumatologyadvisor.com/wp-content/uploads/sites/18/2023/11/Man.Sitting.On_.Table_G_sb10069531b-001.jpg.

Furthermore, the biopsychosocial model emphasizes the need to address psychosocial problems in conjunction with biological treatments and that optimal treatment interventions incorporating psychological support are likely to be more successful in occupational and health performance (Burton et al., 2008). The interaction of the psychological symptoms with the physical health not only complicates treatment but also demands interprofessional collaboration between healthcare workers, patients, and, where possible, employers. The identification and treatment of these common psychological symptoms are necessary to improve overall patient care and promote recovery (Figure 12.1).

12.1.2. Relationship between Chronic Pain and Mental Health

Chronic pain, particularly of rheumatic diseases, is directly related to mental disorders, typically forming a vicious cycle of worsening physical and psychological state. Evidence indicates that a large number of patients with chronic musculoskeletal pain, approximately 74.7%, also have their mood disorders undiagnosed, particularly in women and widows (Salazar et al., 2013). This contact aggravates not only the pain experience but also increases the likelihood of access to healthcare services, stressing the necessity for integrated care approaches. Moreover, the psycho-social impact of rheumatic illnesses cannot be neglected as the impact of chronic pain encompasses significant socio-economic burdens and compromised quality of life (Chipping et al., 2016). As such, there is a need to tackle the psychological dimensions of chronic pain because improving mental health dramatically enhances compliance with treatment and overall patient health outcomes for patients who are addressing these multifaceted problems.

12.1.3. Anxiety and Depression Prevalence

Prevalence rates of anxiety and depression among rheumatic disease patients are far too high, affecting both physical and psychosocial function. Research has indicated that musculoskeletal pain patients have a high prevalence of anxiety and depressive disorders, particularly in females, in whom there is a high prevalence of arthritis and rheumatoid arthritis. Specifically, it was noted in one research that the overlap between musculoskeletal pain and chronic mental illness was common, noting the complex interrelation between physical and psychological conditions (Agüera et al., 2014). In addition, mounting evidence suggests that the alterations of gut microbiota can also contribute to elevated anxiety and depression among rheumatic disease patients, which indicates the multidimensional nature of these diseases (D'Amelio et al., 2016). An understanding of the prevalence of these mental illnesses is significant as it calls for a holistic treatment plan comprising both physical rehabilitation and psychological support, finally improving the patient's quality of life (Figure 12.2).

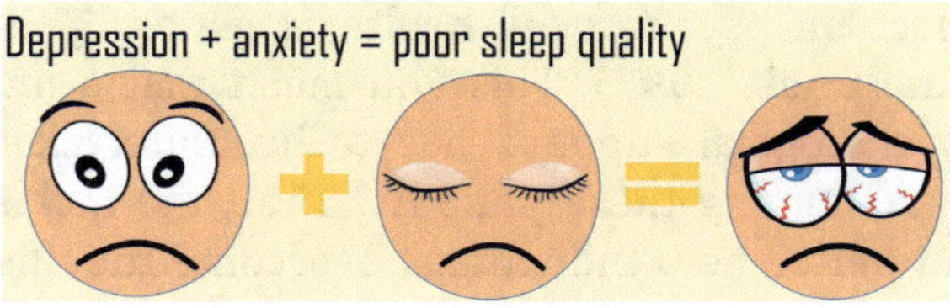

Figure 12.2. The prevalence of anxiety and depression among individuals with rheumatic diseases is alarmingly significant, influencing both physical and psychosocial well-being.

Source: https://pub.mdpi-res.com/medicina/medicina-59-01633/article_deploy/html/images/medicina-59-01633-ag.png?1694169222.

12.1.4. Coping Mechanisms Among Patients

Patient coping patterns with rheumatic diseases are a critical component of surmounting the psychological and physical barriers of the diseases. Adapting and employing effective coping can have a significant impact on health and quality of life. Research has identified that patient education interventions, e.g., group patient education programs based on social learning theory, have enhanced the self-efficacy and self-management behaviors among patients.

For instance, these interventions have yielded significant positive outcomes in targeted domains, e.g., functional disability and knowledge retention, as quoted from studies evaluating group education among rheumatoid arthritis patients (Taal et al., 1993). However, it is fascinating that even while physical gains are typically reported within overall patient groups, psychosocial gains will not automatically improve to the same extent, and therefore, there is a deficit that has to be addressed by interventions (Taal et al., 1997). Last but not least, coping skill development through training and support can empower patients to handle their disease more effectively.

12.1.5. Role of Psychological Support in Treatment

The importance of psychological support in the management of rheumatic illnesses is critical in improving patient outcomes and promoting self-management. Psychological constructs like social support and self-efficacy have a significant impact on an individual's ability to stay on treatment protocols and control their symptoms. A highly significant study affirms that sense of dependency and pain can detract from health quality of life, emphasizing the necessity to consider emotional well-being as much as physical treatment (Taal et al., 1993). Furthermore, while group education classes have been demonstrated to advance patient knowledge and some facets of behavior, their effect on psychosocial health is generally limited, particularly in rheumatoid arthritis patients (Taal et al., 1997). This will mean that a multi-dimensional approach, both education and good psychological support, has to be undertaken to sustain early gains and improve global health status among these patients. Thus, the inclusion of psychological support in treatment regimens can better help individuals overcome the obstacles related to their conditions (Figure 12.3).

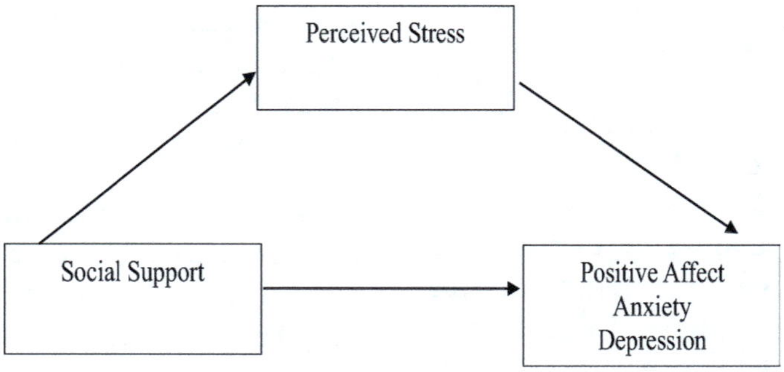

Figure 12.3. Psychological factors , such as self-efficacy and social support, significantly influence an individual's ability to adhere to treatment regimens and manage symptoms effectively.

Source: https://www.frontiersin.org/files/Articles/1330720/fpsyg-15-1330720-HTML/image_m/fpsyg-15-1330720-g001.jpg.

12.1.6. Impact of Disease Severity on Mental Health

The severity of rheumatic disease also plays a vital role in the mental health of the involved patients, often resulting in comorbid mood disorders. Research highlighted that approximately 74.7% of patients with chronic musculoskeletal pain, a common symptom of rheumatic disease, suffered from undiagnosed mood disorders, emphasizing the need for enhanced diagnostic processes in primary care (Salazar et al., 2013). Furthermore, symptoms like pain intensity and sleep are found to aggravate these psychological issues, indicating a causative relationship between physical and psychological health (Salazar et al., 2013). Although education programs would optimize disease management ability and physical health, they are of limited intervention on psychosocial health in most instances, particularly in the case of rheumatoid arthritis patients. This means that while physical care is essential, there is a pressing need for integrative interventions that also intervene in mental health problems to improve overall patient outcomes for rheumatic disease management.

12.1.7. Stigma associated with Rheumatic Diseases

Stigma associated with rheumatic diseases predominantly aggregates the psychosocial problems of the patients, adversely affecting their overall well-being. These patients can also become socially isolated and stigmatized due to a lack of knowledge regarding rheumatic diseases and their latent presentation.

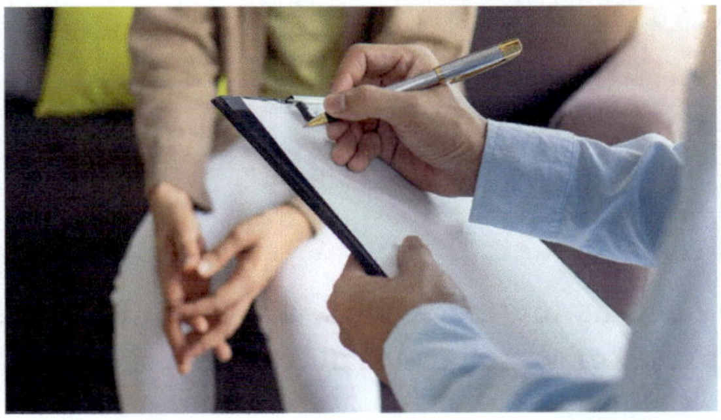

Figure 12.4. The stigma associated with rheumatic diseases significantly exacerbates the psychosocial challenges that patients face, hindering their overall quality of life.

Source: https://www.asterhospitals.in/sites/default/files/styles/webp/public/2024-11/psoriasis.jpg.webp?itok=3gvfAPfZ.

Stigma can influence self-esteem and lead to anxiety and depression, which, as per a study, can lead to a substantial decrease in physical quality of life scores in such patients (Ben-Shlomo et al., 2002). In addition, social interaction between the patients is often limited as they move through the social attitudes that devalue their experiences and capabilities. Addressing this stigma is significant because the interventions not only need to address the physical regulation of rheumatic disease but also psychological health and the enablement of supportive networks of social support (Bee et al., 2016). By reducing stigma, we can improve both quality of life and coping for patients affected by these chronic diseases (Figure 12.4).

12.1.8. Influence of Psychological Factors on Disease Progression

The interactive dynamic of psychological factors influences disease progression in patients with rheumatic diseases, particularly rheumatoid arthritis. Psychological distress, such as depression and anxiety, is prevalent among these patients and has been shown to have a negative effect on treatment outcomes and overall coping with chronic disease. The interaction between psychological well-being and disease activity suggests that individuals with rheumatoid arthritis may be at increased disease burden if psychological distress is not recognized and not treated adequately. There is evidence that identification and treatment of these psychological factors can enhance the effectiveness of treatment and adherence, leading ultimately to improved outcomes for the patient.

Also, resiliency or positive psychological attributes, such as adaptive coping styles and optimism, may have potentially protective functions in relation to disease progression; however, these are not so well supported in rheumatic disease. Thus, the integration of psychological care within the extended therapeutic model is imperative to achieve enhanced health outcomes and respond to the intricate nature of rheumatoid arthritis (Geenen et al., 2015; Mechling, 2020).

12.1.9. Importance of Mental Health Screenings

Mental health screenings in rheumatic diseases are critical in uncovering and treating emotional distress that is typically accompanied by chronic illness. Individuals suffering from chronic pain, for instance, low back pain, are at greater risk of suffering from mood disorders , such as depression and anxiety that will exacerbate their physical condition and hinder recovery (Gouveia et al., 2015). Moreover, the overlap between mental and physical health is considerable; dispositional optimism, for example, will improve quality of life related to health by provoking health-inducing behavior and augmenting symptom management self-efficacy (Treaster et al., 2021). As such, universal screening for mental health will contribute to early intervention measures, with integrated care being administered for both physical and mental health. This dual approach not only contributes to the mitigation of some of the symptom load of rheumatic diseases but also contributes to better overall patient outcomes, underscoring the need for mental health screenings in this population (Figure 12.5).

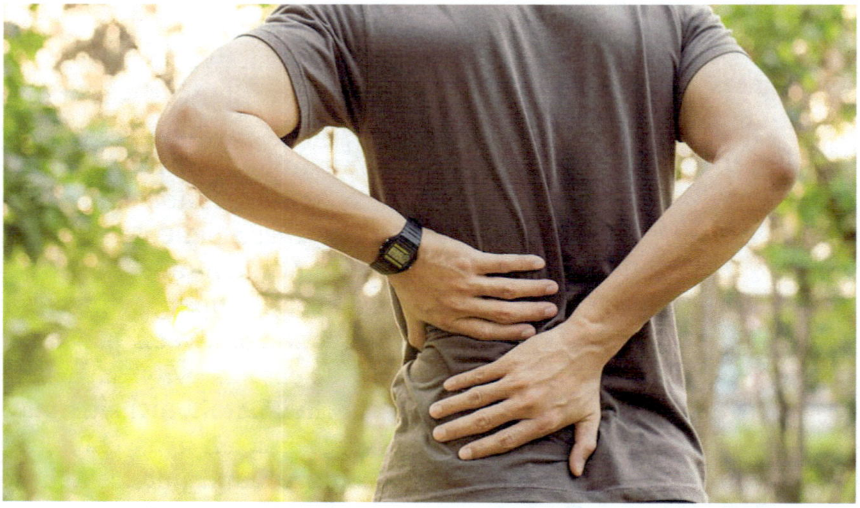

Figure 12.5. Individuals suffering from chronic pain, such as low back pain, are at an increased risk for developing mood disorders like anxiety and depression, which can exacerbate their physical symptoms and hinder recovery.

Source: https://www.recoveryranch.com/wp-content/uploads/2020/03/shutterstock_607977332.jpg.

Test Your Knowledge

1. How does chronic steroid use affect mood and cognition?
2. How does fatigue in rheumatic diseases affect mental status and functional ability?

12.2. Social Implications of Living with Rheumatic Diseases

Learning Outcome

1. Understand social relationship and support system effects;
2. Recognize challenges in maintaining employment;
3. Describe the impact on family relationships;
4. Understand social isolation and its impact;
5. Highlight the role of a community support group;
6. Discuss the role of societal opinions in affecting self-esteem;
7. Describe barriers to social participation;
8. Understand the importance of social networks to adjustment;
9. Acquire methods for enhancing social support.

Living with rheumatoid diseases extends much more deeply than never-ending physical suffering and profoundly impacts social relationships and developmental processes. In adolescents and young adults, the diseases not only restrict physical activity but also disrupt socialization and autonomy. This results in an intense sense of isolation in major developmental stages (Chaplin & Cai, 2019). Such social isolation has the potential to aggravate anxiety and depression and lead to a suboptimal quality of life. Further, children with rheumatic diseases also have complex issues that create pressure on family relationships and necessitate reassessment of the social roles in the family environment (Ballabeni et al., 2017). Adequate control of the disease, accompanied by supportive health systems, must be facilitated to provide physical and psychological well-being. By establishing social constructs that are focused on social support and useful healthcare interventions, society can mitigate the adverse social impacts of rheumatic diseases, thus improving the overall psychosocial welfare of sufferers.

12.2.1. Effects on Social Relationships and Support Systems

In addition to physiological effects, rheumatic diseases do have significant effects on social relationships, support systems. The patients usually experience debilitating pain and disability that causes them to isolate themselves from social interactions and prefer staying alone. As observed in research, the psychological weight of these diseases triggers emotional stresses , such as frustration and anxiety, further straining family and friends' relationships (Oliveira et al., 2012).

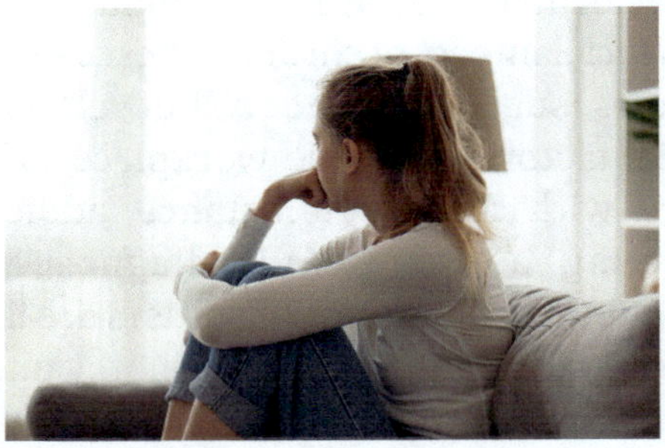

Figure 12.6. Patients often experience debilitating pain and disability, which can lead to withdrawal from social interactions and a sense of isolation.

Source: https://www.verywellhealth.com/thmb/LvIwCWDwyN_kWdjvpWPV59zQvf4=/1500x0/filters:no_upscale():max_bytes(150000):strip_icc()/upset-woman-sitting-on-couch-alone-at-home-1063392686-398bb41f1f2146c5b6abeea6257e1d0b.jpg.

However, their effects can be moderated through the presence of an efficient support system, as illustrated by studies attributing the importance of patients' families and friends to their support of their well-being. Psychological distress, which also prevails among individuals with rheumatoid arthritis, not only interferes with response to therapy but also depletes patients' resources to engage meaningfully with their social support (Geenen et al., 2015). As a result, the establishment of robust support systems can form an integral part of the management of the physical and psychological consequences of rheumatic diseases (Figure 12.6).

12.2.2. Challenges in Maintaining Employment

Continuing work in the face of a rheumatic disease poses serious issues, particularly due to the multifaceted nature of such diseases. They usually suffer from crippling fatigue and pain, which may be debilitating and affect task performance as well as productivity. The psychosocial impact of chronic illnesses, as noted by studies, suggests that social development is a crucial factor within the workplace for those afflicted with them. For instance, adolescents and young adults (AYAs) diagnosed with rheumatic musculoskeletal disorders are likely to experience challenges with autonomy and peer relationship development, both of which play a crucial role in work stability and satisfaction (Chaplin & Cai, 2019). Moreover, women living with rheumatoid arthritis predominantly experience limitations that adversely affect their body image and subjective quality of life, also increasing their challenges to navigate the labor market (Carradice et al., 2011). These interconnected challenges underscore the necessity of addressing physical and mental health in an effort to develop a supportive work environment that aids in promoting and retaining work for individuals with rheumatic disease.

12.2.3. Impact on Family Dynamics

Rheumatic disease diagnosis tends to reverberate through family structure, creating role and responsibility changes, as well as emotional climate. Where one of the family members is suffering from chronic pain or disability linked to conditions like rheumatoid arthritis or lupus, the care and support may fall on someone else in the family. The switch may result in disturbance of the traditional family structure, with the necessity for adjustments that might turn out to put strain on relationships and challenge good communication. There is evidence that chronic disease tends to provoke guilt and shame in suffering parents as they attempt to fulfill parenting roles in addition to their health, influencing the well-being of their children and the entire family (Sauder et al., 2016). In addition, the psychological effects of such diseases, such as anxiety and depression, may also intensify conflict within the family, ultimately requiring a joint effort to promote resilience and empathy (Cardona et al., 2016). Such changes illustrate the complex interdependencies of family members dealing with the psychosocial issues caused by rheumatic diseases (Figure 12.7).

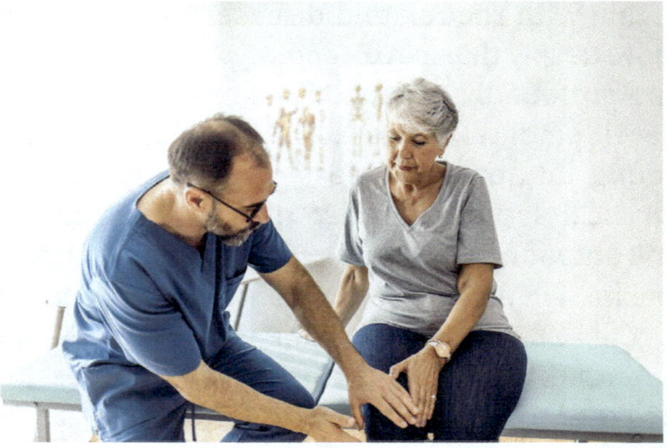

Figure 12.7. The diagnosis of rheumatic diseases often reverberates through family dynamics, leading to shifts in roles, responsibilities, and emotional climate.

Source: https://www.verywellhealth.com/thmb/BoD91m_Kg3QqCQTviFUOEffSb8Q=/1500x0/filters:no_upscale():max_bytes(150000):strip_icc()/GettyImages-1325014006-90421ccba6a74586adf120927a8a6e2d.jpg.

12.2.4. Social Isolation and Its Consequences

Social isolation typically manifests as a deep-rooted result of rheumatic diseases, severely affecting patients' psychosocial health. Ongoing physical limitations that accompany diseases like chronic chikungunya and juvenile arthritis not only decrease daily functions but also cause social withdrawal, thus feelings of isolation and hopelessness. They usually complain of mood changes, and these may be depression or anxiety, hence increasing isolation (Bailey et al., 2023). The isolation is not just for the patient alone but extends to family and community relationships, creating a trend of dependency and low social support (Bruns et al., 2010). The ramifications of such social isolation can be an extremely diminished quality of life, increased healthcare utilization, and increased caregiver burden, and the importance of addressing these psychosocial concerns in comprehensive treatment plans for rheumatic diseases is illustrated.

12.2.5. Role of Community Support Groups

The role of community support groups is crucial in addressing the psychosocial issues of rheumatic disease patients. These support groups offer an environment of shared experience, allowing members to empathize with one another through comparable challenges and develop coping strategies. Through group sessions, members often report greater emotional resilience, which is required due to the chronic pain and disability present in these conditions. Furthermore, support groups can offer access to relevant information and resources regarding treatment, thereby allowing individuals to make informed choices regarding healthcare. The incorporation of peer support not only reduces perceptions of loneliness but also promotes compliance with medical advice, as indicated by the focus on patient outcomes in clinical guidelines (Williamson et al., 2017) and the value of integrated care to maximize treatment effectiveness (Kirchhof et al., 2016). This community-based system of health and well-being demonstrates the crucial role that support networks play in the control of chronic disease , such as rheumatic diseases (Figure 12.8).

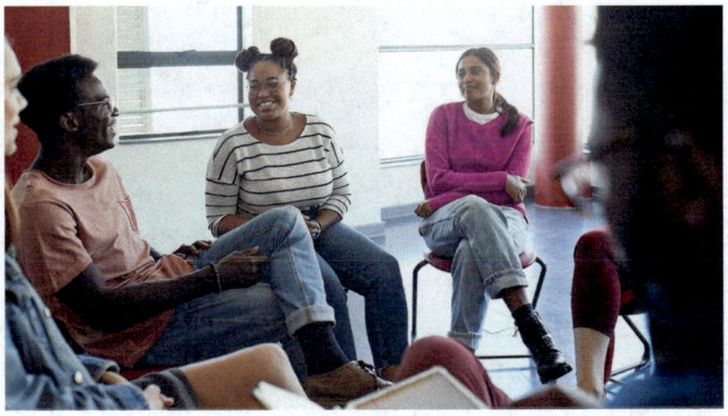

Figure 12.8. Community support groups play a vital role in addressing the psychosocial needs of individuals suffering from rheumatic diseases.

Source: https://i0.wp.com/post.healthline.com/wp-content/uploads/2020/04/therapy-group-therapist-talking-1296x728-header.jpg?w=1155&h=1528.

12.2.6. Influence of Societal Perceptions on Self-esteem

Societal perceptions significantly affect people's self-esteem, particularly for those with rheumatic diseases. Consider chronic diseases; they are sure to be stigmatized, and the outcome is that individuals with them feel less worthy and inadequate. All the misconceptions and judgments that end up occurring around rheumatic diseases enhance psychological distress, which passes through the route of increased anxiety or depression. These social attitudes can be internalized by patients with rheumatic diseases, and in turn, create a vicious cycle of negative self-image and poor quality of life related to health. (Treaster et al., 2021) quote that people with chronic diseases have a low quality of life due to the psychiatric sequelae of their conditions, which further fixes their low self-esteem. Besides, as stated in Benelli et al. (2015), mental health help-seeking barriers may prevent individuals from expressing such emotions, leading to unmet psychological needs that have a detrimental effect on self-esteem, thus rendering them more difficult to achieve an overall psychosocial well-being.

12.2.7. Barriers to Social Participation

Social participation is critical for individuals with rheumatic diseases because it determines their psychosocial well-being, yet there are various barriers to their social participation. Chronic pain and physical disability associated with such conditions are likely to induce social isolation affecting self-esteem and quality of life. The social and developmental context of AYAs with chronic rheumatic musculoskeletal disease needs to be clarified since they influence their disease management and overall psychosocial outcome (Chaplin & Cai, 2019).

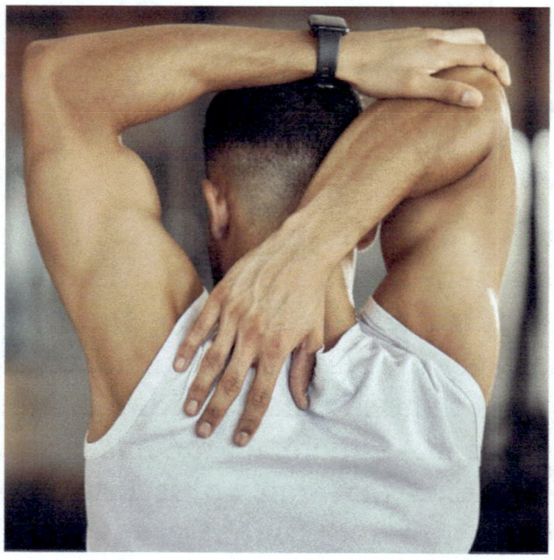

Figure 12.9. Chronic pain and physical limitations associated with these conditions often lead to social isolation, negatively affecting self-esteem and quality of life.

Source: https://www.qntsport.com/img/cms/Design%20sans%20titre-10.png.

Further, system issues, such as the lack of culturally competent healthcare professionals, contribute to barriers to participation, particularly in marginalized communities. For instance, Aboriginal Health Workers (AHWs) are essential to connecting these groups with health care systems, yet they get their skills underutilized due to lack of recognition as well as access to training opportunities (Reath et al., 2025). Breaking these barriers is necessary for facilitating social inclusion and enhancing the overall well-being of individuals with rheumatic illnesses (Figure 12.9).

12.2.8. Importance of Social Networks for Coping

The contribution of social networks in managing rheumatic diseases like rheumatoid arthritis (RA) cannot be overemphasized since they have a significant bearing on patients' emotional and psychological status. Social support plays an important role as a buffer against the distress that in most instances is reported to occur with chronic conditions, promoting coping and enhancing effective self-management practices. Individuals with strong social relationships are likely to possess better quality of life and healthy coping behaviors, which are significant factors in overcoming RA adversity. Furthermore, significant gender differences are reported in terms of experiences and coping methods, particularly related to the psychosocial impact of RA and the effectiveness of support mechanisms. As identified in recent literature, a majority of them so with men, there exists a disturbing lack of knowledge about their specific support needs within the context of RA (Flurey et al., 2015; White et al., 2015). As such, the improvement of social networks is a crucial component for the augmentation of psychosocial outcomes among individuals with rheumatic diseases.

12.2.9. Strategies for Enhancing Social Support

Effective interventions for enhancing social support for patients with rheumatic disorders are crucial to enhance their overall psychosocial well-being. Among the promising ways is to organize group education programs that facilitate community and shared experiences among patients. These programs have been found to enhance participants' health knowledge, through which patients can improve their management of disease. However, while group education improved physical health status, it sometimes fell behind the improvement of psychosocial health outcomes and therefore needed increased research on individualized intervention to sustain early gains (Taal et al., 1997). Psychological distress recognition and management are also important since symptoms like depression and anxiety can significantly hamper treatment outcome and coping capacity (Geenen et al., 2015). By attending to both educational and affective types of support, health care providers can create more comprehensive systems that better equip patients to deal with the subtleties of living with rheumatologic disease (Figure 12.10).

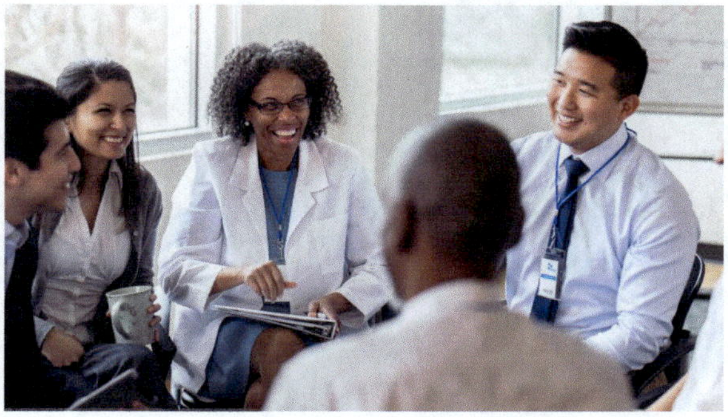

Figure 12.10. Implementation of group education programs that foster community and shared experiences among patients.

Source: https://jnj-connectivity.brightspotcdn.com/dims4/default/1a87f8e/2147483647/strip/true/crop/1400x787+0+73/resize/1000x562!/quality/90/?url=https%3A%2F%2Fjnj-brightspot.s3.amazonaws.com%2Fjnj-connectivity%2Fbe%2F28%2F9e8092b94f2484c61e4b0386bcfb%2Fgettyimages-1134043603.jpg.

Test Your Knowledge

1. How might stigma surrounding invisible diseases (e.g., lupus, fibromyalgia) impact social interactions?
2. What are the effects of rheumatic disease on caregiving and parenting roles?

12.3. Economic Burden of Rheumatic Diseases

Learning Outcome

1. Understand the direct medical cost of treatment
2. Explain indirect cost due to lost productivity;
3. Focus on the monetary burden on families;
4. Explain insurance coverage and access;
5. Know the economic impact on health systems;
6. Describe the cost-effectiveness of psychosocial treatments;
7. Discuss the government and policy role in support;
8. Learn financial planning for patients in the long term;
9. Know the significance of financial counseling.

The financial contribution of rheumatic conditions extends beyond straightforward health expenditure, playing a significant role in affecting the quality of life of patients and their productivity in society. Rheumatoid arthritis and juvenile arthritis are conditions that often generate functional disability and may be associated with increased utilization of healthcare, often manifested as high rates of attendances and hospitalization (Salazar et al., 2013). For instance, the high rate of undiagnosed comorbid mood disorders among chronic pain patients hastens such financial burden, as comorbid patients are bound to overuse healthcare services and thus incur more costs (Salazar et al., 2013). In addition, juvenile arthritis also has not only the physical impact on children but also the emotional and social dysfunction that continues into adulthood, and the economic burden to individuals as well as to families becomes even more difficult. Therefore, addressing the economic cost of rheumatic disease needs a multidisciplinary approach with not only medical treatment but psychological support as well as socioeconomic considerations.

12.3.1. Direct Medical Costs Associated with Treatment

The immediate medical expenditures for the treatment of rheumatic conditions are considerable and complex, including costs related to medication, physician appointments, and hospital care. Patients often suffer a range of physical difficulties, including pain and disability, that may complicate their ability to comply with regimens of treatment. For instance, a study noted that self-efficacy plays a crucial role in health-related concerns, where poor adherence to health recommendations is normally blamed on patients' coping expectations rather than their clinical conditions (Taal et al., 1993).

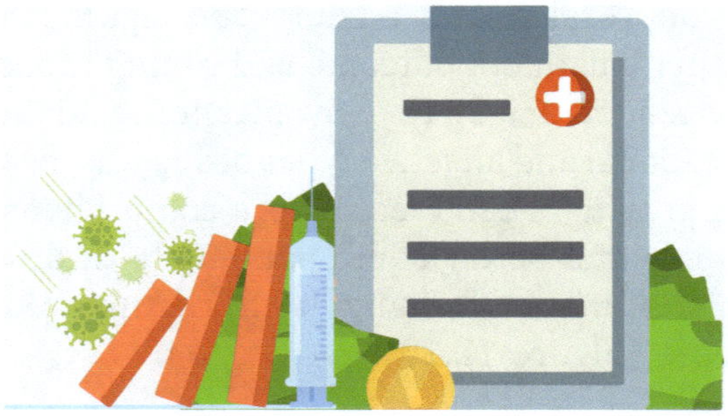

Figure 12.11. The direct medical costs associated with the treatment of rheumatic diseases are significant and multifaceted, encompassing expenses related to medication, physician visits, and hospitalization.

Source: https://ihf-fih.org/wp-content/uploads/2023/11/YEL-2023-Deliverables-1.png.

Additionally, the majority of chronic musculoskeletal pain patients also experience high rates of occult mood disorders, which complicate their management further and boosts healthcare consumption (Salazar et al., 2013). Therefore, having knowledge of and managing both the psychosocial as well as physical needs of these patients is a requirement in the designing of effective treatment plans that not only reduce direct medical costs but also enhance overall patient outcomes (Figure 12.11).

12.3.2. Indirect Costs Related to Lost Productivity

Rheumatic diseases, and rheumatoid arthritis in particular, have elevated indirect costs in terms of lost productivity among the afflicted. These are not only due to absenteeism but also presenteeism, when workers report to duty but are unable to perform at their optimal abilities due to sickness. Workers with such conditions often acquire functional limitations that make them unable to work optimally within their capabilities, leading to lower productivity and creative outputs (Voskuyl et al., 2012). The psychosocial effects of emotional distress and social impairment due to chronic disability and pain also increase the productivity loss (Bruns et al., 2010). When these patients strive to conquer the double challenge of dealing with their illness and doing well on the job, economic costs of lost productivity extend outside the workplace and spillover into families and society at large. Being able to manage these indirect costs with special interventions at the workplace could enhance overall productivity with some respite from the emotional and social costs incurred by the patients with rheumatic diseases.

12.3.3. Financial Strain on Families

The financial impact on families with rheumatic illnesses is a critical concern that is entrenched in psychosocial problems. Conditions like arthritis not only result in substantial medical expenses but also lead to loss of earnings for caregivers and patients alike, upon which there is the need for adjustments in budget by families (Smedley et al., 2014). Moreover, in mothers with chronic illnesses, the weight of carrying out parenting responsibilities also adds to feelings of incompetence and guilt when they perceive their own ill health to be an impediment to quality care (Sauder et al., 2016). These twin dangers of economic pressure and emotional distress can potentially make family lives stressful because families must inhabit a time of dissolution of such boundaries between doctor's office and home life. Thus, it is essential to understand the psychosocial dimensions of cost burden as it evokes the need for support mechanisms oriented towards the needs of the patient who can alleviate the cost burden and also address the broader emotional implications of managing chronic diseases (Figure 12.12).

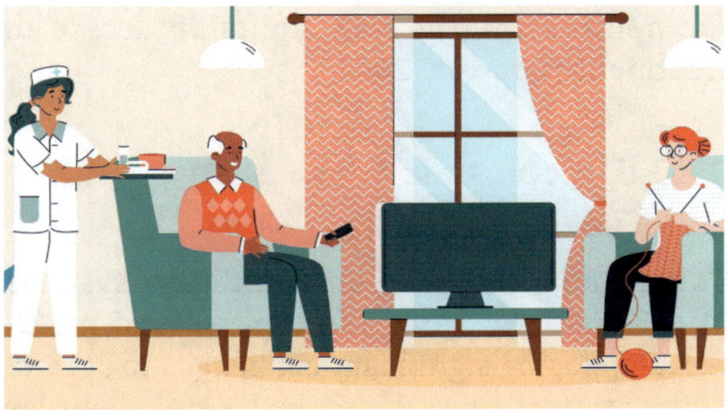

Figure 12.12. Chronic conditions , such as arthritis not only incur substantial medical expenses but also lead to a loss of income for caregivers and patients alike, necessitating adjustments to family budgets.

Source: https://irpp.org/wp-content/uploads/2023/10/Long-Term-Care-Financing.jpg.

12.3.4. Insurance Coverage and Access to Care

The interaction between insurance coverage and access to care is a critical aspect in the management of rheumatic diseases, as it affects treatment response and the quality of life of patients. Restricted insurance coverage can impede access to appropriate healthcare services, adding further burden to the psychosocial problems of individuals with chronic illness. For instance, rheumatic diseases patients may require intensive care, such as frequent consultation and alternative treatment modalities, which are not fully reimbursed by their insurance plan. As a result, care gaps may occur, particularly at transitions of care, such as the transition from pediatric to adult rheumatology, where disease status and treatment management might be poorly managed if access is restricted (Ravelli et al., 2009). Furthermore, the psychological and emotional stress of coping with insurance complexity can reinforce the sense of vulnerability and loneliness among patients, stressing the need for policies that deliver equitable access to treatment (Loprest, 2007).

12.3.5. Economic Impact on Healthcare Systems

The economic impact on healthcare systems of rheumatic diseases is extensive and multi-faceted, posing significant challenges to society and patients alike. Musculoskeletal disorder patients are at risk for chronic pain and disability, which leads to increased medical costs associated with treatment, drug therapy, and rehabilitation. Crucially, the burden of disease is not just clinical presentations but also involves relevant socioeconomic consequences in the form of absenteeism and presenteeism at work, which undermine productivity and economic independence (Gouveia et al., 2015). Further, research identifies interrelated psychosocial factors whereby mental health conditions , such as depression and anxiety, have been linked to exacerbating the physical condition felt by rheumatic patients (Chipping et al., 2016). Hence, the economic burden must be addressed through an integrated solution that addresses both medical measures and psychological intervention mechanisms to prevent costs and promote the overall health of affected populations (Figure 12.13).

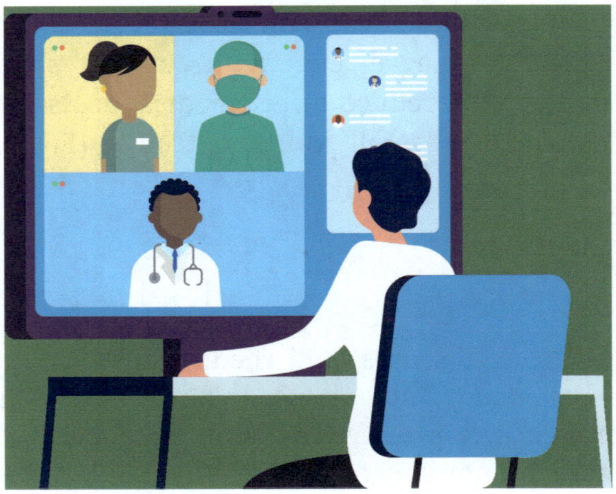

Figure 12.13. Individuals suffering from musculoskeletal conditions often experience chronic pain and disability, which leads to increased healthcare costs associated with treatment, medication, and rehabilitation.

Source: https://i0.wp.com/spritehealth.com/wp-content/uploads/2020/07/Supportive_2.png?ssl=1.

12.3.6. Cost-effectiveness of Psychosocial Interventions

Psychosocial interventions for the management of rheumatic diseases increasingly receive acceptance as an essential component of enhancing patient treatment and work outcomes. It is contended that research shows that the sole use of biomedical treatments for such conditions as upper limb disorders may not be adequate, as these approaches are not tackling the multifaceted experience of patients. Multimodal treatments that integrate psychosocial support and traditional medical treatment have proven to deliver significant improvement in the management of pain as well as workplace retention (Burton et al., 2008). Similarly, the undervalued significance of foot problems in rheumatoid arthritis demonstrates that psychosocial-based comprehensive care has a profound benefit in advancing the quality of life in patients (Chapman et al., 2010).

Interventions like these can create a culture of integrated care among patients, employers, and health professionals, which eventually results in improved management taking into account the interactions among biological, psychological, and social factors affecting rheumatic diseases.

12.3.7. Role of Government and Policy in Support

Government plays a key role in developing policy to sustain persons with rheumatic diseases, most importantly in supporting the psychosocial aspects of these diseases. Policy success to deal with rheumatic diseases relies on the recognition of intricate interrelatedness among physical health, mental health, and socioeconomic status, as indicated in current research. For instance, rheumatology clinics are encouraged to provide integrated psychosocial care, highlighting the importance of integrating mental health care into clinical practice (Chipping et al., 2016). Furthermore, the example of Aboriginal Health Workers demonstrates the importance of culturally relevant care in addressing the specialty challenges faced by marginalized populations, where socioeconomic disadvantage greatly impacts health outcomes (Reath et al., 2025). By favoring collaborative approaches that engage multiscalar healthcare professionals and drawing on community resources, government policy can enhance holistic treatment of rheumatic diseases, ultimately leading to improved patient compliance, effectiveness of treatment, and overall quality of life (Figure 12.14).

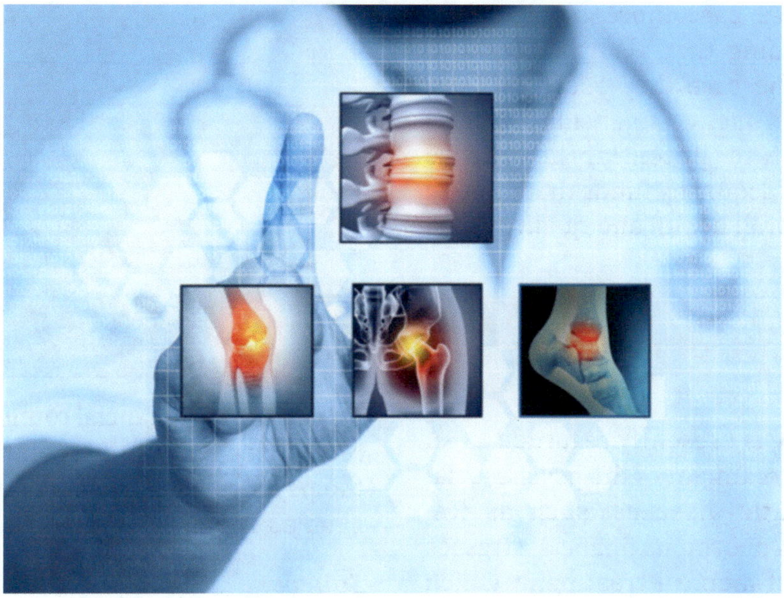

Figure 12.14. The government plays a critical role in shaping policies that support individuals affected by rheumatic diseases, particularly in addressing the psychosocial aspects of these conditions.

Source: https://m.economictimes.com/thumb/height-450,width-600,imgsize-1393742,msid-108681086/the-research-emphasizes-the-importance-of-discussing-family-planning-and-tailoring-medical-care-for-individuals-with-rheumatic-diseases-to-reduce-risks-during-pregnancy-representative-image.jpg.

12.3.8. Long-term Financial Planning for Patients

Good long-term financial planning is necessary for rheumatic disease patients because the persistent nature of such a disease is likely to lead to enormous medical bills. Long-term conditions like rheumatoid arthritis not only incur costs in terms of treatment and medication but also affect the working capacity of the patient, therefore his or her income, and even his or her savings plan. As emphasized in recent discussions on the psychosocial impact of rheumatic diseases, managing such diseases must consider the social and economic settings of the patients, particularly among young adults and adolescents who are seeking to navigate development (Chaplin & Cai, 2019). Secondly, restricted access to basic services , such as orthotic care makes care more burdensome on patients, something that also manifests in grievances about the care they receive (Ross, 2012). Therefore, proactive financial planning needs to incorporate potential healthcare expenses and aim at acquiring funds that directly benefit patients' overall health and quality of life in the long term.

12.3.9. Importance of Financial Counseling

Financial counseling is presently regarded as an integral part in the treatment of the psychosocial aspects of rheumatic diseases, such as RA. Patients end up with enormous financial stresses from the expense of medical treatment, which aggravates psychological distress and makes treatment regimen adherence complicated. Handling this fiscal issue is important because running out of enough finances leads to more stress, further endangering a patient's state of health. Evidence demonstrates that self-efficacy is maximally relevant in self-managing medical illnesses, and economic advice can enhance self-efficacy by providing patients with information and skills to make healthy financial choices (Taal et al., 1993). In addition, notification of the economic implications of treatment regimens can abate fear and allow for enhanced adherence to health recommendations and guidelines, ultimately improving quality of life (White et al., 2015). Thus, the integration of financial counseling in the care continuum of rheumatic disease patients is imperative to complete management and improved psychosocial outcomes (Figure 12.15).

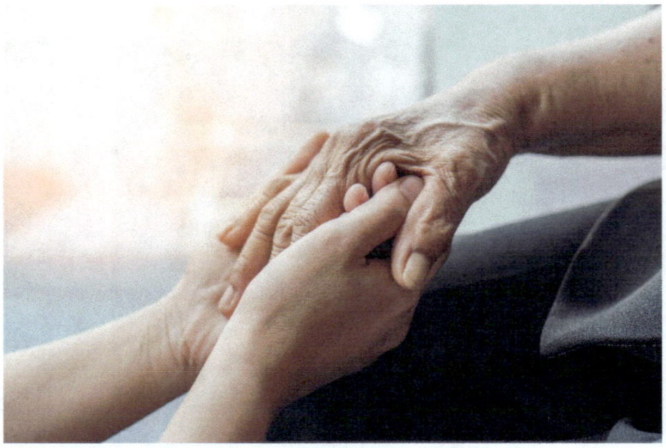

Figure 12.15. Financial counseling is increasingly recognized as a critical component in managing the psychosocial aspects of rheumatic diseases, such as rheumatoid arthritis (RA).

Source: https://medizinonline.com/wp-content/uploads/2023/10/iStock-1218464621-1920x1280.jpg.

Test Your Knowledge

1. What are the financial barriers to accessing biologic therapies in rheumatology?
2. How do insurance limits affect continuity of care in chronic autoimmune patients?

12.4. Interventions and Support Strategies

Learning Outcome

1. Give an overview of psychosocial interventions;
2. Understand the role of a multidisciplinary care team;
3. Know the role of patient education;
4. Discuss the effectiveness of cognitive-behavioral therapy;
5. Explain stress reduction and mindfulness strategies;
6. Highlight support groups and peer counseling;
7. Describe the physical therapy role in psychosocial health;
8. Highlight family involvement in treatment plans.

Optimal control of rheumatic diseases necessitates an overall understanding of both medical and psychosocial management, as these patients may present with significant issues that cannot be readily addressed through physical symptoms. Interventions involving group education have been demonstrated to be an encouraging tool for intervention, having been found to enhance patient knowledge and maintain positive behavior change over time if somewhat variably successful in improving psychosocial health status (Taal et al., 1997). Moreover, a biopsychosocial response is crucial here, recognizing that treating only biological factors would be inadequate; psychosocial factors tend to be central in recovery and job retention (Burton et al., 2008). Combining all these varied strategies of support not only enlists the patient's strength but also promotes a unified effort by healthcare professionals, family, and employers, thus bringing overall treatment outcomes closer. Future research must focus on refining these interventions and testing for long-term efficacy to allow for the sustained improvement in the quality of life of individuals with rheumatic disease.

12.4.1. Overview of Psychosocial Interventions

Psychosocial interventions are key to the management of rheumatic diseases because they address both the psychological and social factors in patient care. Group education programs, for example, have been found to enhance patients' knowledge about their condition, health behaviors, and health status. Research highlights that while such a program of education may lead to improved physical health outcomes, it does not often translate to improved psychosocial well-being, particularly in the case of rheumatoid arthritis patients (Taal et al., 1997). Also, successful management of upper limb disorders illustrates the significance of adopting a biopsychosocial perspective, which acknowledges that psychosocial factors are key to establishing occupational health outcomes (Burton et al., 2008). Hence, an interdisciplinary care process integrating medical, psychological, and social support systems is required to improve the quality of life of rheumatic disease patients, in turn leading to improved long-term health outcomes (Figure 12.16).

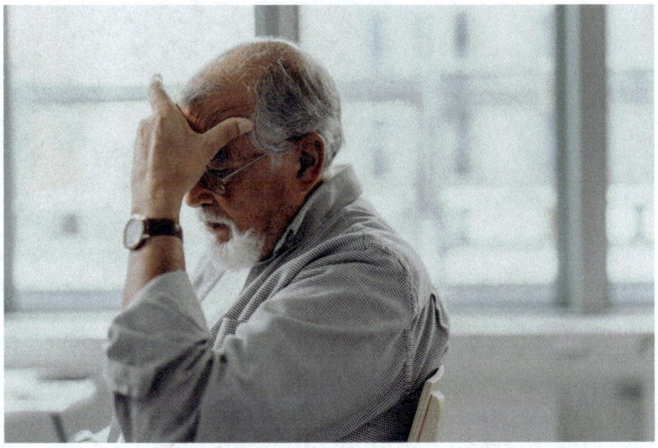

Figure 12.16. Psychosocial interventions play a crucial role in managing rheumatic diseases, addressing both the psychological and social dimensions of patient care.

Source: https://www.rheumatologyadvisor.com/wp-content/uploads/sites/18/2024/10/Stressed.Older_.Man_G_1765296829.jpg.

12.4.2. Role of Multidisciplinary Care Teams

The multicomplication of rheumatic disorders calls for the implementation of multidisciplinary care teams to treat the various psychosocial aspects of the disorders. Most often, these teams comprise rheumatologists, physical therapists, occupational therapists, psychologists, and social workers, thus promoting an integrated approach to patient care. Through integrating various specializations, care teams are capable of creating specialized rehabilitation programs emphasizing pain management, joint function protection, and facilitation of active participation in daily activity. The relevance of this approach is underscored by a growing amount of literature that identifies the positive impact in relation to multidisciplinary rehabilitation in rheumatic disease patients, including improved quality of life and enhanced psychosocial well-being (Alnaimat et al., 2023). Besides, discourse on transitional care for the situation of adolescents with conditions , such as juvenile idiopathic arthritis points out the significance of collaborative strategies in providing appropriate transition to adult health care (Camfield et al., 2018). This collaborative model not only enhances clinical outcomes but also creates a supportive environment for patients who need to go through the hassles of chronic disease.

12.4.3. Importance of Patient Education

The role of educating the patient in the management of rheumatic disease cannot be overstated, as it allows patients to become actively involved in their own care. Patient education regarding his or her condition results in enhanced adherence to treatment programs and lifestyle modifications and leads to improved health outcomes.

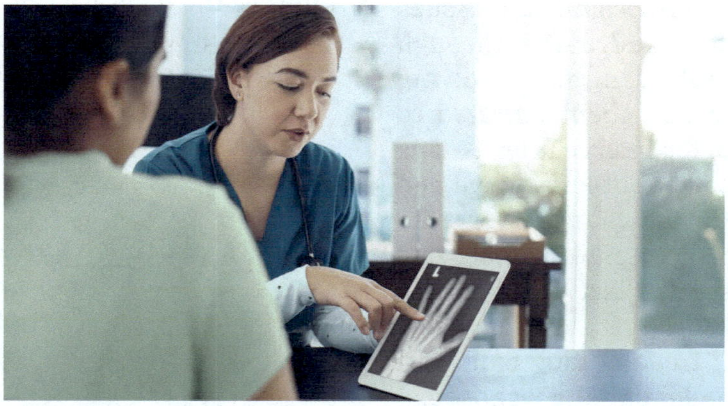

Figure 12.17. The significance of patient education in the management of rheumatic diseases cannot be overstated, as it empowers individuals to actively participate in their healthcare.

Source: https://images.everydayhealth.com/images/2025/understanding-disease-progression-in-ra-1440x810.jpg.

A study highlighted that educational group programs proved to be very effective in improving the participants' knowledge, though maintenance was inconsistent, particularly among RA patients (Taal et al., 1997). Moreover, the connection between compliance and self-efficacy with health is vital; compliance issues are common among most RA patients, which are more about patients' perceptions of self-efficacy than the functional inability or pain (Taal et al., 1993). Therefore, educational interventions must target development of these self-efficacy expectations, which not only improve health recommendation compliance but also enhance psychosocial functioning in patients with rheumatic diseases (Figure 12.17).

12.4.4. Cognitive-behavioral Therapy (CBT) Effectiveness

The success of CBT in managing the psychosocial aspects of rheumatic diseases is well-documented, particularly in enhancing patient outcomes. CBT addresses the cognitive processes underlying pain and emotional distress, consequently resulting in enhanced coping for patients. There is evidence to support the fact that CBT can lead to remarkable improvements in physical as well as psychological well-being among different groups, but its effectiveness could vary based on some conditions. Specifically, while group education-based interventions strengthen patient knowledge and can enhance physical health status, their impact on psychosocial health is less in patients with RA alone (Taal et al., 1997). Moreover, successful management interventions within the biopsychosocial framework highlight that psychosocial interventions must be combined with biological treatments keeping in mind the reality that a multidimensional approach can yield the best result in supporting a return to work as well as general well-being (Burton et al., 2008).

12.4.5. Mindfulness and Stress Reduction Techniques

Mindfulness and stress reduction techniques are now significant components in managing the psychosocial implications of rheumatism, giving patients general benefits outside of symptom management. These techniques, such as Mindfulness-Based Stress Reduction (MBSR), encourage people to cultivate awareness of their emotional and cognitive states and, by doing so, sense mastery over what they feel. Research indicates that MBSR has the potential to enhance patients' emotional well-being who are suffering from illnesses like systemic sclerosis because it allows individuals to become more aware of and respond to their stimuli, thus reducing stress (Pollina et al., 2023). Besides, the use of psychological interventions like mindfulness has been identified to alleviate pain and emotional distress in neurological rehabilitation environments to the advantage of the demand for multidisciplinary treatment planning (Castelnuovo et al., 2016). In general, such approaches not only improve improved health outcomes but also assist in allowing patients to manage the complex psychosocial climate that comes with chronic diseases (Figure 12.18).

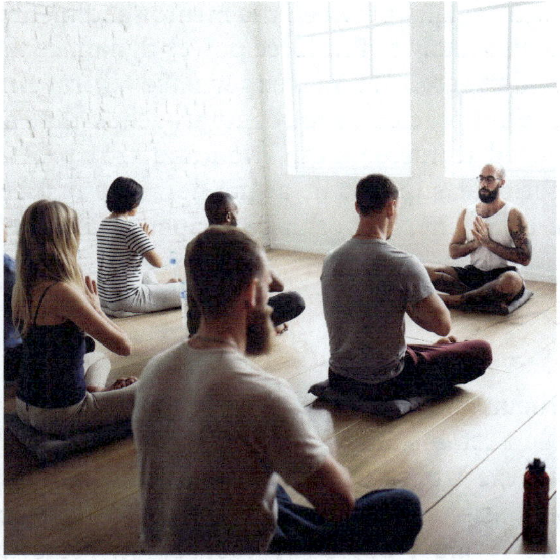

Figure 12.18. Mindfulness and stress reduction techniques have emerged as significant components in managing the psychosocial aspects of rheumatic diseases, offering patients holistic benefits that extend beyond physical symptoms.

Source: https://files.nccih.nih.gov/files/yoga-class-meditation-ThinkstockPhotos-637955386-square.jpg.

12.4.6. Support Groups and Peer Counseling

Peer counseling and support groups are also vital in alleviating the psychosocial challenges that dominate individuals with rheumatic diseases. These interventions foster a sense of community and shared understanding and provide emotional support that can assuage distress and feelings of isolation. These programs are only as effective as the participants' motivation levels permit, however. Evidence further indicates that low motivation to engage in self-management programs heavily limits their impact on health behavior and overall results, especially when their participants witness declines in their health or stress due to life events (Bode et al., 2008). In addition, while peer support is likely to create equality between the mentor and mentee, it is also likely to reinforce power dynamics that can detract from the experience. Unraveling these intricacies requires approaches that are tailored to foster motivation and that provide emotional support in a manner that respects the uniqueness of each participant's process.

12.4.7. Role of Physical Therapy in Psychosocial Health

In rheumatic diseases, physical therapy plays a key role in establishing psychosocial health through both the treatment of physical and emotional domains of patient well-being. Although physical therapy most obviously focuses on restoring function and mobility, its influence extends beyond the body into psychosocial outcomes to a wider extent. For instance, group education courses, which are most often a part of physical therapy, can have a beneficial influence on knowledge and disease management behavior. However, research indicates that although such programs have a beneficial influence on physical health status, they do not positively contribute to psychosocial health, particularly for those patients with rheumatoid arthritis (Taal et al., 1997). Additionally, the interplay between self-efficacy and adherence to health recommendations underscores the importance of psychosocial support in the treatment settings. Augmentation of self-efficacy expectations through specialized education may lead to improved pain and disability management, ultimately fostering increased psychosocial resilience among patients (Taal et al., 1993). Physical therapy is thus a critical component in the overall management of rheumatic conditions (Figure 12.19).

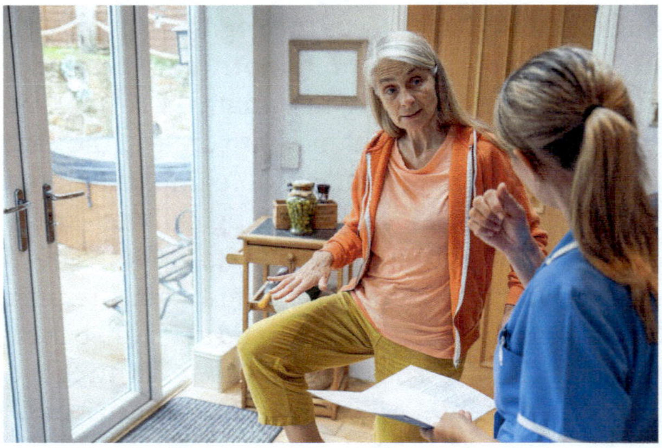

Figure 12.19. Physical therapy plays a crucial role in enhancing psychosocial health by addressing both physical and emotional dimensions of patient well-being.

Source: https://www.rheumatologyadvisor.com/wp-content/uploads/sites/18/2022/06/standing-on-one-leg_G_1356376815.jpg.

12.4.8. Family Involvement in Treatment Plans

Family involvement in treatment plans is a significant element in treating rheumatic diseases, particularly among AYAs battling both their illnesses and socialization. Engaging families makes it possible to ensure treatment strategies are tailored to the individual's own psychosocial circumstances, something that is crucial in adherence and outcomes. It is the responsibility of healthcare providers to make this relationship viable by building up the family's capacity to support the AYAs autonomy so that they can make decisions about care in an informed manner (Chaplin & Cai, 2019). Apart from that, studies have shown that structured transition care, as it is emphasized by the call for patient-centered treatment, enhances communication among patients' family members and healthcare professionals, eventually culminating into self-advocacy and self-management for adolescent patients. Thus, including family participation in treatment programs not only makes treatment environments friendly but also results in improved health outcomes among patients dealing with the challenges of rheumatic conditions.

Test Your Knowledge

1. What is the role of multidisciplinary care teams in the management of complex rheumatic disease?
2. How may occupational therapy help to cope with joint deformity or stiffness in everyday life?

Summary

The psychosocial dimensions of rheumatic diseases, and particularly rheumatoid arthritis (RA), need a more subtle response that is sensitive to gender inequalities and their impact on patient management. Recent research highlights the glaring differences in the psychosocial life of RA in men and women, illustrating the inclination for studies with mixed genders to ignore the specific needs of male patients. This dearth is vindicated in findings, which substantiate the need for single-purposed study of coping mechanisms and support networks particularly beneficial for men with RA (White et al., 2015). Further, emotional distress and self-management differ according to gender, which demands that therapeutic interventions aimed at improving quality of life and social support be tailored to every patient (Flurey et al., 2015). Compelling extensive future research is essential in order to close these gaps and optimize therapeutic measures based on the different psychosocial needs of patients with rheumatic diseases.

The psychosocial analysis of rheumatic diseases discovers significant findings with regard to the interaction between psychosocial and biological determinants in the management of these conditions. Such an observation is that biomedical care and ergonomic modification are insufficient; rather, multimodal interventions with a biopsychosocial orientation are most supportive of occupational outcomes, particularly return to work and work maintenance (Burton et al., 2008). This is an indication for joint effort among employers, healthcare professionals, and patients in establishing a culture that acknowledges the high contribution of psychosocial factors to rehabilitation. Foot issues that are prevalent among rheumatoid arthritis patients also lead to disability and tend to remain underdiagnosed in clinical practice. This is a cry towards increased incorporation of podiatric care into rheumatology in order to provide holistic care and better patient outcomes (Chapman et al., 2010). These findings underscore the critical need for an integrative treatment approach that addresses both the medical and psychosocial components of rheumatic illnesses.

KEY TERMS FROM THIS CHAPTER

- biopsychosocial model
- inclusion
- physical health status
- exercise
- group education programs
- chronic mental illness
- functional disability
- biological demands
- psychosocial care
- psychosocial factors
- rest
- anxiety
- social learning theory
- knowledge retention

Critical Thinking Questions

1. Which of the following psychosocial variables is most commonly associated with disease activity and poor outcomes in rheumatoid arthritis patients?

a. Use of social media

b. Depression

c. Marital status

d. Educational level

2. Which of the following mental health conditions is most vulnerable in chronic rheumatic disease patients?

a. Bipolar disorder

b. Attention deficit disorder

c. Anxiety and depression

d. Schizophrenia

3. Which of the following is an intervention that has been found to be helpful to both physical and mental health in rheumatic disease patients?

a. Isolation and rest

b. Strict immobilization

c. Cognitive behavioral therapy (CBT)

d. Antibiotic therapy

4. Fatigue in rheumatic disease is typically best managed by:

a. Increasing immunosuppressive medications

a. Promoting light physical activity and psychosocial support

b. Reducing fluid intake

c. Increasing caffeine intake

5. Which of the following is TRUE regarding the effect of chronic pain on quality of life in rheumatologic patients?

a. It tends to improve with tolerance of pain over time

b. It has little impact on sleep or function

c. It often leads to mood disorders and social withdrawal

d. It is rarely a problem in autoimmune arthritis

Short Answer Questions

1. What is the prevalence of depression and anxiety among patients with chronic rheumatic diseases?
2. What is the cause of emotional distress in individuals with rheumatoid arthritis due to chronic pain?
3. In what way do rheumatic illnesses affect social interactions and family function?
4. What are the challenges for rheumatic patients to remain in the workforce?
5. What are the direct and indirect costs of treating rheumatoid arthritis?
6. How do productivity loss and absenteeism contribute to the economic burden of lupus and chronic illness?
7. What are the most useful psychosocial strategies for improving the quality of life for patients with rheumatic diseases?

Answers to Critical Thinking Questions

1. (b); 2. (c); 3. (c); 4. (b); 5. (c)

References

1. Castelnuovo, G., Giusti, E. M., Manzoni, G. M., Saviola, D., Gatti, A., Gabrielli, S., Lacerenza, M., Pietrabissa, G., Cattivelli, R., Spatola, C. A., Corti, S., Novelli, M., Villa, V., Cottini, A., Lai, C., Pagnini, F., Castelli, L., Tavola, M., Torta, R., Arreghini, M., ... Tamburin, S. (2016). Psychological Treatments and Psychotherapies in the Neurorehabilitation of Pain: Evidences and Recommendations from the Italian Consensus Conference on Pain in Neurorehabilitation. *Frontiers in psychology*, *7*, 115. https://doi.org/10.3389/fpsyg.2016.00115 (accessed on 17th June 2025).
2. Agüera, A., Agüera-Ortiz, M., Asghari, M., Astin, F., Bravo, J., Breivik, H., Campbell, P., et al. (2014). Association of painful musculoskeletal conditions and migraine headache with mental and sleep disorders among adults with disabilities, Spain, 2007–2008. https://core.ac.uk/download/161360208.pdf (accessed on 17th June 2025).
3. Alnaimat, F., & Barukba, H. (2023). Rehabilitation in rheumatic diseases. https://core.ac.uk/download/621136279.pdf (accessed on 17th June 2025).
4. Bailey, A., Doran, C., Duits, A., Gerstenbluth, I., et al. (2023). "It's very saddening, you keep on wondering when the symptoms will be over": A qualitative study exploring the long-term chikungunya disease impact on daily life and well-being, 6 years after disease onset. https://core.ac.uk/download/597498374.pdf (accessed on 17th June 2025).
5. Ballabeni, P., Fonjallaz, B., Gueniat, C., Hofer, M., et al. (2017). Impact of a nurse-led telephone intervention on satisfaction and health outcomes of children with inflammatory rheumatic diseases and their families: A crossover randomized clinical trial. https://core.ac.uk/download/90251631.pdf (accessed on 17th June 2025).
6. Bee, P., Lovell, K., MacFarlane, G. J., McBeth, J., et al. (2016). Managing chronic widespread pain in primary care: A qualitative study of patient perspectives and implications for treatment delivery. https://core.ac.uk/download/77614574.pdf (accessed on 17th June 2025).
7. Benelli, E., & Bianco, F. (2015). Models of collaboration between psychologist and family doctor: A systematic review of primary care psychology. https://core.ac.uk/download/80154468.pdf (accessed on 17th June 2025).
8. Ben-Shlomo, Y., Camfield, L., & Warner, T. (2002). What are the determinants of quality of life in people with cervical dystonia? https://core.ac.uk/download/2771617.pdf (accessed on 17th June 2025).
9. Bode, C., Emons, P. A. A., Galetzka, M., Laar, M. A. F. J. van de, et al. (2008). Limited results of group self-management education for rheumatoid arthritis patients and their partners: Explanations from the patient perspective. https://core.ac.uk/download/pdf/11474838.pdf (accessed on 17th June 2025).
10. Bruns, A., Skarin, A., Hassett, A. L., Amine, B., Duarte-Salazar, C., Petersen, C., Gerhardt, C. A., et al. (2010). Burden of childhood-onset arthritis. https://core.ac.uk/download/pdf/8437352.pdf (accessed on 17th June 2025).
11. Taal, E., Riemsma, R. P., Brus, H. L., Seydel, E. R., Rasker, J. J., & Wiegman, O. (1993). Group education for patients with rheumatoid arthritis. *Patient education and counseling*, *20*(2-3), 177–187. https://doi.org/10.1016/0738-3991(93)90131-f(accessed on 17th June 2025).

12. Burton, A. K., Kendall, N. A., Pearce, B. G., Birrell, L. N., & Bainbridge, L. C. (2009). Management of work-relevant upper limb disorders: a review. *Occupational medicine (Oxford, England)*, *59*(1), 44–52. https://doi.org/10.1093/occmed/kqn151(accessed on 17th June 2025).

13. Cai, R. A., & Chaplin, H. (2019). Impact of rheumatic disease on social development in adolescents and young adults. https://core.ac.uk/download/286268267.pdf Chaplin, H., Cai, A. (2019). Impact of Rheumatic Disease on Social Development in Adolescents and Young Adults. In: McDonagh, J., Tattersall, R. (eds) Adolescent and Young Adult Rheumatology In Clinical Practice. In Clinical Practice. Springer, Cham. https://doi.org/10.1007/978-3-319-95519-3_3 (accessed on 17th June 2025).

14. Camfield, P., Campbell, F., Department of Health, Kirkham, J., Arnott, J., Burke, L., Peak, M., et al. (2018). The transition of adolescents with juvenile idiopathic arthritis or epilepsy from pediatric health-care services to adult health-care services: A scoping review of the literature and a synthesis of the evidence. https://core.ac.uk/download/146494407.pdf (accessed on 17th June 2025).

15. Cardona, F. C. G., Cox, C. J., Cunningham, M. W., Orefici, G., et al. (2016). Pediatric autoimmune neuropsychiatric disorders associated with streptococcal infections (PANDAS). https://core.ac.uk/download/54531412.pdf (accessed on 17th June 2025).

16. Carradice, A., Hakkinen, A., Williams, A. E., Oppenheim, A. H., Greco, A. J., et al. (2011). "I could cry, the amount of shoes I can't get into": A qualitative exploration of the factors that influence retail footwear selection in women with rheumatoid arthritis. https://core.ac.uk/download/pdf/8612900.pdf (accessed on 17th June 2025).

17. Chapman, J., Dalbeth, N., Gow, P., Rome, K., et al. (2010). Podiatry services for patients with arthritis: An unmet need. https://core.ac.uk/download/1662153.pdf (accessed on 17th June 2025).

18. Chipping J, Mooney J, Macgregor AJ (2016) The Benefits of Syndication of Mental Health Nurses within Rheumatology Out-Patient Departments: A Narrative Discussion. Ann Nurs Pract 3(5): 1062(accessed on 17th June 2025).

19. Creemers, M. C. W., de Brouwer, S. J. M., Evers, A. W. M., Kraaimaat, F. W., et al. (2010). Experimental stress in inflammatory rheumatic diseases: A review of psychophysiological stress responses. https://core.ac.uk/download/pdf/8435859.pdf (accessed on 17th June 2025).

20. D'Amelio, R., Laganà, B., Rosado, M., Picchianti Diamanti, A., et al. (2016). Microbiota and chronic inflammatory arthritis: An interwoven link. https://core.ac.uk/download/54535728.pdf (accessed on 17th June 2025).

21. Geenen, R., Jacobs, J. W., Pereira da Silva, J. A., Santiago, M. B., et al. (2015). Psychological factors associated with response to treatment in rheumatoid arthritis. https://core.ac.uk/download/75985969.pdf (accessed on 17th June 2025).

22. Gouveia, N. S. A. (2015). *The Burden of Chronic Low Back Pain in The Adult Portuguese Population: An Epidemiological Population-Based Study Under the Scope of Epireumapt.* https://core.ac.uk/download/157632323.pdf (accessed on 17th June 2025).

23. Kirchhof, P., Benussi, S., Kotecha, D., Ahlsson, A., Atar, D., Casadei, B., Castellá, M., et al. (2016). 2016 ESC guidelines for the management of atrial fibrillation developed in collaboration with EACTS. *European Heart Journal, 37*, 2893–2962. https://doi.org/10.1093/eurheartj/ehw210 (accessed on 17th June 2025).

24. Loprest, P. (2007). Strategic assessment of the state of the science in research on employment for individuals with disabilities. https://core.ac.uk/download/71340960.pdf (accessed on 17th June 2025).

25. Mechling, C. (2020). Rheumatoid arthritis: A literature review and comprehensive treatment analysis. https://core.ac.uk/download/304929451.pdf (accessed on 17th June 2025).

26. Oliveira, A., & Sá, M. C. (2012). Psychological and social factors in rheumatic diseases. https://core.ac.uk/download/542333201.pdf (accessed on 17th June 2025).

27. Pollina, A., Pezzutto, A., El Aoufy, K., Rasero, L., Matucci Cerinic, M., Guiducci, S., Bellando-Randone, S., et al. (2023). *Systemic Sclerosis Patients Experiencing Mindfulness-Based Stress Reduction Program: The Beneficial Effect on Their Psychological Status and Quality of Life.* https://core.ac.uk/download/610288296.pdf (accessed on 17th June 2025).

28. Taal, E., Rasker, J. J., Seydel, E. R., & Wiegman, O. (1993). Health status, adherence with health recommendations, self-efficacy and social support in patients with rheumatoid arthritis. *Patient education and counseling*, *20*(2-3), 63–76. https://doi.org/10.1016/0738-3991(93)90122-d(accessed on 17th June 2025).

29. Taal, E., Rasker, J. J., & Wiegman, O. (1997). Group education for rheumatoid arthritis patients. *Seminars in arthritis and rheumatism*, *26*(6), 805–816. https://doi.org/10.1016/s0049-0172(97)80024-8 (accessed on 17th June 2025).

30. Ravelli, A., Hersh, A. O., Milojevic, D. S., Lotstein, D. S., von Scheven, E., Falcini, F., Fantini, F., et al. (2009). The challenges of transferring chronic illness patients to adult care: Reflections from pediatric and adult rheumatology at a US academic center. https://core.ac.uk/download/pdf/8299511.pdf (accessed on 17th June 2025).

31. Reath, J., Abbott, P., & Deshmukh, T. (2025). 'It's got to be another approach': An Aboriginal health worker perspective on cardiovascular risk screening and education. https://core.ac.uk/download/pdf/30674167.pdf (accessed on 17th June 2025).

32. Ross, K. (2012). A call to action: Providing better footwear and foot orthoses for people with rheumatoid arthritis. https://core.ac.uk/download/9844219.pdf (accessed on 17th June 2025).

33. Alejandro Salazar, María Dueñas, Juan Antonio Mico, Begoña Ojeda, Luis Agüera-Ortiz, Jorge A. Cervilla, Inmaculada Failde, Undiagnosed Mood Disorders and Sleep Disturbances in Primary Care Patients with Chronic Musculoskeletal Pain, *Pain Medicine*, Volume 14, Issue 9, September 2013, Pages 1416–1425, https://doi.org/10.1111/pme.12165(accessed on 17th June 2025).

34. Sauder, L. (2016). *Das Erleben von Frauen im Spannungsfeld von Mutter- und chronisch Kranksein*. https://core.ac.uk/download/55329690.pdf (accessed on 17th June 2025).

35. Smedley, C., Fisher, K., Wong, M., Kayess, R., & Bates, S. (2014). Arthritis and disability. https://core.ac.uk/download/pdf/30673486.pdf (accessed on 17th June 2025).

36. Treaster, M. (2021). Optimism and physical health-related quality of life in chronic illness: Mediating effects of control beliefs and health behaviors. https://core.ac.uk/download/346382397.pdf (accessed on 17th June 2025).

37. Voskuyl, A. E., Gommer, A. M., Bruce, B., de Zwart, B. C., Mancuso, C. A., Noben, C. Y., Boot, C. R. L., et al. (2012). An intervention program with the aim to improve and maintain work productivity for workers with rheumatoid arthritis: Design of a randomized controlled trial

and cost-effectiveness study. https://core.ac.uk/download/pdf/15477540.pdf (accessed on 17th June 2025).

38. White, A., Baczyk, G., Beck, A. T., Behnam, B., Brownhill, S., Flurey, C. A., et al. (2015). Men, rheumatoid arthritis, psychosocial impact and self-management: A narrative review. https://core.ac.uk/download/29018487.pdf (accessed on 17th June 2025).

39. Williamson, P., Altman, D. G., Bagley, H., Barnes, K. L., Blazeby, J., Brookes, S., Clarke, M., et al. (2017). *The COMET Handbook: Version 1.0. Trials, 18.* https://doi.org/10.1186/s13063-017-1978-4 (accessed on 17th June 2025).

INDEX

E

F

G

H

I

J

K

L

M

N

O

P

Q

R